HOW TO BE YOUR OWN DOCTOR

by Carl E. Shrader, M.D.

Acacia Publishing, Inc.
2004

First Edition
Copyright 2003 by Carl E. Shrader, M.D. All rights reserved.

Acacia Publishing, Inc.
1366 E. Thomas Road, Suite 305
Phoenix, AZ 85014

ISBN: 0-9671187-8-6

Published by Acacia Publishing, Inc., Phoenix, Arizona
www.acaciapublishing.com
Printed and bound in the United States of America

*This book is dedicated to George Sprague and Tom Geiler,
two of the best friends a man ever had.*

To Bob Steele, my Hoosier basketball compadre.

*To Chick Warnock, the brother I never had
"My buddy, my buddy... Your buddy misses you!"*

And to Nomney, whose love transcended all understanding.

ACKNOWLEDGEMENTS

Grateful thanks to the following people, who have helped to bring this book to successful publication:

Vicky Graves, pharmacist and friend, who helped with some of the drug savings suggestions in the book and as a colleague providing advice and information for all manner of medication-related questions for over twenty years.

Jessica Curran, gifted photographer, who figured out what I really look like and took a picture of it before I knew what was happening.

Bradford Larson III, who spent *days* finding us an acronym toll-free phone number (1-866-SAVE-$$$) for marketing this book.

Ellin Dodge, author and friend, who taught us a lot about the logistics and pitfalls of publishing.

Ruth Ann DeLap, my office nurse for 28 years, who helped make me a better and more effective doctor, and who will remember quite a few of the anecdotes herein.

My wife and partner Margaret, for copy editing, suggestions, cover art work, and general encouragement during the past five years of writing efforts.

My publisher, Karen Gray, a creative and dedicated editor, who has organized my manuscript into a cohesive and, we hope, enjoyable book.

And to the American Academy of Family Physicians for keeping me at the top of my profession throughout my career.

TABLE OF CONTENTS

Additional reliable and accurate medical information can be obtained from the American Academy of Family Practice web site: www.familydoctor.org

CHAPTER 1 -- INTRODUCTION

When was the last time you spent sixty dollars or more to see a doctor for a condition, only to be told that you need to eat more fiber, take two aspirins every four hours, take 1000 milligrams vitamin C, drink lots of fluids, stop smoking, whatever? Did you feel that you had wasted your money? Did you ignore the advice you just paid for? After you read this book, you will feel that your medical dollar is much better spent.

One of my patients bled to death unnecessarily in another town after an auto accident. A friend bled to death in a hospital ER waiting room. A young woman took a single bite of a substance she was allergic to and would have died without the quick assistance of a nearby nurse. A man was choking and was saved by the quick action of someone who knew what to do. Some medical conditions can be fatal if not recognized quickly by someone nearby. With the knowledge I will share with you in this book, it won't happen to you or your family.

By reading and referring to this book you will be able to provide a higher standard of medical care for yourself and your family, without <u>ever</u> consulting a physician, than the founding fathers of our country enjoyed with the aid of all their physicians throughout the 18th and 19th and into the early 20th century. And you will know how to get far more for your money when you <u>do</u> need to consult your doctor in this 21st century.

Although, in over 40 years of practice, I have encountered <u>almost</u> everything in medicine at least once, I know more about some conditions than others. They will be addressed at greater length here.

Everything you will read here is my own opinion, based upon my own personal experience in a still very active medical practice in most cases, along with my own personal research through dozens of medical journals and lectures to try to present information here as up to the present minute as possible.

In this book I will mention some names of companies, brand-name drugs, specific other brands that I like and have used. I have not, nor will I ever receive any payment for anything I mention in this book. I mention them only because I have found that what I mention by name works better than almost every other item of a similar nature. I believe that you can trust what I mention by name.

I was a GP (general practitioner) when I started practice, which meant to me and to most of my patients that I had some degree of acquaintance with, if not complete expertise in, almost all of areas of medicine, "from the erection to the resurrection," one of my colleagues once said, although I think he was stretching it a little. After that I was an FP (family practitioner) because the American Academy of Family Practice, to which I have belonged since 1961, felt we could achieve more respect by making a public statement that we care for whole families. And we do. Before delivering babies cost too high malpractice premiums (an extra $36,000 per year) and too little sleep, I had the pleasure of delivering several second generations and just recently could have had yet a third generation to deliver.

Now HMOs and politicians have demoted us to PCPs (primary care physicians) or gate-keepers. (I'd like to be the gate-keeper at Heaven's Golden Gate for the HMO executive who thought that one up!!)

And recently during contract negotiations with a group of us physicians, the medical director of one of the largest HMOs in the country, who wanted to pay us as little as possible, said that we're the "product" his HMO is selling.

If you find a GP, FP, PCP, gate-keeper, or "product" that you like, cherish her or him, send the occasional thank you note, the occasional pie, or jar of blackberry jelly from your garden, the photo of the little child he or she delivered to put on his bulletin board. Let him know he or she is appreciated by some real people and isn't just a "product" sold by an insurance company.

We all know how many times your child has been ill all day at the baby sitter's or day-care center, but you didn't find out until you picked her up after work. Doctors know and expect this. Call your doctor then and that will give him some leeway about having a warm dinner with his family (I can't tell you how precious that is!) and still being able to see your child or phone in a prescription before the pharmacy closes.

Calling your (or any) doctor at 3:00 a.m. for something that started yesterday morning won't get you a very enthusiastic nor wide awake response. However, if something that has seemed minor undergoes a sudden turn for the worse, by all means call him. Don't just go to the emergency room, as that, at best, doubles the cost and the doctors there don't know you.

You are at more risk when treated by a tired doctor at 3:00 a.m.; and most pharmacies, at least in my area, close at 9:00 p.m. so to be sure to have a coherent response and adequate medicine, try to at least talk to your doctor (or the doctor covering for him) by 8:00 p.m. If you are going to an Urgent Care facility, be there by 7:00 p.m.

If your doctor, or any doctor about to treat you or a member of your family has alcohol on his breath or seems impaired in any way, find another doctor. You can always go to the ER instead. This is one time when I give you absolute permission to go to the ER if you can't find another physician who you feel confident is not impaired.

To fully understand this book you will have to learn a <u>very</u> few medical names for parts of the body, plus only a <u>few</u> more medical terms. Some of these follow.

<u>Aorta</u>, the biggest blood vessel in the body, comes out of the heart upward then quickly curves around and goes down into the back of the abdominal cavity beside the front of the backbone (spine), sending out branches all along the way to arms, brain, lungs, heart (the coronary arteries that produce a heart attack when they get blocked), liver, spleen, stomach and intestines, kidneys, reproductive organs, and legs.

<u>Trachea</u>, this airway leads from the Adam's apple or <u>larynx</u> (as in laryngitis) where the vocal cords we speak with live, down into the <u>bronchial tubes</u> (as in bronchitis) of the lungs, which then branch out in all directions in the lungs, getting smaller and smaller until they are only one cell thick in tiny air sacs called <u>alveoli</u> (al vee o lie).

These alveoli are the first things damaged by smoking. When enough have been destroyed, you have emphysema (or COPD). So now is the time to quit smoking, because the alveoli will repair themselves a lot when you quit, even if pretty badly damaged. Don't wait too long.

<u>Esophagus</u>, the food tube from the back of your throat to the <u>stomach</u>, passing through a small hole in the diaphragm (where <u>hiatal</u> hernias occur) along the way. Food, especially bread, sometimes get stuck there in older people and people who don't chew their food well, either because they are in too much of a hurry or because they don't have very good teeth, or take bites that are too big. Also safety pins, pennies, quarters, beads, rocks, nails -- you name it and it has probably found its way into a little kid's esophagus.

<u>Duodenum</u>, the first part of the small intestine. The stomach empties into it. So does the <u>gallbladder</u>, sending in bile to digest fat. Right at the entrance to the duodenum is the place where peptic ulcers form. About 25 feet (really!!) later the <u>small intestine</u> (small bowel) winds its way into the <u>large intestine</u> (large bowel) down in the lower right side of your abdomen. Right at that spot, about two inches from the small bowel opening, is the <u>appendix</u>, right at the tip of the first part of the large bowel. It can vary in size from perhaps one inch upward. I once personally took out an inflamed appendix that was 7 inches long!

Then the <u>ascending colon</u> goes up -- ascending -- got it? to under the right side of the liver (our factory for manufacturing almost everything that keeps us alive and warm), turns left, and becomes the <u>transverse colon</u> which travels left over to the area of our <u>spleen</u> (which filters and stores unneeded blood while producing antibodies to fight infection, among other things), then turns south as the <u>descending colon</u>, then the <u>sigmoid colon</u> (which supposedly looks like a Greek letter s -- don't you believe it!), into the <u>rectum</u> and out the <u>anus</u>, passing behind the <u>prostate</u> along the way.

Thus ends our anatomy lesson. That wasn't too bad, was it? A very few other terms will come up later, but I will carefully explain them. Words like penis, vagina, thyroid, ovary, testicles, most of which you have heard about (though some were only whispered when you were a teenager).

CHAPTER 2 -- WORDS and PHRASES to WATCH OUT FOR

"As long as you're here, ..." could mean that something expensive, not related to your office visit, and possibly unnecessary in your healthcare is forthcoming. Or it could mean that you are overdue for your Pap smear or prostate check, and you will actually be saving both time and some money by doing it now. It depends on the doctor.

"He's very thorough," means he does a lot of tests. Not necessarily all bad for your physical health, but may be bad for your wallet.

"We don't need to bother with a consultation." These are the words of a doctor who thinks he knows everything. <u>Run</u>, don't walk, to the nearest exit. These are the words of a doctor who is afraid that his opinion will be contradicted by a consultant, and one who probably needs a <u>lot</u> of help from consultants.

"Let's try this natural diet supplement we have right here." This means that you are about to supplement his or her income, but may not supplement any particular good feelings in your body. He or she is selling it at high retail price.

I had a lady in my office last week who was happily paying a naturopathic practitioner $20 per month while barely meeting her mortgage payments. That's $240 per year for the same exact vitamins and minerals she could get at Walgreen's for $15.99 for a whole year's supply! I've had other patients paying two or three times that. The body doesn't care where the chemicals come from, just that they are pure. If the label says "USP approved," then they are pure.

"Let me just try some manipulation here to take away the numbness and pain on the outside of your leg and foot," means you're probably about to have a ruptured lumbar disc made worse.

"Be sure to apply antibiotic ointment to the wound three or four times a day" means that the wound will literally take twice as long to heal because the ointment kills body cells at the edges of the wound, prevents oxygen from getting to the injured tissues, and causes maceration (tissues stay moist, turn white and may pucker). Wounds that heal the best are those that are cleaned out well before repair, then kept clean and dry, with no ointment. I have seen many a wound that was inadequately cleansed to the depths and got infected in spite of antibiotic ointment and oral antibiotics. Doctors who are too busy to fully cleanse a wound often think these measures will substitute for proper cleansing. They are wrong! And you will pay the price in extra office visits and/or complications.

"You need surgery immediately!" Maybe. Definitely so if you have appendicitis. But a bowel obstruction: maybe, maybe not. It may depend upon who makes that statement. Be aware that doctors tend to think in terms of the way they are trained. A surgeon tends to think of surgery first, but most good surgeons will also consider and discuss with you possible non-surgical alternatives, if indeed there are any.

> *"I won't be responsible for your life if you leave this office without agreeing to..." In the case of my wife over twenty years ago a "society" urologist wanted to operate on one of her kidneys for kidney stones. Her thoughts were that, in the first place, she was pretty sure that some alternatives existed for her fairly small stones; and in the second place, she wouldn't trust him to treat even a wart on her rear end, or something perhaps a little more graphic. You get the idea. What happened was that she saw another doctor, passed some stones, which were then analyzed, and then went on a diet low in oxalates from then till now. I've known her for 18 years, during which she has never required further treatment for kidney stones. P. S. She does drink a lot of water, and I only rarely have to caution her to stay away from some of the oxalate foods she used to love.*

CHAPTER 3 -- ABDOMINAL PAIN

The abdomen contains the stomach, small intestines, large intestines, liver, gall bladder, pancreas, spleen, great blood vessels (the aorta and its many branches, and the inferior vena cava and its many tributaries), and the uterus, fallopian tubes and ovaries in women. The urinary bladder often feels as though it is in the lower abdomen, especially when it is full, but it is actually in a sort of pouch outside of the peritoneum lining just under the pubic bone. Likewise the kidneys are technically within the abdominal muscle structure but outside of the peritoneal covering of most of the abdominal interior.

Here we will discuss various conditions located or felt in the abdomen, along with how they feel and how to treat them. Then we will talk about pain in these areas.

Mid Upper Abdominal Area (epigastrium or pit of the stomach, solar plexus, above the navel or belly button):

Peptic Disease (see the chapter). This is usually described by those who suffer from it as a burning pain. It may be simply irritation of the walls of the stomach or duodenum (the first part of the small intestine into which the stomach empties). Or it may be an actual ulcer or raw sore in the walls of those organs.

Antacids or certain bland foods taken into the stomach to counteract the acid will usually put out the fire. Reducing the production of stomach acid is also necessary for healing. Avoiding tobacco, caffeine, including even decaf coffee, and alcohol is absolutely essential because they are the worst for causing acid production.

If you get no relief from either of these, along with a few doses of Zantac, Pepcid, Axid, or Tagamet, then other conditions must be considered.

In recent years we have found that many, perhaps most, ulcers are caused by infection with a germ called Helicobacter pylori (H. pylori), which can be cured by massive doses of multiple antibiotics. More about that in the chapter on **Ulcers**.

If an ulcer is penetrating deeply into the back wall of the duodenum, then it may irritate the adjoining pancreas (a large digestive gland) and cause pain straight into the back similar to an actual attack of Pancreatitis (see below).

If the ulcer perforates through the front wall into the abdominal cavity, then it produces a sudden onset of very severe pain as the stomach acid hits the peritoneum (the thin glistening lining of the inside of the abdomen. That is what is inflamed when you get peritonitis -- a very bad and still often fatal condition). One minute you are well, and the next minute you have severe pain. In a perforated ulcer, the pain may start very suddenly in the epigastrium and then spread downward as the acid seeps out farther and farther.

Appendicitis (see below) also often starts with pain in the epigastrium, but it starts more slowly than the ulcer hole pain, and moves gradually down into the right lower quadrant of the abdomen. With a perforated ulcer, one minute you are well and the next you have a terrible pain.

Gall Bladder Disease. This can be severe and incapacitating if a gallstone is trying to pass down the bile duct into the duodenum. Most of the time the gall bladder itself, when inflamed, will produce pain and tenderness in the area just under the right ribs (see below).

Pancreatitis. This is usually a very severe pain that bores straight through into the middle of the back. You don't want to move. Your abdominal muscles become hard as a board. You may go into shock because there may be severe bleeding into the body of the pancreas as it digests itself. This is called Acute Hemorrhagic Pancreatitis and is life-threatening. There is little that can be done to cure this aside from treating shock with fluids and certain minerals, along with medication to stop the production of digestive juices.

I well remember the autopsy of a patient of mine who wouldn't believe me when I told him what was going to happen to him. When the pathologist and I examined his pancreas, we found that it had turned into calcium soap. You could have washed your hands with it! (The process, for those of you who have been exposed to organic chemistry, is called saponification.)

Alcohol abusers are those most likely to develop this condition. It can recur in its non-hemorrhagic form over and over. Each time the pancreas is further damaged, until it finally causes death.

Sometimes an ulcer will perforate on the back side of the duodenum straight into the body of the pancreas. This produces pain similar to that of regular Pancreatitis, but less intense because the area of inflammation is relatively small, and usually is not life-threatening because the hole in the small intestine soon seals off.

I vividly remember a patient and friend who had a CT done in an eastern city while he was on vacation, and nothing abnormal was found. A month later we repeated it in Flagstaff, and this time found a pancreatic cancer. Nothing could be done for him except "palliation" with pain meds.

Cancer of the Pancreas. This can be difficult to diagnose, even now, with all the exotic imagery we have available. Symptoms depend on whether the tumor is located in the head, body, or tail of the pancreas. The first symptom may not be pain, but rather yellow eyeballs from obstruction of the common bile duct leading from the gall bladder past the head of the pancreas, where even a small tumor can push against it enough to close the tube and cause the bile to back up, ultimately into the bloodstream. The outlook here is better than for a cancer in the body or tail of the gland, which grows without producing any symptoms until eventually there is enough pain to make one go to the doctor. Then it may be diagnosed, or at lease suspected from various imaging studies, such as CT, MRI, or ultrasound. Even those may not pick it up very early.

Any cancer of the pancreas carries a grim prognosis. Although there are reported survivals, I have never known one. My father was one who didn't. If pain is the presenting symptom, even an accurate diagnosis the next day will not enable a cure.

This is one of the most painful of all cancers, and makes the patient and his or her family appreciate the hospice folks more than words can ever tell. If you ever see a case of pancreatic cancer in someone you love, you will become an advocate for legalized assisted suicide (euthanasia). I don't want to get into that here, as I am a fairly religious person and feel "conflicted" about this subject.

For sure this is one condition where any and all pain control medications are appropriate, including the most addicting narcotics.

Heart Disease. Occasionally discomfort or actual pain from heart disease is felt in the upper mid abdomen. It is more likely to be felt as a pressure or cramp in the pit of the stomach rather than anything sharp. Also there is no tenderness to pressing on the area with the hand if it is heart disease, and heart disease does not usually improve if you take antacid.

But, if you have history of heart disease, have your doctor evaluate that upper abdominal pain.

Gas in the bowel. If you place a finger on your abdominal wall and tap on it with the tip of a finger of the other hand, it will sound hollow, like a drum. Usually when there are no complicating factors, there will be a lot of noise inside the stomach wall. You can put your ear against the wall of someone with this problem, and it will sound almost like a washing machine, with constant noise throughout the whole abdomen. Relief comes with repeated passing of gas from the rectum. Mylicon or Mylanta anti-gas pills can be chewed as treatment for this condition.

Small bowel obstruction. This pain tends to come in waves, accompanied by very active bowel sounds limited to just the area behind where the bowel is blocked. It is different because the sounds aren't heard all over. Also after the first little while there is no gas passing from the rectum. One of the main causes of this condition is an adhesion from previous surgery that makes a band around part or all of a nearby part of the small intestine. Sometimes it is just a partial obstruction and slowly subsides if nothing but clear fluids are taken into the GI tract for awhile. Sometimes one has to be admitted to the hospital for naso-gastric suction (a tube through the nose down into the stomach with suction attached to it). Pain that feels like something is pulling on the inside of your belly button and milder pain around that area is usually from something wrong with the small intestine.

Food poisoning. After the pain has been present for not very long, there will usually develop vomiting and/or diarrhea. But not always. Sometimes it just hurts until your body can fight it off, and the things above have to be considered. Again, a dose of antacid and/or Pepto-Bismol may help a lot. See the chapter on **Food Poisoning** for more.

Gastroenteritis, the most common cause of all abdominal pain, is very often a result of food poisoning (see the chapter on **Food Poisoning**). It usually eventually produces diarrhea, and may or may not be accompanied by vomiting.

Treatment of vomiting. When you vomit, you not only lose fluids, but also electrolytes (especially sodium and potassium chloride). These need to be replaced, along with the fluids.

If you can keep just a swallow or two down, then take a 75 mg Zantac, chew and swallow it. Wait a half hour and repeat it until you keep two tablets down. Or take a 10 mg Pepcid AC chewable tablet and do the same. These will help to overcome the very severe inflammation of the walls of the stomach.

After you have kept down one of those meds for an hour, then you can start to try some fluids. But very slowly. Start with 1 tablespoon of dilute Gatorade (your favorite flavor), wait ten minutes, take two tablespoons, then increase by a teaspoon every ten minutes if you are keeping it down. If you vomit, drop back to the amount that you did keep down and increase as before. Ice chips are often good and tolerated well, but you still need the salt and potassium.

Don't even think of anything solid. After awhile you can add Jell-O water and clear soup, such as chicken noodle soup without the noodles. In twelve hours you can add the noodles, as well as salty crackers, and maybe some applesauce and mashed ripe bananas. If all is well with these, then just gradually add other foods that you know always agree with you. Continue to take the Zantac or Pepcid for three to four days, because the stomach normally takes about that long for the inflammation to go away in an uncomplicated case. Milk, oddly enough, is often not tolerated until about the third day for those who normally tolerate it quite well because the enzyme lactase can't be produced in adequate quantities by an inflamed stomach.

Pedialyte is the preferred solution for kids. Gatorade is too strong for them. If you use Gatorade for kids, it must be diluted, using 1 part Gatorade to two parts water.

You can do your own home-made electrolyte "1-2-3 solution" by mixing 1 cup of orange juice, 2 cups of water, 3 tablespoons of sugar, and 1/2 teaspoon of table salt. Mix and chill. For adults start with a tablespoon, and increase by a tablespoon every ten minutes. If you vomit, then drop back to the dose where you didn't, and increase again ten minutes later. For kids, start with a teaspoon and increase as above.

Right Upper Quadrant Pain

(Divide the abdomen into four parts by drawing mental lines vertically and horizontally through the navel.)

The conditions that are likely to produce pain here are:

Inflammation of the gallbladder (Cholecystitis) This condition is usually associated with gallstones, which can be made mainly of cholesterol or calcium. They can be as tiny as grains of sand (and those that size which are made of cholesterol can be dissolved with medication over time). The largest one I have seen was almost two inches in diameter, and that person just had a little intolerance to fat as a symptom.

Bile is stored in the gallbladder, and is squeezed out into the duodenum in small or large quantities to aid digestion when you eat a meal that has fat in it. If the gall bladder is sick, as with stones or inflammation due to infection, for examples, then not enough bile can reach the small intestine to help digest the fat, and you get indigestion whenever you eat fat. We call that fat intolerance, and it is a frequent symptom of gallbladder disease.

Sometimes a gallstone passes from the gallbladder down the cystic duct. That usually causes pretty severe pain. If it then passes into the common bile duct, which includes bile excretion from the liver, and hangs up there in a smaller tube, then you have pain, but also very soon yellow eyeballs, and clay-colored stools. The reason is that the bile (AKA bilirubin) soon backs up into the blood stream when it can't drain into the duodenum normally.

Acute inflammation of the liver (Hepatitis) usually hurts in the right upper quadrant because the right lobe of the liver is the larger one by far. That doesn't mean it won't also hurt on the left also. It is more likely to just be an ache rather than something severe.

Very light-colored stools and yellow eyeballs are common symptoms of liver inflammation, as well as cirrhosis of the liver (which usually doesn't hurt and isn't tender when you press on it). Hepatitis A or B are by far the most common causes of liver inflammation in this country. Common causes elsewhere include the very serious malaria and yellow fever, which are transmitted by mosquitoes.

If you want to get an idea about whether your liver may be enlarged, lie on your back and draw up your knees to relax your stomach muscles. Then put the tips of the fingers of your left hand around just below your right ribs, pointing approximately toward your right shoulder. Press downward with your fingers as you take a really deep breath. If your liver is not enlarged, you may feel the slightly sharp edge of it slide down against your fingers. It is not normally tender when you touch it. It normally does not slide downward more than one finger's breadth below the rib margin. Also it is normal to not feel it at all if your abdomen is soft (and not fat). Those with diseased livers may feel the liver edge to be rounded and extending downward as much as two or three fingers below the ribs. Those that are enlarged and also tender usually have a relatively new inflammation, whereas those that are enlarged but not tender usually have a condition that has been there for awhile.

An enlarged liver accompanied by fluid in the abdomen is a very bad condition, and must have all the medical help the person can get.

Left Upper Quadrant Pain

Ruptured spleen. This usually starts with some kind of trauma to the left lower ribs. Blood is a pretty irritating substance to the tissues of the body when it is outside of the blood vessels. So when blood gets into the peritoneal cavity, it hurts. Just ask a woman who has pain with ovulation, where just a few drops of blood spill out when the egg breaks loose each month in some people.

If the spleen is swollen, as it usually is for awhile in Infectious Mono, it doesn't take much of a jar to cause a tear in its exceedingly delicate wall. A broken rib in that area can penetrate it. So

One ruptured spleen I successfully diagnosed in time to save a life early in my career was caused by a rubber ball thrown by the woman's two-year-old child two or three days before she began to feel faint when she stood up, and she didn't even remember it happening until after the operation.

it is a really good idea for football players to always wear rib pads. Unfortunately we aren't usually wearing rib pads when we are involved in auto accidents or other contact sports, such as falling off of mountains, or crashing while snow skiing. I will confess, however, that I ordered a football rib belt through the trainer of our football team for skiing after my second set of ski-related rib fractures, and I wear it to this day when I ski. It makes falling far less painful.

The pain usually starts in the left upper quadrant and spreads down the gutter of the left side of the back wall of the abdomen before spreading all over if bleeding is really profuse. Another case I saw acted like a ruptured ectopic pregnancy because the first symptoms she had were down in the pelvis around the uterus. The clue was that her husband had been overseas on a TDY mission for the US Air Force for three months, and she swore that she had been faithful to him.

> *If you have abdominal pain and begin to feel faint when you stand up, that is a truly life-threatening emergency, and you must get to a hospital immediately. Unless there is a hospital nearby and you have someone to drive you there quickly, call 911. The feeling of faintness with abdominal pain, especially if accompanied by an increase in your heart rate of fifteen or twenty or more beats per minute on standing (e.g., from a sitting rate of 70 to a standing rate of 85 to 90), often means that you are bleeding internally. You must go to a hospital to find out.*
> *As quickly as possible!*

An **obstruction of the large intestine** at the corner by the spleen, where the bowel turns south toward the rectum, can cause some severe cramping there as the bowel contents, especially gas, try to pass. In that situation there would be swelling and the hollow drum-like sound when you tap the wall of the pit of the stomach (epigastrium).

And you wouldn't be able to pass gas after the first hour or so.

Right Lower Quadrant Pain

This is the most difficult area to figure out before surgery. The most likely diagnosis, percentage-wise, is probably not appendicitis, but it is the one that is most important to think about, because even in this day and age people still occasionally die from a ruptured appendix.

In women of the childbearing ages who are sexually active, especially with more than one partner, the pain is often found to be an inflamed Fallopian tube. A pelvic exam will usually find that the tube on the left side is also tender, along with the sore right one. Fever can be quite high in these, particularly if there is a pelvic abscess. This condition is called **P. I. D.** (for Pelvic Inflammatory Disease) or acute salpingitis.

The bacteria which cause by far the most of the P. I. D. cases in this country are gonorrhea and chlamydia. Gonorrhea tends to be more dramatic as to severity of symptoms, but chlamydial infections are just as bad where sterility is concerned.

P. I. D. causes the Fallopian tubes to scar, shrink, lose their little cilia for attracting the eggs to come in from the ovary after the monthly ovulation, or become totally closed forever so that pregnancy can't occur. P. I. D. is by far the greatest cause of infertility, in this country at least.

Older sexually active women can certainly contract this condition, but it is less likely after the menopause.

Ruptured tubal pregnancy. P. I. D. scarring of the tubes is also the cause of most of the tubal (or ectopic) pregnancies because the fertilized egg is bigger than the sperm that fertilized it and often can't get through the little hole that the sperm wiggled through in its trip up from the vagina.

Thus, when the egg comes to rest against the tube wall instead of that of the uterus, it just attaches itself there and starts to grow blood vessels to supply the growing ovum. Since the tube wall is very thin, this soon becomes a problem, either with not enough blood coming to the embryo so that it dies, or with too many blood vessels, so that it ruptures from the tube and bleeds, often heavily. Emergency surgery is needed if it ruptures. If it doesn't rupture, there is a medicine that will help the body to absorb the dead tissue. Your doctor can help you with that.

Appendicitis. The classic history of a case of this is that the patient begins to have some discomfort in the epigastric area of the upper abdomen some time, perhaps even a day or two, before coming in to see the doctor.

The patient's appetite diminishes, and there may be some nausea, but usually little or no vomiting.

Then after a time the pain leaves the upper abdomen and moves down to the lower right side, where it stays and gradually or rapidly gets worse. The patient typically lies on his side and doesn't want to move.

Pressing on the area where the pain is produces marked tenderness at that point if the appendix is located near the inner abdominal wall, as it often is. Releasing the deeply pressing fingers suddenly may produce a reflex pain which we call rebound tenderness. If that is present, then we can be pretty sure that something is irritating the peritoneum (the inner lining of the abdominal wall). That something is usually an inflammatory process such as appendicitis produces.

The pain of appendicitis may get worse and worse, then suddenly get much better for several hours before getting much worse over a wider area. When that happens, it often means that the appendix has ruptured, releasing the swelling that was causing one type of pain (as when we lance an abscess). But then the released pus begins to move out away from the area, inflaming the surrounding bowel and lining of the abdominal cavity, with resulting peritonitis. In addition to the pain, you get sicker, with vomiting often starting. The bowel sounds will go away as the peritonitis gets worse. If the doctor is called when the pain has just gone away, the diagnosis becomes even more difficult than usual, and he may feel he has to observe the patient for awhile when he really would be operating if he could just see under the skin.

> *Appendixes generally average about 3 inches in length, but I personally operated on one that was 7 inches long and hung down beside the rectum. That one certainly had non-typical symptoms, suggestive of prostatitis!*

One thing that usually won't happen is diarrhea at this time. Also it is very unusual for diarrhea to actually cause the appendicitis. I have seen only one such case. But, if you have diarrhea, and develop right lower quadrant pain, then see a doctor, because the pain of uncomplicated diarrhea is much more likely to be located in the middle or left side of the lower abdomen.

Appendicitis symptoms vary considerably depending upon the location of the appendix, that is, which way it is pointed from its attachment to the cecum (the first part of the large intestine). If it is pointed toward the back, there may be no right lower quadrant pain at all, but rather pain in the right lumbar area of the back (a retrocecal appendix). If it bends down into the pelvis and is fairly long, the pain will be identical to an inflamed Fallopian tube in women.

In this situation, as well as others where right lower quadrant or pelvic pain is involved, it is often not possible to make an accurate diagnosis pre-operatively. The diagnosis that must be made is whether this is an "acute abdomen" that requires surgery.

Surgeons often feel a little embarrassed to have to report to patient and family that the appendix was found to be normal. But they shouldn't because it is far better to remove a normal appendix than to not operate and have the appendix rupture.

Left Lower Quadrant Pain

The symptoms that occur in the right lower quadrant with ectopic pregnancy and P.I.D. are identical on the left side. These, of course occur only in women.

Diverticulitis is often called the left-sided appendicitis, and may have similar symptoms if an inflammation occurs. This condition usually occurs in people of both sexes sometime after age 50. Some people age faster than others, however, and I recall seeing one lone case in someone at age 36.

This condition without inflammation is called **diverticulosis.** It is a condition where little weak spots develop in the large intestinal wall. These are a result of the aging process to a considerable degree, but also they are a result of high pressure in the bowel over the years. After a while they become little, then larger, pockets pooching out from the main bowel wall. Solids in the bowel may become deposited in the pockets; and, if they aren't able to get out regularly, the stool materials (which are teeming with bacteria) cause that area to become inflamed. An abscess may result, with almost the same symptoms as appendicitis. Some people have a lot of these diverticulae and eventually have to have part of the left side of the bowel removed surgically to cure them. Others have their inflammations cleared up by antibiotics (something we can't do with appendicitis).

Treatment of this condition after the inflammation subsides is simple. The same thing will go far in totally preventing diverticulosis from developing in the first place. **Just keep your stools soft and avoid constipation** so that the pressure inside the bowel never gets very high. This is usually easy to accomplish and does not require the use of laxatives (which are mostly very undesirable -- see below). (See also the chapter on **Constipation**, some of which is reproduced below.)

A high fiber diet does wonders for our bowels. This consists of all kinds of raw fruits and vegetables, as well as whole grains in the form of cereals and whole grain breads.

Raisin bran with a cut-up banana and milk is a particularly good fiber breakfast. Popcorn is the highest fiber of all. The high fiber retains more water and prevents the stool from becoming hard.

Drinking enough water daily will help enormously to keep the stools soft. **FYI**: the water in the upper GI tract is absorbed by the last portion of the bowel. If you are not taking in enough water, the bowel will take out more and more water from the stool, making it harder and harder (constipated).

For the average person drinking at least eight 8-oz glasses of water (and little or no caffeine) will totally prevent hard stools. And you'll save a wad of money on over-the-counter methods for "keeping regular."

Laxatives and constipation. Constipation refers to a hard stool, not how often we have a bowel movement. Some people, for example, have a bowel movement only once a week. If the stool is soft, then they are not constipated.

Constipation can cause **anal fissures** (tears in the mucous membrane of the anus), which can be cured by applying Vitamin A&D ointment twice a day and softening the stools. Constipation also increases the pressure on the bowel wall and, over a period of time, leads to the development of diverticulosis.

The time when it is most natural to have a BM (bowel movement) is after a meal, when peristalsis is most active in moving the food along down the GI tract.

When you feel the urge to go, do it. Don't wait several hours, because the longer the stool is in the rectum, the harder it will get as all the water is absorbed by the bowel wall.

The use of laxatives will, again over a period of time, lead to chronic loss of the ability to move the digested food wastes along. Soon you will be unable to have a bowel movement without stronger and stronger laxatives. The safest laxative is a high fiber one like Metamucil. That one softens the stools and preserves normal bowel function.

If you are constipated and a high fiber diet hasn't helped in a few days, feel free to take a warm water enema, consisting of warm water right out of the tap, about a quart of it. Every pharmacy has an enema kit, with instructions how to use it. Hang the enema bag with warm water in it from the shower rod or top of the shower stall with a coat hanger. The best way is to lie on your left side and insert the nozzle into your rectum by pointing it toward your belly button. That is the direction your anal canal runs, and a nozzle lubricated with Vaseline or K-Y Jelly will slide right in. Then release the catch that controls the flow of water and let the bag empty.

After the bag is empty, gently remove the nozzle and lay it on a paper towel you have put there in advance. (Don't worry about making a mess. It's unavoidable, and it's just another human frailty that doctors and nurses deal with on a daily basis. Also mothers of little children. Just wash your hands thoroughly afterwards.) Lie there for 15 or 20 minutes if possible, so that the water can soften the stool somewhat for a foot or more above the rectum. Then, when you feel a pretty good urge, go ahead and sit on the toilet and let it come out.

Sometimes older people who are physically inactive complain of lower abdominal pain as they develop what we call an **impaction**, where the stool is hard as a rock and has to be dug out with a gloved finger. You can do it yourself, if necessary. In this case, after a regular enema has failed, give yourself or the person you are caring for a mineral oil enema. Let the oil stay in place for several hours, all night if possible. Then try one more warm water enema before going further. If still no results, then lubricate your finger and insert it into the rectum. Press the finger into the firm or hard fecal mass and always push toward the tailbone. That will avoid any possible damage to the bowel. Then just dig bits of it out at a time. This is no fun, and having done it dozens of times doesn't make it any better. But the person with the impaction will be <u>very</u> grateful. See the chapter on **Constipation** for further discussion of this and other bowel elimination problems.

CHAPTER 4 -- ACNE

Acne affects almost every teenager to some extent as a result of hormone changes going on in the body that especially affect the oil glands of the skin. It is usually more severe in boys. Certain birth control pills sometimes cause acne to flare up again for women after the teenage years. It usually subsides by age twenty, but may persist to some degree in a few people into their thirties.

*Acne prevention is difficult due to the hormone influences, but you can greatly reduce the severity and improve the self-image of your teenagers by cleaning out the blackheads at home and having them cleanse their acne areas twice a day.

For the milder forms of acne Revlon has a great blackhead remover which can be purchased at many pharmacies for only about $3.00. There are holes of different sizes at each end for different sized blackheads. You use it by first washing your face thoroughly, then putting the clean instrument on the blackhead so that the blackhead is centered in one of the holes. Then just push straight downward until the blackhead pops completely out. I've seen blackheads that were fully an inch long, so don't be surprised at your results.

Then cleanse again, either with alcohol, which I prefer, or just regular soap and water, which is probably just as good as the alcohol. An ideal time to do this blackhead removal is after a hot shower, when the skin is especially soft.

It takes several weeks for the blackheads to fill back up again, and each time you clean them out, they come back smaller. As long as you are the only one using the instrument, just washing it carefully with soap and water and then dipping it for a few minutes in alcohol after each use will be adequate disinfection. If your brother or sister is also using it, then you really should also pass it through a flame briefly before use. A cigarette lighter works well, as does a gas grill starter. Just be careful where you use the fire. Catching the house on fire while you are supposed to be saving money by cleaning out your own blackheads is not an acceptable option.

Most doctors don't have time to clean out the blackheads or just don't want to fool with them. Dermatologists will charge $50 or more for doing this. So this is **a real money-saver.** In those with especially oily skins, I recommend using a detergent on the acne areas. Not everyone's skin will tolerate detergents; so if a rash develops, stop the detergent.

Retin-A gel is often prescribed for use after washing in the evening. It causes the surface layers of the skin to turn a little red and peel, thus opening up the clogged pores. Its chief disadvantage is that you can't go out in the sun with it on your skin or damage will occur. So if you use this, be sure to wash it off in the morning before leaving the house.

Accutane is essentially Retin-A in pill form and, because of possible side effects, is reserved for only the worst cases of acne, those with the cystic nodules and potential scarring, plus those with poor response to other treatments. And we try to limit its use to boys because it will cause damage to your baby if you take it when pregnant (even when you haven't yet missed a period). No doctor will order it for girls unless they are on at least one, but preferably two reliable birth control methods and sign a statement that they understand the risks and will not allow themselves to become pregnant while taking the medication. Also, if you are a girl, your doctor should require that you have a negative pregnancy test before giving you a prescription for it.

Its effects on the fetus disappear soon after you stop it. So you can feel safe in getting pregnant when you have been off of it for three months or more.

Oxy-10 is a pretty good over-the-counter medication to put on the skin to reduce the number of acne pimples. Use as directed after first cleansing the skin.

Benzoyl peroxide (BP), 5% applied daily reduces plugging of the pores 100-fold in only two days.

Antibiotics are often necessary in moderate to severe cases, with pus pockets in the tissues. If you are in the sun quite a bit, you must tell your doctor because the tetracycline family, especially doxycycline and minocycline increase your risk of sunburn. He will be more likely to use erythromycins in that case.

Someone who has been using these broad-spectrum antibiotics for quite awhile may become more susceptible to yeast infections of the acne areas, vaginal area, and intestinal tract. The normal bacterial flora in the bowel get severely disturbed and may need supplemental acidophilus capsules periodically, or perhaps even daily. Occasionally systemic yeast treatment with nystatin (pretty cheap) or Diflucan (much more effective in only 1-3 days, but also much more expensive) is needed, and that can have a dramatic effect in those whose cysts are growing yeast in them.

CHAPTER 5 -- ADDICTION TO LEGAL DRUGS

My mother was addicted to legal drugs, and a close medical colleague of mine accidentally died of an overdose; so this has always been a source of special concern to me in my medical practice. When I was still in medical school, I had some wisdom teeth pulled. The dentist gave me a drug for pain called Nembudiene, which was a combination of Nembutal, a barbiturate sleeping medication, and codeine, a strong pain drug. Boy, I want to tell you, I felt no pain! In fact, I felt so wonderful that I decided then and there that I had better suffer a little pain and never take those again. Otherwise I might easily get hooked on them. The next narcotic I took was one shot of Demerol a few hours after my appendectomy about 40 years later.

Addiction does happen to doctors all too often, and the DEA no longer allows a physician or dentist to prescribe most of these drugs for themselves or their families. All the state medical societies now have committees which attempt to rehabilitate physicians impaired by drug abuse. That includes alcohol, which of course is also a drug but not a controlled one since the repeal of Prohibition. Most, if not all, state licensing boards now require that all physicians who suspect another of being drug-impaired report that physician to them for investigation and appropriate action.

Patients who suspect a physician of substance abuse should also contact their state licensing board. Also refuse to allow that physician to continue to care for you or your family.

> *Recently in my clinic I had three such people come in within an hour, a man and two women. The man showed me a skin abrasion which he said had been inflicted on him two days before by someone hitting him with a piece of rebar. I was certainly sympathetic to him until I looked closely at the "wounds" and saw that they were almost healed and thus didn't fit his story. Also, when his attention was diverted, he had no tenderness. Furthermore, when I checked with the front office girls, they said that he had been walking straight upright when he walked in the front door but was stooped in pain when I walked into the examining room. So he didn't get his drugs of choice but did get a program for getting well without them.*
>
> *One of the women had pelvic pain which was unbearable and got worse when under stress, a not unusual problem, especially if there has been an abusive relationship at any time back to childhood. But drugs only make the problem worse over time. Counseling is essential here, but some doctor had let her sad story cloud his judgement and had allowed her to become addicted to Percocet. I couldn't cure her problems at our urgent care clinic, but for sure I didn't feed her addiction. I gave her some good alternatives, none of which she listened to. Two hours later we got a call from one of our other clinics, where she had come with a slightly different story but still a drug-seeking one that the bright young female doctor had instantly recognized. I don't know where that patient is today. Perhaps she has returned to the "doctor" who helped her get hooked in the first place.*
>
> *The third young woman had nothing wrong with her. She merely wanted drugs to give to her boyfriend and asked for the same thing he wanted.*

If you note alcohol on the breath of a physician who is caring for patients, refuse to allow his care, complain to the hospital nursing supervisor, the hospital administrator, and the medical chief of staff. We know that our reflexes are impaired by an average of 10% by just one drink of alcohol and by 25% after the second drink in less than an hour. I have seen the actual testing being carried out. And the blood levels of these people are not high enough to be considered legally drunk in most states! I'll be frank: if the reflexes are impaired, then the thinking processes are too. Most of us in practice no longer have even one drink when on call for patient care. And that's as it should be. Those who can't control their stress levels in other ways, such as exercise or meditation or relaxation tapes, should not be in a position to damage someone through impaired thought processes. And doing surgery or delivering babies is absolutely criminal conduct.

Goodness knows, there are sufficient ways in which medical judgement can be clouded without involving drugs. Having to care for a sick person at 3:00 AM, for example, then having to treat 25 to 40 patients the next day when tired.

There are a whole host of so-called controlled substances which require a certificate from the DEA (Drug Enforcement Administration) for a doctor to prescribe or dispense. The reason they are "controlled" is because they have great potential for producing addiction in susceptible people. The most common ones that get people into trouble are sleeping pills, anti-anxiety pills (which some call "happiness pills"), and pain pills.

My rule of thumb for narcotics and other potentially addicting substances is to prescribe them for no more than two weeks. After that the patient must have some other way of controlling pain, or just tough it out. People with chronic pain should never be given addicting drugs, but rather one or more of a number of alternatives.

The use of antidepressant medicines often helps to raise a person's pain threshold enough that something non-habit forming can be used, such as aspirin or Tylenol, instead of the stronger stuff.

Couch potatoes don't handle pain as well as those who have at least a small degree of fitness. Almost any kind of exercise, especially one lasting 30 minutes or more at a time, goes a long way toward raising your pain threshold, and should be started almost immediately after an injury.

Smokers tend to feel more pain than non-smokers, possibly because not enough oxygen is getting to the injured tissues, but possibly also because one of the hundreds of chemicals in tobacco smoke is poisonous to inflamed or irritated tissues. Yet another reason to stop smoking.

Those under stress have lower pain tolerance, as do people who aren't getting enough sleep. Relaxation exercises are good for both types of problems. Please see the chapters on **Insomnia** and **Staying Well Mentally** for help in these areas.

Those who are hooked on drugs play all kinds of games and become great actors and actresses in order to persuade doctors to prescribe habituating and addicting drugs.

A favorite time for these people to come in is just a few minutes before closing, when everybody is tired after a twelve hour shift and ready to go home. They assume that we will give them what they want just to get rid of them. Wrong!

Pharmacists are very good about calling and letting us know when a person is getting pain meds from multiple doctors.

People with migraine headaches are tough. Narcotics actually cause rebound headaches in them so aren't a good idea for multiple reasons. True migraine patients are miserable, and we all want to help them. Some people claim to have a migraine and

> *One man was so incensed when I wouldn't give him his oxycontin (a particularly addicting drug) at closing time that he reached down and untied my shoestring before he stalked out of the door. I'm not sure -- would that be considered assault, or battery?*

ask for a specific drug. That is usually a tip-off for a drug seeker.

I really feel sorry for people in pain, and I give as much pain medication as a person needs for an acute injury or for cancer patients. But I won't add to the problems by allowing those with an injury to become addicted.

I don't care if the cancer patient becomes addicted as he or she nears death. But it is surprising how few do. Many want to be in full command of their thinking processes as long as possible but just want to know they can have pain meds if they need them. We even use IV morphine which the patient can control to take as much or as little as he or she wants. Rarely does one take as much as I would order. These are mostly very courageous people.

CHAPTER 6 -- AIDS (Acquired Immune Deficiency Syndrome)

What It Is

- It is caused by a virus called HIV (human immunodeficiency virus).
- Being HIV positive does not mean one has AIDS.
- AIDS is fatal.

In June, 1981, the Centers for Disease Control and Prevention (CDC) included in their weekly report the fact that five gay men in Los Angeles had died from a very rare parasitic lung infection called pneumocystis carini pneumonia. It was soon discovered through careful study of further cases that those afflicted with this condition had abnormally low immune systems. Initially all cases were in the gay community, but it didn't take long for some to appear in people who had had a blood transfusion and those who shared syringes and needles to "shoot up" drugs.

Early requests for funds to study what was apparently a new and very deadly disease were mostly met with a deaf ear by Congress and the President. After all it was probably just God's way of punishing people for being gay. Never mind that God made them that way from birth. But the so-called Moral Majority (in my opinion they are neither!) exerted enough influence for the first several years to seriously restrict funding. So a lot of people died who didn't need to because the cause of the pneumocystis carini infections was slow in being found. A virus was always suspected, but it was hard to find. Once found, it was hard to evolve a test for it. It began to turn up in other parts of the world, particularly in Africa, where it was strictly a disease of heterosexual people.

Finally the Human Immunodeficiency Virus (HIV) was nailed down as the culprit. There are at least two subtypes now known. Now for a vaccine. No way Jose! It mutates too rapidly for a vaccine to be developed so far. In that way it is like the flu viruses, which produce at least one new strain for which we need a new vaccine every year. But new medications are constantly being tested and approved on a fast track by the FDA. The protease inhibitors are the ones which have allowed people like Magic Johnson, the famous Los Angeles Lakers basketball star, to live as long as ten years after being diagnosed and still show no signs of deterioration.

As soon as a blood test for it was developed, our blood bank supplies became more secure again, after thousands who had been transfused in the early 1980s became infected with HIV. Arthur Ashe, the famous and well-loved tennis star was the most visible of those.

In the twenty years since the CDC first reported those deaths over 22 million people around the world have died of AIDS, over 438,000 in the U. S. Currently in our country it is estimated that about 900,000 people are HIV positive, and 1/3 of them don't know it because they haven't been tested. Another 1/3 have AIDS now. Worldwide approximately 36 million people are HIV positive, 25 million in Africa, where it apparently originated.

The gay community continues to lead the numbers of new cases of AIDS victims. One gay spokesman said recently that the reason is that young gay men feel that either it's not around any more or that there is a cure since there are so many HIV-positive guys around who look so good.

Right now in the U. S. about 15,000 die from AIDS each year (down from 40,000 three or four years ago), but there are still 40,000 new cases being reported each year, almost exactly the same for the last ten years. At least the numbers are no longer rising exponentially as they did in the 1980's.

Want to know in what group the infection rate is growing the fastest, percentage-wise, though not in total numbers? The old folks! Believe it or not, with or without Viagra, there is a sex life after 65! These older people no longer need fear unwanted pregnancy, so they don't practice safe sex. But they need to!

The second fastest growing HIV positive segment of the population is the young heterosexual boys and girls between the ages of 15 and 21. Not surprising since those are also the ones with the majority of other sexually transmitted diseases.

The following lists are being passed out to interested people in various walks of life by health departments and others who are helping to slow the spread of this terrible disease. This happens to be the one I have been using in my office. I don't know the origin of it, and I have modified it somewhat as further information has become available.

Symptoms of AIDS

(may not appear for 10 years after infection with HIV).
- Swollen glands
- Chronic diarrhea
- Severe weight loss
- Night sweats or fever
- No appetite (anorexia), always tired (but see also the chapter on **Depression**)
- White patches in the mouth (yeast infections)
- Purple bumps and blotches

- Dry coughing that doesn't go away

If you have any of these symptoms, see your doctor.

How It Is Spread or Transmitted

Transmitted through:

- Sexual contact with an HIV-infected person.
- Blood transfusion with infected blood or blood products.
- Syringes and needles previously used by an infected person -- also tattoo needles.
- Infected blood, and other body fluids to a lesser degree, coming in contact with mucous membranes of the eyes, nose, mouth, anus and rectum, and vagina.
- The mother to the child, transmitted during pregnancy or through mother's milk after delivery.

<u>Not</u> transmitted by:

- Doorknobs
- Toilet seats
- Insect bites
- Handshake
- Plain kissing
- Sneezing/coughing
- Casual contact with HIV-positive individuals, e.g., shaking hands, hugging
- Sharing of food

How to Prevent It

Folks, we all should know that the only ways to be sure that you won't contract HIV are, first and foremost, don't have sex with anyone until after you are married and you both have negative tests for HIV. Second, don't use IV drugs. Third, don't have a situation where you have to have a blood transfusion. Fourth, don't become a health care worker, where you may accidentally come into contact with HIV-infected blood. That pretty much covers it.

BUT, if you are going to have sex, be sure the guy wears a condom and knows how to put it on so that it isn't likely to break. The way you do that is to put it on after he has an erection (hard-on) and allow some room at the end for further expansion during lovemaking. And be very careful to avoid spilling semen on the skin or sheets on removal of the rubber. See the **Condoms** part of the **Contraception** chapter for more explicit instructions.

Don't floss your teeth before going out on a date. Any little break in the mucous membrane of the mouth can make you more susceptible to blood-borne disease from someone you kiss. And if you already have AIDS, the small amount of blood in your mouth could infect your date if you kiss. (Kissing normally isn't likely to transmit the HIV virus.)

Wash your hands, as well as the penis and vagina and the surrounding areas, before and after having sex. This makes for good foreplay. But be sure to put on the rubber as soon as the penis is hard.

What To Do If You Are Exposed

An all too common exposure which we see in our clinics is one where a health care worker is stuck by a needle that has been used on a patient. If the patient is known, then the risk can be judged by simply asking the patient whether he or she has AIDS or any other blood-borne diseases and/or getting the patient's permission to do lab tests on a sample of his or her blood. I have yet to know of a patient who did not answer truthfully or readily agree to the blood tests for AIDS and Hepatitis B and C at the least.

If you have a needle stick injury from a patient known to you to be HIV positive, then you must as quickly as possible wash and disinfect the wound with surgical soap (or just plain soap), Betadine, dilute bleach, or whatever. Drop everything to do that. Then get immediately to a doctor who deals with these injuries, because if you can get started on the prophylactic agents Combivir or Indavir within two hours, you have at least a 90% chance of staying free of the infection. The sooner the better. Maybe your hospital pharmacy can give you one pill to start on while the paper work is being done. This is an emergency even more than a laceration is.

Theoretically we have to pretend that everyone is infected until proven otherwise. That is why we use Universal Precautions. But sometimes we know that the patient is in the hospital with pneumocysitis carini infection, which is caused by AIDS, and we might hurry a little faster. The biggest problem arises when the needle is among others in a container for disposal, so that the patient it was used on cannot be identified. The Centers for Disease Control (CDC) in Atlanta, have suggested a protocol for these and other types of exposures which we almost all follow. It is briefly outlined here. It also requires that you get the prophylactic medication as soon as possible.

Lab tests after exposure include blood tests for HIV, Hepatitis B, and Hepatitis C, along with liver function tests and antibody tests to determine whether anyone who has been immunized against Hepatitis B needs a booster series. A week later the lab tests are discussed with the person, and a Hepatitis B booster is given, if indicated. Another will be given in a month, and a third in six months. The patient is then given appointments for the next year for follow-up labs as well as the immunizations.

CHAPTER 7 -- ALCOHOLISM and the EFFECTS of ALCOHOL

Alcoholism is a disease in addition to being a social disorder. Many people who abuse alcohol and drugs have a hereditary defect in their bodies which makes them more likely to become addicted.

How does one know that he or she is an alcoholic? All alcohol abusers deny that they have a problem. I frequently have patients who report that they don't drink very much, "just one or two (six-packs) of beer per night." Or "I just drink white wine." CAGE is one way to evaluate whether you have a problem.

Some simple questions to ask are:

- Do you <u>ever drink to excess</u>? The definition of excess can be bent to fit one's own situation as the observer or the drinker. There is general agreement that you drink to excess if you ever drink enough to have a blood alcohol at or above the legal limit for your state. That amounts to no more than two drinks in three or four hours for most people. An occasional such episode (e.g., New Year's Eve) need not be serious, provided you are not driving. But it may be a warning signal. More than once is a big red flag.

- Drinking to excess also includes whether you drink every day. Do you <u>need</u> a drink every day, or even once a week?

- Do you get "the jitters" if you don't have a drink? Some people think they are not alcoholics if they don't delirium tremens (DTs) when they have not had a drink for a few days. Nothing could be farther from the truth. I have known and treated literally hundreds of alcoholics during my career but less than two dozen patients with DTs. But I have had <u>several</u> dozen patients with cirrhosis of the liver, which occurs almost exclusively in alcoholics. Having DTs even once, however, is diagnostic of alcoholism.

- Has anyone in your family or circle of friends, or a doctor, ever suggested to you that you are drinking too much?

- After drinking the previous evening or day, do you sometimes have trouble remembering everything that happened after your first drink?
- Do you ever feel the need for an "eye-opener" in the morning?
- Do you ever sneak a drink at work?
- Have you ever gone on "a bender" that lasted several days or more?
- Do you ever have trouble resisting the urge to drink?
- Have you ever felt you might possibly have a drinking problem?
- Has alcohol ever affected your work or an interpersonal relationship?

The answer of "yes" to any of these questions means that you are probably an alcoholic.

The younger that a person is first exposed to alcohol, as in an 8 or 10 or 12-year-old that is allowed by the parents to drink wine at holiday occasions, or in a teenager allowed a drink at dinner, the more likely he or she is to become a problem drinker later.

There is a good reason why there are laws against under age drinking and that is that alcohol has a much more profound effect on their minds and bodies before they reach full maturity. In my opinion that doesn't occur until about age 20 to 23.

I well remember a 17-year-old fraternity brother of mine who had never had a drink before he came to college as a freshman. He (illegally, of course) began to drink at parties on weekends, then before going to bed at night, then as soon as he got out of class. By the end of his freshman year he was a hopeless alcoholic and dropped out of school with cirrhosis of the liver. In my medical career I have known only two with cirrhosis who were younger.

The Native Americans of the Southwest either drink to the point of alcoholism or they don't drink at all. No Indian is a social drinker. There appears to be an enzyme deficiency, probably in the liver, that leads them to become addicted. There is some speculation that the same enzyme deficiency may be related to the extremely higher rates of diabetes, particularly in the Pima Indians, who have a diabetic rate of 50 percent or more in their tribe. The carbohydrate metabolism seems to be affected.

There is speculation that the same or a related enzyme deficiency may be present in people who are carboholics -- that is, people who binge on refined carbohydrates and get fat, especially in the abdomen, but don't drink alcohol. It's as though they are addicted to sweets instead of alcohol. The "sugar high" occurs when the blood sugar rises quickly above your baseline after you eat or drink something sweet. In response to the higher blood sugar, your body then puts out extra insulin, which causes the blood sugar to fall below your baseline. That lower blood sugar causes you to be hungry. So you eat more refined carbohydrates and the blood sugar goes up again. These cycles occur repeatedly all day long, forcing sugar into fat storage and increasing your weight.

Complex carbohydrates, on the other hand, are absorbed much more slowly so that the sugar peaks and valleys are much smaller and can be metabolized without going into fat storage.

Enough of that.

Alcohol removes our inhibitions, layer by layer, with each drink. After a few drinks people often do things they would never do if they were sober.

Just one or two drinks will loosen our tongues and the guy who's normally a wallflower may become the life of the party -- often to his or her embarrassment the next day.

There probably isn't too much harm in becoming the life of the party once, just so long as you don't try to drive home, or ride with somebody who's been the doing the same as you. Doing it on a regular basis, however, is not a good plan.

States are clamping down more and more on drinkers who drive. Many have reduced the legal limit in the blood to 0.08, and it is likely that some will go on down to 0.05 in the next few years, the same as many foreign countries. There are a very few countries who have zero tolerance -- if you even have a blood-alcohol of 0.01, you'll be arrested. By no coincidence those countries have minuscule alcohol-related fatality rates compared to us.

In the U.S. alcohol is involved in more than 50 percent of fatal accidents. (Sometimes cell phones seem to be involved in the other 50 percent.)

Falling asleep at the wheel is common enough when just the oxygen in your blood is reduced. Even a little alcohol greatly increases that risk.

There been some medical studies suggesting that you should take two drinks of alcohol every day to improve your blood fat profile. Many doctors now accept the studies as facts.

Don't believe them! It has been well known for years (and confirmed many times in my own practice) that "excessive" alcohol will raise your cholesterol and triglycerides. It will also

High altitude greatly accentuates the drowsy effect of alcohol, especially for those who don't normally live at high altitude. I cared for an emergency room patient from Chicago who had one drink early in the evening in a town located 3000 feet below Flagstaff. About 15 miles outside of Flagstaff, at 7000 feet, he fell asleep at the wheel, went off the road and rolled over several times.

His injuries were severe, but fortunately he had remembered to put on his seat belt and he survived.

raise your blood pressure and may you push over into type II diabetes if you're possibly susceptible.

The main reason for the blood fat abnormalities is that they are processed in the liver, and alcohol is a poison, especially to the liver. If alcohol "in excess" can (and does) have those effects, doesn't it make sense that smaller quantities (and I'm not saying the two drinks is a small quantity -- in some people that is enough to make them legally drunk!) will also have a smaller but still bad effect on the liver?

> *Within a year after those articles began popping up in the popular literature I had several people in my practice who were faithfully drinking two glasses of red wine every night. Some, of course, used the studies as an excuse, while others really believed it would be good for them. At least five of those people turned up with abnormal liver function tests that indicated that the alcohol was killing some liver cells and making the others sick. Two or three others showed up with high blood pressure. One had become diabetic.*

If you want to drink with little risk to your body, limit your intake to no more than two drinks no more than two nights a week, and never drive after drinking even one, nor ride with anyone who has had a drink. Allow your body several days to detoxify with no alcohol in the body each week and take a good multivitamin that is high in vitamin B-complex.

Also remember, alcohol is empty calories and contributes to obesity.

Alcohol Consumption During Pregnancy

Alcohol consumption during pregnancy is now the chief cause of preventable mental retardation in the U. S. **We now know that even one drink of alcohol during your entire pregnancy is too much.**

In Conclusion

Most people won't get into trouble if they drink no more than two normal strength drinks no more than twice a week and they never drive after any drinking. But some will.

Everyone's metabolism is different. Everyone should have some days when there is no alcohol at all in the body. For alcohol is a poison, a mild and pleasant one in moderation, but still a poison. A few liver cells are damaged and/or die with each drink. Since we all have billions of liver cells, that is not usually a problem. The difficulties begin to arise when there is always some alcohol in the body so it can't heal the damaged cells. Or when there is a large quantity of alcohol in the body at times. I guarantee you that you kill at least 100,000 liver cells every time you get drunk, and millions if you really go on a bender. People with alcoholics or drug addicts in their families should never drink alcohol, or the odds are overwhelming that they will become alcoholics. It is hereditary.

CHAPTER 8 -- ALTERNATE THERAPIES

Forget Homeopathy. It isn't approved by the FDA, but mainly it flies in the face of reason and just plain <u>doesn't work</u>. It is a terrible waste of money.

Healing by energy fields. This is a distinct possibility. Our bodies each have unique and measurable energy fields surrounded by invisible auras. The Russians 40 or 50 years ago developed a method for picturing these fields called Kirlian Photography. And UCLA's Department of Kinesthesiology at one time had a machine that could measure auras.

Research at the Rhine Institute at Duke University indicates that about one in every 10,000 people can actually see another person's aura. I know two such people. One of them played first violin in a symphony orchestra for about twenty years. Her husband told me that they had been married for almost forty years before she told him she could see auras, because she was afraid he would think she was crazy.

Zinc and the common cold. Only zinc gluconate in the lozenge form has been shown in well-designed studies to shorten the duration of a cold. However it shortens the duration by only one day. None of the zinc formulas have any beneficial effect on the severity of cold symptoms.

For those, try 1000 mg of Vitamin C daily, lots of fluids, extra sleep, and one of the Alka-Seltzer formulas.

For herbal remedies, see the extensive chapter on **Herbal Remedies.**

Acupuncture is an ancient (6,000 years old) Chinese therapy which uses tiny, almost hair-sized needles which are inserted into various spots in the body corresponding to the maps of the body's energy fields. I have no idea how it works on those energy fields, but it often does. If you decide to go this route, be sure you go to someone who has been trained by a Chinese therapist. The stuff that many chiropractors try to persuade you they can do with "acupressure" is mostly just a means of separating you from your money. However, acupuncture really does work for a lot of things when used by experienced and well-trained hands.

The day before I started writing this a very nice older lady came into our clinic complaining of abdominal pain of several months duration. She also had become aware of a hard lump on the right side of her abdomen several months ago. She was concerned about this but told me that she had been seeing her **"microscopist"** every six months for several years. He had been taking a blood sample from her each time, at $50 a visit, and then displaying what he alleged was her blood, highly magnified, on a computer screen. He would then study the display and tell her what was going on in her body. I asked what his qualifications were, and she told me that "he is very highly educated," with all kinds of certificates on his walls. But he was not a doctor, not even a Ph. D.

When she had last seen him several months ago with the abdominal symptoms, he looked at her blood and told her that she just had "a problem with yeast." Now I have seen at least several hundred patients who have had yeast infections, and I am not aware of any conceivable test where anyone can look at a blood smear and make that diagnosis, unless, perhaps, the patient is desperately ill with yeast growing in the blood stream just before death. I also have never before heard of "a microscopist" who is allowed to practice medicine.

The reason that my patient finally sought help from a doctor was that she had not been able to keep any solid food and very few fluids down for three days. On physical examination I found that she was dehydrated and had two huge rocklike tumors in the abdomen which were almost certainly far-advanced cancer. That "microscopist" should be strung up by his testicles! Because of his scam and his ability to sell himself as a knowledgeable professional, this nice lady is going to die very soon without ever having a chance for treatment. We all know that cancer is a bad diagnosis, but almost every one of those has a chance for cure if found in time. The "microscopist" with his scam assured that she would never seek legitimate health care providers in time.

So, add "microscopist" to the long list of people who prey on an unsuspecting public, and spend your health care dollars somewhere else.

CHAPTER 9 -- ANEMIA

Anemia simply means not enough red blood cells in the body.

What tests tell us we are anemic? The simplest ones are the best usually. First a CBC (complete blood count) can tell us a lot of other things besides just whether a person is anemic or not. Also it is very economical.

There are three main ways we measure your blood cells in a CBC: counting the number of red blood cells in a small measured amount of blood and multiplying that by a factor to obtain a number for you, which is then compared to a reference range for other people who have been determined to be "normal." The second is to measure the amount of hemoglobin (the chemical inside our red blood cells which carries the oxygen). The third is to measure the percentage of red blood cells in the liquid blood by what is called the hematocrit. Other evaluations include the size of the red cells, and whether they are smooth and round with normal color and nothing visible inside them.

For those who live at high altitude, the normal ranges are somewhat higher than for those who live at sea level, because we need more oxygen-carrying capacity in the reduced oxygen of 7,000 feet, where I have lived for most of my life. At that altitude our hemoglobins and hematocrits and total red cells increase an average of about 15% within three months of moving to the mountains. The other adaptation that occurs is in the lungs, where chemical changes begin to occur almost overnight to allow the smaller oxygen level to be absorbed more efficiently.

A hemoglobin of 12 grams percent at sea level, for example, might be considered normal, but at altitude would be anemic.

Second is a total serum iron test. You may have a normal serum iron and still be developing iron deficiency anemia. An abnormal serum ferritin test often precedes the eventual fall in total iron, and this test is particularly helpful in athletes.

A reticulocyte count will tell us whether the bone marrow is responding properly to the blood loss by cranking up the production of red cells.

Last of the common tests is the TIBC (total iron binding capacity). These can all be done at your neighborhood laboratory, and you can have an answer by the next day. Usually the CBC and/or ferritin will suggest a problem, and then it can be confirmed by the other tests.

Then the detective story begins, with the search for the cause of the loss of blood.

Several substances are necessary for proper production of new red blood cells to occur in the bone marrow. The most important of these are iron (ferrous, the valence two form, for those of you who are chemistry students), vitamin B 12, folic acid, and protein. Other vitamins and food substances are also needed for completely normal cell development, but these are the most important.

There are many different types of anemia. The most common, however, is Iron Deficiency Anemia, and that is the only one we will discuss here.

Iron Deficiency Anemia is caused primarily by loss of blood faster than it can be replaced by the body. Red blood cells normally live about four months before they begin to break down and be filtered out by the spleen to be then dissolved and recycled by our bodies.

Women who menstruate lose red cells each month, especially if their periods are long and heavy, and thus need to be especially sure that they provide enough of the raw materials mentioned above to the bone marrow red cell factory.

It is very unusual for men to become anemic from iron deficiency unless they are losing blood from the intestinal tract.

Athletes, particularly runners, who overtrain sometimes have this problem, because too many older red cells are damaged when their feet strike the ground for them to keep up with. They may complain of feeling tired, with loss of energy. Thus an abnormal serum ferritin level, may be the first sign that it is time to back off, take some iron and vitamins and protein, and generally let their bodies catch up. Usually a couple weeks will suffice to have them feeling exceedingly fit again.

Other situations where iron deficiency anemia occurs are people with a lot of nosebleeds, bleeding hemorrhoids, ulcerative colitis, post-surgery where more than a pint of blood was lost during the operation, people who donate blood frequently, pregnant women who must provide the materials for their baby's blood, and people with blood loss from diseased kidneys. Some people don't have enough acid in their stomachs to dissolve the iron for proper absorption. Sometimes these folks are benefited by taking iron along with citrus juice.

Babies, particularly if not breast-fed, may need iron supplementation starting about the third month as the iron stored in their livers from their mothers is depleted with increasing blood production in growth. Also babies who eat a lot of mashed potatoes seem to be more susceptible to this type of anemia.

Mead-Johnson makes a vitamin-iron formula called Fer-in-sol which I like to add to the diets of these kids by the end of the third month. It has to be given when there is no milk in the stomach or it won't be absorbed enough.

Those who have something in the GI tract that bleeds, such as a peptic ulcer, bleeding polyps, or a bleeding cancer will often become anemic. Such bleeding can be usually be confirmed by a stool specimen that is tested for occult blood. You just take a small dab with the little stick, like a small tongue blade, break open the stool which you have caught in some paper or fished out of the toilet, spread it thinly like butter on the small square of specially treated paper which your doctor has given you, and take or send it back to his office. He will put some drops of a test chemical on it and see if it turns blue, indicating blood.

When red cells are lost, there is no recycling of the materials in them to maintain the equilibrium. Therefore we must adjust our diets, with more protein, vitamin and mineral intake to allow for the needed extra production by the marrow. Extra iron in the form of ferrous sulfate is cheap and readily absorbed if there is no milk in the stomach at the time you take the pill.

Feosol is the oldest, cheapest, and

I had a lady patient one time who had bleeding hemorrhoids, to the point where she finally gave up and had them removed surgically. The bleeding had caused her to develop this anemia. I ordered her to take three Feosol tablets daily. A month later her blood count was even lower, though she wasn't bleeding any more than before. She was feeling lousy. I asked her if she had been taking her iron, and she assured me that she was. Another two weeks went by, and her count was still lower. Finally I asked her if she was taking Feosol. She said that she had asked for it at the drugstore, but the pharmacist had assured her that another cheaper brand was also ferrous sulfate, and therefore just as good. NOT SO! She then went back and got Feosol. By the end of a week her blood count was up 20%, and in three weeks it was back to normal! Then she had her surgery.

still one of the two or three best iron products on the market. But take the *Feosol* brand, not a generic substitute.

Not every stomach can tolerate the Feosol tablets. So the company offers Feosol Spansules -- a lot of tiny time-released granules. Taking them with citrus juice helps absorption.

There are also a couple of other iron formulas for those with sensitive stomachs made by good drug companies, but only a couple. ***This is one very important medication that** *always* **requires the brand name.** Fortunately, with iron we aren't talking big bucks.

Red meat has all the materials needed to produce healthy red blood cells, but red meat has certain drawbacks for some of us; so we may not be eating the one food that has everything and thus need to provide ourselves with supplements.

CHAPTER 10 -- ANKLE SPRAINS

The most common by far is the lateral sprain, where the foot turns in and overstretches one or more of the ligaments around the outside bone of the ankle (which we call the lateral malleolus). It is very unusual for any of the ligaments to be totally torn through. The sprain can vary from a mild but still painful stretch, with possibly some microscopic tears in the muscle, just as a newspaper gets little tears before all the fibers come apart as you pull on it, to a gross tear where there is almost instant swelling due to bleeding from torn blood vessels. You can have a pretty good idea that your sprain isn't a bad one, no matter how much it hurts, if there is little or no swelling. The milder ones you can treat yourself and **save money doing it.**

If your injured ankle swells a lot right away, then you need to see a doctor. If he determines, possibly with the aid of X-rays, that it is a sprain, then these suggestions that follow will help you get well faster. Obviously the same things work if you did not have to see a doctor.

Follow the acronym RICE (Rest, Ice, Compression, Elevation).

First and fourth, get off the foot and elevate the whole leg. That will help reduce the total swelling, and swelling is our enemy for a rapid recovery.

Second, get ice on it for 20 to 30 minutes as soon as possible. Keep applying ice at least two or three times a day for at least the next five days. There is some discussion among us sports medicine doctors about whether and when heat has a place in musculoskeletal injuries, but we all agree that <u>you should use ice, and nothing but ice, for at least the first 24 hours after any injury.</u> Heat causes more swelling initially, and I personally think that we should wait at least five days before using it. Then I like to use ice for 10 minutes, heat (medium heat from a heating pad -- never use the high setting -- we want to warm it, not cook it!) for 10 minutes, and ice again the last 10 minutes. Always wind up with ice.

Third, put something soft, like a horseshoe of foam, Kleenex, or whatever you can think of, around the lower part of the bone, with the opening in the U up. Wrap it in place with an elastic bandage as follows: Start wrapping on your foot just behind the toes, and take two or three turns pretty tightly around the foot before going around behind the ankle and then back around the heel and instep. Keep wrapping, like a figure-8, still pulling it pretty tightly, as you cover the area of soreness and swelling three or four times. I've been asked many times how tight to wrap an ankle. The answer is, as tight as you can unless the toes turn dark, and the foot goes to sleep. In that case, it is too tight and must be loosened. What you are trying to do is to both put enough external pressure on the torn and bleeding blood vessels to stop the bleeding, and to prevent other fluid from moving into the area and slowing down the healing process.

If bearing weight is pretty painful, then crutches may be required for up to three days, with minimal assisted weight bearing as tolerated.

After three days it isn't going to bleed any more, and it is time to start exercising, within limits, to help promote healing. From this moment on you must work to overcome the muscle atrophy that begins almost instantly when an injury occurs. Even without an injury our muscles begin to lose strength, or wither, or shrink, or atrophy within two or three days of not using them. So your exercise must begin on or before the third day to avoid atrophy, which can take a lot longer to overcome than it takes for the injured ligaments to heal. Even pretty badly torn ankle ligaments are usually healed back together in three weeks. But rehabilitation must continue much longer than that in all but the mildest of sprains.

Proper use of crutches: They must be adjusted so that your hands, not your armpits, support all of your weight when you walk. (There are large nerves in the armpit which must not be damaged.) You may need to put some additional padding on the handgrips. Put the tips of the crutches out in front of you and swing your body forward so that your good foot lands, not too far, out in front of you. Then just alternate the foot and crutches as you swing forward. Going up, and especially downstairs, can be a real challenge. For going down, especially for older people, it is a really good idea to have a strong belt somewhat loosely around your waist or chest for someone behind you to grasp and help steady your balance. Better yet, don't do stairs with crutches. When you are ready to quit the crutches, walk for a day with one crutch in the opposite hand. (Use it, or a cane, in the opposite hand because when one foot goes forward in walking, the opposite hand and arm swing forward to maintain your balance.)

You can take care of a sprained ankle yourself and **save yourself a lot of money** if you pay close attention to what I am describing here.

If you are an athlete or have unlimited funds (in which case you might not have bought this book), then having a physical therapist or athletic trainer work on your ankle every day with ultrasound, muscle stimulation, and other modalities plus exercising with therabands and other activities, will provide you with the quickest recovery. But you can get well pretty quickly even if you are entirely on your own. Always remember **only with faithful exercise will your ankle return to full normal function.**

I well remember one female patient I had back in Warsaw, Indiana who had sprained her ankle six months before she came to see me. It still hurt, and she still walked with a limp! The calf muscles of the injured leg were smaller than the other calf, and her shoe size had been reduced by a full size by the shrinkage of the small muscles of her foot.

She "had taken care of it" herself. First, she told me, she used heat on it because it felt better than ice. Then she borrowed someone's crutches and used them for two weeks. Then she used a cane for another three or four weeks, always being careful not to move the foot any more than she had to. She was horrified by my outline of treatment, but, bless her heart, she followed my instructions and after about three more months had a normal foot and ankle.

As soon as you are able, you should start the exercise where you rise up on your toes with both feet at the same time, then rock back on your heels with your toes up in the air. Do ten to start with, maybe three times a day. Gradually increase the number of repetitions until you are doing 100 without stopping on a flat surface. Then get a one-inch thick board. Go up on the board on the balls and toes of your feet and back off the board on your heels. Work up to 100 in a row on the one-inch board; then advance to a 2X4 or other two-inch thick board. Or you can just use a stair step. It is a little easier to regulate how much you are doing with the boards, but, since the main purpose of this book is to help you save money, use whatever is readily available.

On about the sixth or seventh day after the injury, it is a good idea to start lateral exercises against resistance. Ideally this would be with about six feet of elastic theraband or rubber surgical tubing. These can be obtained inexpensively from medical and physical therapy supply stores in big cities. In smaller communities, try using some tie-down bungee cords that you get at Checker Auto or Auto Zone stores. Just string some together to get the right length. Put the elastic cord around your foot just behind your toes. Then put it under your other foot and pull up on it with your opposite hand. Then turn your foot outward, keeping the heel on the floor and allowing it to rotate as the toe portion turns outward. Work up to at least 100 in a row every day, while pulling a little harder with the opposite hand to increase the resistance.

You can also stand with your foot against the wall, or your desk, and turn the toes part of your foot strongly against the wall for a slow count of twenty several times a day.

The last exercise which is absolutely necessary is one that teenagers especially do well with. That is standing up and balancing with almost all your weight on the injured foot all the time and every time you are talking on the telephone. This exercise strengthens the small muscles of the inside of your foot and completes the rehab program after three or four weeks.

As noted above it takes three weeks for an injured ligament (and most other wounds) to knit. The normal ligament has then been replaced by scar tissue, which is never quite as strong and elastic as the uninjured one. Therefore we work very hard to build up all the surrounding ligaments and muscles to more than make up for the injured one. If you do the exercises faithfully, your ankle will be just as strong and useful as it ever was in the past. **As with so many other conditions in your body, it's up to you!**

CHAPTER 11 -- ARTHRITIS

There are many types of arthritis. The most common is <u>osteoarthritis, or degenerative arthritis</u>. This begins anytime after about age 25 and is accelerated by wear and tear on particular joints. Obese people and those who do a lot of lifting tend to have more of the degenerative processes in the weight-bearing joints of the spine, hips, knees, and, to a lesser degree usually, the ankles.

Rheumatoid arthritis is the most disfiguring and crippling type, and you really need ongoing medical assistance for RA.

No matter what type of arthritis you have, making the muscles surrounding those joints as strong as possible will relieve a lot of discomfort and infirmity through graded exercise and <u>gentle</u> stretching. Always the key word is gentle. There are a number of books that you can get at a bookstore or the library that will guide you through a program for any joint. A single session with a physical therapist, who will teach you a program, is always a really good investment that you will get more out of if you have read a book first.

Medications that are helpful for this type of arthritis include most of the so-called non-steroidal anti-inflammatory medications (also called NSAIDs), such as ibuprofen and naproxen, which can be obtained over the counter, the newer COX-2 inhibitors, such as Celebrex, Bextra, and Vioxx, and the supplement Glucosamine.

The older NSAIDs adversely affect the stomach and intestinal tracts of about 20% of those who take them, so always take them with meals. Even when taken with meals, you should stop immediately if you develop heartburn, indigestion, stomach cramps, loose bowels, diarrhea, or bloody or black tarry stools. If you have ever had a peptic ulcer or GERD, stay away from these.

The newer COX-2 drugs have a <u>much</u> safer profile but still can affect the stomach in 2-5% of those taking them. They don't cause drowsiness, and their effects on liver and kidneys are kinder. But their <u>cost is exorbitant</u>, and they require a prescription. (See the chapter on **Saving Money on Drugs**.)

Glucosamine is the best bargain of the group, with no significant side effects in most people. Since it is classed as a dietary supplement it is not regulated by the FDA; so really accurate figures on side effects are hard to find. It is often combined with chondroitin at double the price. **Save money.** Buy the glucosamine alone. The studies that indicate the beneficial effects of glucosamine alone do not show any additional benefits from adding chondroitin. The dose of glucosamine is 500 to 1,500 mg daily. They can be found in capsules, tablets, or powder. Watch for sales of 20 to 40% off at your neighborhood pharmacy, and stock up at those times.

> *I have had four people in the hospital with gastrointestinal hemorrhages from these older medications. Also, if you take them for long periods of time, you must have your liver and kidney functions tested periodically for possible ill effects. And they can cause drowsiness.*

There are many arthritis publications advertising companies that specialize in making or selling various types of aids for weak and misshapen fingers and other joints.

> *Van Cliburn, the world famous pianist who specialized in the music of Tchaikovsky, developed such severe arthritic changes in his fingers from the heavy dramatic striking of the keys that Tchaikovsky requires if played correctly, that he had to have joint replacements before he was 40. I got to hear him play as beautifully as ever here at Northern Arizona University a year after joint replacement surgery.*

The most important thoughts I can leave you with here are to exercise as much as possible on a daily basis within the limitations of your condition, read books, check out catalogs with arthritis aids, and consult a physical therapist at least once, even if you have to pay for it yourself.

CHAPTER 12 -- ASTHMA

Asthma is a disease of the lungs in which the air tubes in the lungs are constricted by the smooth muscle in their walls and the flow of air is thereby limited. Other things that occur are swelling of the mucous membranes of the bronchial tubes, and formation of dry mucous plugs, which cause even more obstruction. Breathing symptoms, such as coughing, chest tightness, wheezing, rapid breathing, and shortness of breath occur as a result. Kids with asthma often are using every muscle in their little bodies in an effort to get enough air into their lungs. The symptoms are likely to be worse in the evening or early morning. Often cough comes before the wheezing or shortness of breath.

Triggers

The symptoms are often made worse, or an attack is brought on by exposure to things that can be a "trigger." These can be playing with a neighbor's new kittens, going out to eat at a restaurant where they still allow smoking, being held by or close to someone with smoke on their clothes, being cared for in a house where someone smokes indoors even when the child is not there, exercise, driving with the car windows open, exposure to something the person is known to be allergic to, and viral infections.

Other triggers include exposure to dust mites or mold spores, animal dander from any warm-blooded creature, cockroaches, and pollen (such as ragweed, Bermuda grass, Russian olive trees, juniper, Russian thistle, rabbit brush, and dozens more in various seasons). Also indoor and outdoor pollutants, such as when big cities announce an "ozone alert" or you can't see the Pasadena mountains from downtown Los Angeles, tobacco smoke, smoke from wood-burning fireplaces, perfumes, and cleaning fluids.

Medications may be triggers, such as aspirin; non-steroidal anti-inflammatory medications, which include ibuprofen in Advil and Nuprin; Naproxen; beta blockers, such as propanolol, atenolol, metoprolol; and several others.

> *My daughter, who was born a little early and weighed about 5 1/2 lbs developed asthma after she contracted pneumonia from measles she had been exposed to in our church nursery when she was about a year old. At the time, I was on active duty in the U.S. Air Force. The pneumonia sensitized her lungs to allergies so that asthma developed much earlier than it might have otherwise. Or maybe she would have been fine all her life. Neither my wife nor I had allergy problems. We'll never know.*
>
> *This was 5 years before the measles vaccine became available. We did, however, have gamma globulin which, if given soon after known exposure, would have made the case of measles <u>much</u> milder.*
>
> *Forgiveness is very much a part of my religious beliefs, but I have often thought how different would the lives of my family have been, if the mother who took her slightly sick child to the church nursery that day had kept it home so that my daughter would not have been exposed. Or if she had had the thoughtfulness to notify everyone whose children were there that day when her own child broke out with a rash!*
>
> *My religious beliefs are pretty strong. My grandfather was a minister, and worshipping God through prayers at meals and at bedtime, along with attendance at weekly church services, was an important part of our lives. I have often recognized that God pulled one of my patients through a terrible illness when I and the specialists I had called in could do no more. I firmly believe that God has answered my prayers for a patient many times.*
>
> *That said, let me tell you to remember this story about my daughter the next time you have a child with a runny nose, and maybe a little cough that you are thinking about taking to church with you. Don't do it.*

Certain physical activities, such as exercise, inhaling cold air, and hyperventilating can bring on attacks.

Certain things going on in your body can trigger attacks, such as stress, upper and lower respiratory infections, and GERD.

Environmental Control

Control of your environment is **absolutely essential**. This includes leaving your normal part of the country during ragweed or other pollen seasons that are included in your allergies, leaving town during smog alerts, or staying indoors in filtered air.

Never ride in a car with the windows open. Remove carpets from your child's bedroom and any other part of the house where the child spends much time. Flooring that works includes linoleum, tile, and wood. Do not use drapes or curtains, at least in your child's portions of the house, and use just shades in his or her room, cleaning them often.

Use no wall hangings or cloth pennants. Remove all stuffed animals and similar things from the child's room. Avoid contact with woolen fabrics. Keep clothing in a closet with the door shut. In other words, what we are trying to do is to reduce all sources of house dust as much as possible, because most asthmatics are allergic to house dust, which inevitably includes mites. The child should not sleep, sit, or lie on any upholstered furniture.

> *If you just can't bring yourself to take away a favorite stuffed toy that the child sleeps with, wash it at least once a week. If you can't wash it, then vacuum it when you clean your child's room, always remembering to keep the child out of the freshly vacuumed room for at least an hour after you finish, to let the dust settle. After you vacuum it, put it in the freezer for several hours to at least kill the dust mites. Microwaving the toys has also been suggested for killing the mites, but I don't know anyone who has tried it and then looked for live dust mites.*

Use special furnace filters to clean the air. Also cover the room air vents with filters to provide additional protection. Wash them or change them every week. What is even better in winter is to use hot water heat, where the hot water circulates through the house without any forced air vents. The only problem with that is that it doesn't allow for summertime air-conditioning.

In summer use air-conditioning to keep from leaving the doors and windows open. That will also help keep down the humidity and reduce mold growth.

Put an air cleaner with an HEPA (high-efficiency particulate air) filter in the child's bedroom; run it 24 hours per day with the door closed, and clean the filter at least once a week. 3-M has a $25 "almost HEPA" filter for furnace and air conditioner which has to be changed every 6 weeks. The best current value for household filtering, in my opinion, is the Eco-air filter, available in all sizes for only $4.95 in most stores, such as Lowe's and Home Depot. It must be changed only every three months. It also is "almost HEPA."

Damp mop and wipe the floors and furniture at least every other day. Use leather or vinyl on wood or metal furniture. Never use the vacuum cleaner when the child is in the room, and keep him or her out of an area where you have vacuumed for at least an hour, because there will always be dust in the air. Use a canister vacuum cleaner. I believe that every major vacuum cleaner company now has an external attachment for an HEPA filter, for less than $20. The filter needs to be replaced every three months. Your doctor may recommend one that he feels is better at trapping dust than others.

Superheated steam cleaning of the areas of the house that still have carpet seems to both kill dust mites and reduce allergens in the carpet.

If you yourself are the asthmatic, always wear a good dust mask whenever you vacuum. Or try to get someone else to do the vacuuming once a week while you leave the house for two or three hours. Some dust masks aren't as good as advertised, so try several. Regular surgical masks may work best. Dust masks are effective for about 30 minutes before they begin to leak a little dust.

In humid climates, use one, or even several, room dehumidifiers. They will pull up to two or three gallons of water per day out of the atmosphere. You are aiming for a household relative humidity of less than 50% in summer, and below 35% in winter. This will considerably reduce the amount of mold and mildew in the house. (These are a problem for the vast majority of asthmatics.) An air-conditioner will also reduce the household temperature and thus slow down mold growth.

Keep pets outdoors, even in winter! All warm-blooded animals have dander, and dander is a bad allergen. Better yet, don't have a pet that has fur. Goldfish are OK. But no turtles. They are often a source of infection, mainly salmonella.

You may feel that you have to try to find a way to keep your beloved pet. ("Do we keep the pet, which we had before the child, or keep the child?" It will probably ultimately be one or the other!)

To try to make your pet less allergenic, you might do the following:

1. Wash it once a week to remove the dander on the skin. This will also remove the allergenic substance in the saliva of cats that dries on their fur when they groom themselves.

2. Shaving or closely clipping furry dogs may possibly cut down on allergies. Hairless breeds produce fewer allergy symptoms, but only a porcelain one is totally allergy free, and that only if dusted at least once a week.

3. Wash the hands after petting animals.

4. Keep them out of the bedroom for sure, and out of the house if you really want to keep them for a long time.

Cats are the worst. They have both dander and dried saliva on their fur as allergens. One of my daughter's worst attacks after we moved to Arizona occurred after she had gone to a friend's house to see her new kittens.

It does little good to try to keep the cat isolated in a room without a carpet. From the time of the diagnosis of asthma, it will take 5 to 6 months of vigorous cleaning to significantly lower the levels of cat allergens in carpets, and they have been found to still be present in mattresses after 15 *years!* **Get rid of the cat!**

Products advertised to reduce a cat's allergens don't work. Save your money. Get rid of the cat!

Wash all bedding once a week in really hot water (above 130 degrees). This will kill the little critters, called dust mites, which live and flourish in our sheets and pillowcases. These are the most common of all allergens (an allergen is a substance which triggers an allergic reaction in anyone) and one of the main ones for asthmatics.

Cover the pillows, mattress, and box springs with special covers. An uncovered mattress will have high quantities of dust mites within four months. Airtight (oxygen-free) vinyl or plastic covers work well but are uncomfortable because of lack of air flow. Some stores and catalogs advertise "hypoallergenic bedding" which may have pores that are too big to keep them out. A finely woven fabric must have a pore size no larger than

0.006 of a millimeter to keep them out. Same size for cat allergens. The zippers should be firmly closed with strapping tape.

Three mail-order companies that have been recommended by one or more allergy specialists for washable allergy bedding, air filters, face masks, air filters, special vacuum cleaners, and other items are:

Allergy Asthma Technology Ltd., Chicago, IL, 1-800-621-5545

Allergy Control Products, Inc., Ridgefield, Conn. 1-800-422-3878

National Allergy Supply Inc., Duluth, GA, 1-800-522-1448

We tried putting our cat out in the garage, with a kitty door she could go in and out through, and a warm bed by the house wall up on a shelf. This actually worked pretty well, but she was a very popular little kitty, and it wasn't long before we found that she had nightly visitors sharing her bed -- and especially her food. One winter night we drove into the driveway, punched the button to raise the garage door, and found there in our headlight glare a large raccoon munching away on her cat food. (We also found a bear cub in the tree outside our front door one summer day, but that's another story.)

I can't stress enough the importance of avoiding all possible sources of tobacco smoke in all asthmatics, no matter what their primary allergies may be. If an asthmatic is also a smoker he or she has a 100% chance of it developing into emphysema (COPD) in later years. That is a terrible way to die. Think of your worst asthma attack ever, and that is emphysema, day after day after day, until death.

So be smart. Stay away from smoking yourself, and also away from any possible sources of second hand smoke.

I highly recommend that your asthmatic person be tested to see what she may be allergic to. Then she will better be able to avoid whatever (in addition to those listed here) may trigger attacks. There is now an **IgE blood test** available for any region in the country, expensive but cheaper than skin tests, and very accurate with no risk whatsoever to the person being tested. Most insurances are now covering it because it is cheaper than skin tests, and your own doctor can order the test.

We have learned that certain things are associated with the initial onset of asthma. These include known allergies, particularly nasal and skin allergies, such as infantile eczema or dermatitis. There is often a family of allergies or asthma. Exposure to tobacco smoke soon after birth (as in a restaurant or country club where they still allow smoking, or a visiting family member, or -- perish the thought -- a close family member). Viral infections, especially in the lungs. Low birth weight.

At the present time asthma affects over 5,000,000 children of school age or younger in our country. The number of pre-school children with it has increased by more than

150% in the last 20 years. The death rate from asthma up to the mid-twenties has nearly doubled in the same period of time, in spite of much new medication and what should be better methods of treatment. Black children are five times as likely as whites to die from asthma.

Some doctors are keeping up with these new treatments, but some are not. **If your doctor does not follow pretty closely the program outlined here, then you <u>must</u> find a doctor who does.** A good family doctor or pediatrician can do a good job of caring for asthma. If possible, try to have a consultation with an allergist, at least for testing to find out what the asthmatic's primary allergies are early in the disease.

Consult the web site of the American Academy of Allergy, Asthma, and Immunology (www.aaaai.org) for excellent information and special products for asthmatics.

Do not allow your HMO to refuse to pay for the latest asthma medicines. Most HMOs won't put any drug newer than three years old on their formularies. Don't let them get away with it if your doctor wants you or your child to start a new medication. Complain long and loud, in writing with copies to your state insurance department and anyone else you can think of. Also complain by phone; ask for supervisors if refused, and get the names of everyone you talk to.

Furthermore, because many who haven't read the story on page 43 will be taking their barely ill kids to the church nursery, I recommend that you pair up with another mother who has a child who goes to the nursery, and one of you baby-sit those kids while the other goes to church, alternating every other Sunday (or Saturday, as appropriate). If you are married, that's easier if neither has to work on your Sunday. Just one of you stay home each Sunday.

How long should you do this? That's not easy, but certainly until your child has received all shots by eighteen months.

For those who work, you have an impossible situation. Many studies have been done on the prevalence of diseases in day care centers, even well run ones. In this situation, exhaust every option you might possibly have and keep your youngster out of one until it is as old as possible. Then try to select one that seems to be the most careful about separating kids who have runny noses and so on from those who are well. Also select one where hand washing by the personnel is emphasized.

What I am leading up to is that moving to a new location, if you can find a job there, may be all that will cure your asthmatic child. You must do careful research, however, because often your child will develop new allergies within a year or two in the new location. Locations above 6,000 feet (Flagstaff is 7,000 feet) are unique because they tend to be dry and free of many kinds of plants that grow at lower elevations. Also smaller cities and towns tend to have less air pollution from autos and trucks and factories.

If you don't make a permanent move, you may find it possible to take your child to the mountains during her allergy season. Leave a week before the season starts, such as the first week of August for ragweed, and come back a week after the season ends. Your doctor can help you with this. In the case of ragweed, you pretty much have to wait till the first frost to be in the clear.

Of course then you run into problems with school starting before the pollen is gone. A number of progressive school systems have gone to an all year quarter schedule, where the parents can select which quarter they want their kids to have their vacations. In cases like that, just select the quarter off that corresponds with your child's main allergy season, and take or send her out of town.

I must hasten to point out, however that I have had many asthmatic patients even in Flagstaff. But probably only ten percent as many as when I was in Indiana and also later in Phoenix.

The program for control of asthma must include patient (and parent, if a the patient is a child) education, avoiding things that trigger attacks, careful testing and recording and follow-up by your doctor (not physician's assistant), and medication. Your doctor must give you a plan for daily management yourself: 1) teach you how to do and record your twice (or more) daily peak flow testing 2) how to use your medications in response to symptoms and peak flow results and 3) when to report symptoms.

Your doctor must give you an Emergency Plan, which will help you to be aware that you are getting a flare-up and tell you exactly how to deal with it. This plan should be given to you in writing after your doctor determines what your own individual needs will be. He may have a "canned" plan for general use, but there must be extra stuff unique to you. One size definitely does not fit all in asthma.

Your doctor must teach you how to use the inhalers and small volume nebulizer correctly. They won't help much if you don't coordinate the inhaling with the triggering of the inhaler. In that case the medicine will all rain out in the mouth instead of in the lungs. Use of a spacer really helps.

Every asthmatic should have a peak flow meter to measure her breathing capability every day of her life. It is the asthmatic's insurance policy. It is better than the ones that insurance agents sell, because it helps prevent problems rather than paying off after problems develop. In the morning blow into it as hard as you can three times and write down the best number. Do the same in the late afternoon or evening, and much more often when you are having problems. After you have done this for a few weeks, when you are having good days and bad, you will be able to recognize, probably with your doctor's help in interpreting the danger zone for you, what numbers mean that a problem may be developing before you actually start wheezing. Then you can simply increase the frequency or dose of your inhaled bronchodilator (such as Proventil or Ventolin or Albuterol) and your anti-inflammatory medicine (corticosteroids such as Advair, Azmacort, Flovent, Pulmicort, or Aerobid, and leukotriene inhibitors, such as Accolate and Singulair) and see if that improves your situation. If the peak flow doesn't improve or gets worse, other medications such as prednisone can and should be added in a schedule, which your doctor <u>must</u> write out for you.

Please be aware that even apparently well-controlled asthma can deteriorate very rapidly and tragically.

People, both big and little, with the following risk factors, are more likely to have sudden deterioration of their asthma.

If the peak flow falls to 50% or less of your best number, that is an emergency and you must see a doctor immediately. If you can't reach one within a short time, then go to an Urgent Care or Emergency Room facility.

1. Past history of at least one sudden, severe flare-up.

2. Having to have a tube put down into your windpipe for asthma at least once.

3. Prior ICU admission to a hospital.

4. Having more than two hospitalizations within past year.

5. Having more than three emergency room visits for asthma in the past year.

6. Having one hospitalization or emergency room visit for asthma in the past month.

A 45 year-old lady patient of mine, whom I hadn't seen for any kind of an asthma attack for some time, went to a picnic. When she came home she told her husband that she was going to go lie down for awhile. He said that she didn't seem to be wheezing. However when he went to check on her in a little while, she was dead. We didn't have peak flow meters in those days.

7. Having to use more than two metered-dose inhaler applications per month of short-acting bronchodilators, such as albuterol (Proventil, Ventolin) or alupent.

8. Current or recent use of non-inhaled steroids (prednisone, Medrol, Decadron).

9. Having difficulty recognizing airflow obstruction or how severe it is. The peak flow meter helps here.

10. Having other potentially or actually serious conditions, such as heart or chronic lung diseases.

11. Having any serious psychiatric or psychosocial problem.

12. Being poor.

13. Living in a city.

According to at least one nationally-known asthma specialist the medications used for asthma fall into two categories: "<u>relievers</u>" or "rescue drugs, which are for symptom relief (your Albuterol inhaler is one such) and may not be needed every day, and "<u>controllers</u>," such as prednisone, corticosteroid inhalers (Azmacort, Aerobid, Flovent (which is combined with salmeterol in Advair diskus), Flonase, and new Pulmicort for use in nebulizers (SVN's) for children one to eight years old), and leukotriene modifiers

(Accolate and Singulair), which need to be used daily for <u>prevention</u> during your patient's asthma season. Serevent was another inhaler, which was a preventative only, but has now been combined with Flovent in the Advair diskus to give everyone a good night's sleep when used, especially at bedtime. Advair is also currently the best one to use to prevent exercise-induced asthma. **Athletes, take note**.

> *In 2001, a little 9-year old girl in Indiana began to wheeze at school and used her Albuterol inhaler. After school, when she got home, she told her mother that she was still short of breath and was going up to her room to use her small volume nebulizer. Within a few minutes she collapsed in her room, and died on life support in the hospital. The newspaper story didn't say whether she had been checking her breathing at least twice a day with a peak flow meter.*

Do not expect your HMO or Medicaid (or AHCCCS in Arizona) to pay for many of these drugs because they are expensive. (See the chapter on **HMOs** for how to deal with that situation). That is one reason why "being poor" is on the high-risk list above.

How can you tell whether your child has asthma?

Three symptoms make us very suspicious:
1. Wheeze, anytime
2. Recurrent cough (more than six episodes in 2 years)
3. Shortness of breath

Now there is a test for IgE antibodies in the blood which tests for inhaled antigens (the stuff we are allergic to) that can be done on kids down even to one year of age. This is just a recent thing, because it used to be recommended only for kids ages six and up. If this test is positive along with the symptom of wheezing, then the chances are 90% that the person has allergic asthma. A positive IgE test with the recurrent cough problem means a 73% chance of having asthma, while positive IgE plus shortness of breath means asthma 80% of the time.

Once you and your doctor have established the diagnosis of asthma, then it is time to start the whole program in motion. Get the Albuterol; get the peak flow meter; get the inhaled corticosteroid. Most HMOs will go at least this far. Then if these provide complete relief of symptoms, stop there. If there are still symptoms, then add as many other parts of the drug program as possible or necessary.

When you or your child is wheezing and/or short of breath, in addition to the medications it is <u>extremely</u> important to push non-caffeine fluids by mouth. The secretions in the lungs get dry and sometimes so thick that you can cut them with a scissors if a lung specialist can pull up a plug through his bronchoscope. A mist small volume nebulizer (SVN) also helps that, as did my daughter's Bird machine.

Work with your or your child's doctor to set achievable goals in the treatment of your or your child's asthma.

Reasonable goals are, first, preventing all attacks during the night. I can really relate to that because I was the one who was up with my daughter 364 nights per year for at least the last two years we were in Warsaw. I read *Heidi* and *Black Beauty* and dozens of other books to her, some several times. In those cases, even before she could read, she would correct me if I read the wrong word. What a memory!

The other night of the year my wife was up with her by herself, probably reading too. So there was never a night when we were all able to sleep through even one night per year.

Prevention of nighttime attacks begins with inhaled corticosteroids, then one tablet a day of Accolate or Singulair (my preference), then one or two inhalations of Advair diskus, if you can afford all that. Your doctor will gladly provide you with drug samples when available. And many drug companies have a free drug program for those who are truly destitute. Your doctor can find out about those if you ask him or her.

The next goal might be "no ER visits" or no hospitalizations, or both.

The next goal should be "no school days missed."

My daughter says that it is very important for even the most severe asthmatic to exercise to the limit of his or her capability every day. So the next goal should be the ability to increase the exercise moderately, perhaps even playing a sport.

Unfortunately, this is the real world, so do the best you can, using these words as a guide. If your doctor doesn't agree with what I am telling you here, then get another doctor, because this is the absolute cutting edge latest and best way to treat asthma. Other drugs and other treatments will come along, but this is where it's at today!

> *I'll never forget that scene in **As Good As It Gets**, where Helen Hunt's little boy was running after her bus as fast as his legs would carry him after the doctor sent by Jack Nicholson had started treating him properly. That really can happen, folks, with good full asthma treatment, uncensored by an HMO or inability to pay for the medications.*

The very idea that such goals are achievable will come as a shock to the families of many asthmatics. They have no idea how good their lives can be.

Continuing the story of my daughter, after I was released from active duty, we went back to northern Indiana to live and practice medicine. She gradually developed more and more attacks of wheezing over the years, till she was basically a shut-in sitting in her room with the Honeywell air purifier, and a dehumidifier out in the hall.

When she was 4, I learned of a new treatment being instituted by Dr. Forrest Bird in Palm Springs, California. I took my daughter out to see Dr. Bird, and we brought back one of his breathing machines. Her breathing treatments kept her going, but we tried allergy shots to no avail. And her condition deteriorated so that during her ninth year she had status asthmaticus three times. Only Decadron and her Bird machine kept her alive. But just barely the last time. Our allergist told us that if at all possible we should try to find a place somewhere in the West above an altitude of 6,000 feet, where the things she was allergic to did not grow. We visited several small and large towns and finally found a spot where they needed another doctor in Flagstaff, Arizona. I had to take some more medical license exams to practice in Arizona, but I was successful the first try and we moved when she was ten.

As Paul Harvey would say, "the rest of the story" is that she got well in the clean, pure mountain air. The little girl who was a shut-in grew up to be on the all-state ski team, and worked in summers leading trail rides and hikes in the North Country of our new home.

Meanwhile the Warsaw Tigers, for whom I was the team doctor for seven years, went on to win the Indiana State Basketball Championship several years later when my younger son was a senior in high school in Arizona. Here he skied in winter instead of playing basketball.

The newer drugs of today might have enabled us to stay in Indiana, but it is doubtful that she would have achieved the good health that she did otherwise in Arizona. So it was a good move for her. She now lives in Alaska, where pollens are few, and there is lots of skiing.

CHAPTER 13 -- AUTO ACCIDENTS

<u>Never</u> carry more people in your vehicle than you have seat belts for. In Arizona and New Mexico it seems that everyone has a pickup truck. Unfortunately most pickup trucks don't have a back seat, and one will never drive very far outside the cities without seeing people riding in the back bed of these trucks. I have personally treated or pronounced dead in the ER several people who were injured when the pickups they were riding in the back of were involved in an accident. The worst case, however, was at 59th Avenue and Bell Road in Phoenix when a drunk driver ran a stop sign and struck a pickup containing ten kids coming back from a picnic with their church youth group. I was the first medical person on the scene. In those days I always carried my medical bag, and I sure needed it there. There were dead and mangled bodies strewn everywhere! The lesson is simple because no one inside the cab with a seat belt on was injured.

Another true story: a patient was brought to me in the ER, and she died there with a massive head injury. She had been in the act of fastening her seat belt as the car she was in was backing slowly out of the driveway at their home. Her car was struck by another car. Her door popped open, and she was thrown out, landing on her head on the pavement and fracturing her skull severely. No one else in either car was injured at all.

In my 40 plus years of practice I have had eleven people (not counting those kids at 59th and Bell) who were thrown out of their vehicles and died of their injuries in low speed accidents when all in the vehicle who had on restraints were totally uninjured.

And tell your school to put seat belts on the school buses. Flagstaff City Schools felt that the padded seats were enough until a bus rolled over, paralyzing one child for life and severely injuring others. I don't know for sure, but I hope, that all Flagstaff school buses now have seat belts. Another such rollover happened elsewhere with one death just three days before I wrote this. The kids should be "encouraged" very strongly to fasten their seat belts before the bus starts again after picking them up. And before the bus leaves the school with a full load at the end of the day, the bus driver should inspect everyone to be sure their belts are fastened, just as the flight attendants do on airplanes. It makes sense since the State of Arizona has a law requiring that all passengers in private vehicles wear seat belts. Kids are therefore mostly taught at home to wear seat belts and can be expected to do the same in buses without much thought.

> **Always put on your seat belt and be sure everyone in the vehicle has theirs fastened before even starting the motor.** *If you have an accident and someone in the car who did not have on a seat belt is injured, you may be legally liable for not making sure that all seat belts were on.*

> *Never talk on a cell phone while driving, not even a hands-free one. Well, possibly if you are on a long wide straight road in the West with no other cars on the road, you might be able to get away with it. But don't do it in city driving. It distracts your attention way too much. I have seen statistics that show that 50% of all auto accidents now involve at least one driver who was using a cell phone. About six months before I wrote this I was almost struck by a young woman driver entering the freeway while talking on her cell phone. Fortunately for us I was watching her and slowed way down to let her in. She never even looked my way!*

Most of the other 50% involve at least one driver who has been drinking alcohol or is on some mind-altering drug.

States are clamping down more and more on drinkers who drive. Many have reduced the legal limit in the blood to 0.08, and it is likely that some will go on down to 0.05 in the next few years, the same as many foreign countries now. There are a very few countries who have zero tolerance -- if you even have a blood-alcohol of 0.01, you'll be arrested. By no coincidence those countries have minuscule alcohol-related fatality rates compared to ours.

I had the good fortune to have Dr. Rollo Harger, inventor of the first drunkometer, as my professor of Biochemistry in medical school. He had us engage in some eye-opening experiments on the effects of even small amounts of alcohol on our ability to react quickly to a situation.

First he called for volunteers to take a timed reaction time test followed by intake of measured amounts of alcohol. Those taking it were given an insulated metal stylus to which a wire was attached. The stylus was rested on a small metal plate in the center of the area. To the right and left about 45 degrees were light bulbs with a metal rail in front of them 12 inches from the stylus start position. One light or the other would go on with no warning. We were supposed to move the stylus as quickly as possible to the metal rail in front of that light. When the stylus struck the rail, the contact was broken, and the light went out. The total time that the light was on was our reaction time.

We got three chances, and the best one was recorded. Then we got one ounce of Jack Daniels, waited 15 minutes, and tested again. Then we took a second ounce of Jack Daniels, waited another 15 minutes, and took the last test.

The test group included one chap who had a beer or two every day, one who drank a beer or two only on weekends, and one who rarely drank alcohol at all. Then Dr. Harger introduced one of his laboratory cleanup men, who, he told us before the man came in, was a full-blown alcoholic. He took the tests, just as we did, drank the two drinks, and was tested after each one again.

The results were consistently the same, percentage-wise, for each of us: a 10% deterioration in reaction time after the first drink, and a 25% deterioration after the second drink. As you might suspect, the alcoholic lab worker's reaction time was much slower than each of the medical students initially, but he had the same percentage of deterioration. With some individual variation, all the medical students were pretty close to the same times, initially and after each of the drinks.

In most states two drinks are not enough to make one legally drunk. BUT, if you are driving 30 miles per hour, and it takes you 120 feet to stop when you have had no alcohol, then with one drink it will take you an additional 12 feet to stop. So if you are able to stop just before hitting someone's rear bumper with no alcohol, that extra 12 feet with one drink puts you all the way into his trunk and then some. And two drinks are an extra two car lengths! Think about it.

Don't drink and drive! Never! Not even one.

CHAPTER 14 -- BABIES

How to Handle Them

Holding a baby properly is very important. Their little neck muscles are too weak to hold up such a large head by themselves until about six or seven months of age. So proper picking up and holding of these little guys is very important if injury is to be avoided.

Their skulls are thin, and the suture lines stay open for a long time to allow their brains to grow without being restricted by the bony skull. The areas that are particularly weak and require the most protection are the front soft part, (called the anterior fontanelle) and the back soft part, which is smaller than the front one and thus closes sooner. (That one is called the posterior fontanelle.) One of the reasons for these soft areas is to give the skull room to mold as it passes down the birth canal.

Always use two hands around the chest area when picking up a baby, and don't jerk it. After the baby is in your arms, you can support the head on the palm of one hand or in the crook of your elbow. Always support the head in some way when breast-feeding.

Feeding Your Baby

Breast-feed as long as possible, a year or more if you can. Breast-feeding confers huge benefits on the baby. And it's good for you, too. See the chapter on **Breast Feeding**.

Foods to Avoid

In the first year (and even later) there are a number of foods that should be avoided for one reason or another.

Chocolate may cause an allergic reaction. It may also start a craving for sweets that can result in obesity.

Candy and all other sweets may start a craving for sweets that can result in obesity. They're guaranteed to increase dental cavities.

Nuts. Allergies can be a problem, especially peanuts and peanut butter. Nuts can also be a choking danger up to ages 4-5 years, and something to put in nose and ears even at school age.

Egg whites. These should be avoided up to age 18 months because they can also stimulate allergies other than to themselves. Cooked egg yolks can be safely given babies by age three months.

Honey. Some contains potentially deadly spores. Botulism has been reported many times from honey, a pretty scary thing. Avoid honey until at least one year of age.

Cow's milk. We used to say it was OK to switch over to cow's milk from formula or breast milk by about age six months. Nowadays that may still be true in most cases, but there is some concern that the casein in the milk can irritate an infant's stomach or intestines, particularly if it has allergies, sometimes causing microscopic blood loss, which of course increases the risk of iron deficiency anemia.

Citrus fruits and juices (grapefruit, lemon, lime, and orange) can cause vomiting. If it does vomit the first time you try it, then hold off on any citrus for a month or so before trying again. Large amounts of undiluted apple or pear juices may cause diarrhea, but are non-allergenic. White grape juice is best of all the juices because hardly any little tykes have a problem with it.

Processed foods, which are high in sodium. I think the best thing is to get a blender (you will save its cost within two months or less) and blend more nutritious and tasty foods for your little one without the use of any salt or preservatives. You can freeze them for later or keep them in the fridge for up to three days.

High-nitrate vegetables. Some areas of the world and our country have a lot of nitrates in the soil, so hold off on home-cooked beets, carrots, collard greens, green beans, and spinach until he is eight months or older. It is said that food canned by commercial baby food makers are less likely to have high nitrates, but I wouldn't rely on that too much.

Allergies in Babies

Non-allergenic foods for infants (for **eczema**)
Enfamil Nutramigen, Enfamil ProSoBee, Enfamil Pregestimil, Isomil, and Baby Basic for milk
Rye-krisp
Grape jelly
Butter
Lamb, veal
Cooked peaches, cooked pears for fruit
Carrots, squash, rice for vegetables
Barley or rice cereals

There is considerable evidence that having our little ones avoid allergy-producing foods for the first 18 months of life may reduce the likelihood of developing allergies as they get older. For sure that approach reduces the skin problem which we call eczema, which is a weeping, red, itching rash which is seen especially in the elbow creases.

Treatment of eczema includes doing everything possible to stop the kids from scratching. That often requires a creative approach. Some actually have to have their hands tied loosely to opposite sides of their beds so they can't reach their bodies. That is a little more extreme than I like.

Trim and file their fingernails down to the quick every day so they can't use them as weapons against themselves. Put mittens on them, day and night. Use Aveeno soaks and soap, coal tar ointment (believe it or not it is white, not black, and _very_ soothing).

Milk substitutes for lactose intolerance
Enfamil ProSoBee LIPIL, Enfamil LactoFree LIPIL, Pediasure

Failure to Thrive

> One infant that I know of was slowly starving, and it had gone from high on the growth chart while still breast feeding to off the bottom of the chart in just two months because of this very mistake.

One infant formula has on the can a picture of someone adding one scoop of formula powder to one baby bottle. This is wrong! Always read the instructions. The correct proportion is one scoop to 2 ounces of water, which would be 4 scoops to an 8-oz bottle.

Other causes of failure to thrive are emotional deprivation, hypothyroid condition, and others. Little ones who aren't getting enough to eat have symptoms such as irritability, can't be consoled, then if hunger persists, withdrawal, listlessness, stiffness when picked up, and constantly searching everywhere with their eyes. These symptoms should be a matter of concern for parents, and you should consult your doctor if they occur.

Use of Walkers

In 1999 about 8,800 children were treated in hospital ERs for injuries caused by the use of infant walkers. By far a huge majority of these also involved stairs, as in pushing the walker to the edge and then falling down the stairs. Most of the injuries were fractures and head injuries. How many more less severe accidents there were that were treated at home, family doctor's office, or urgent care facility can only be guessed at. But there were probably a lot more than 8,800.

Most walkers are used with the idea of getting the child to walk sooner. Although this may seem logical, a number of studies have conclusively shown that those who use walkers show sitting, crawling, and walking capability _later_ than those who do not use walkers.

Preventing Walker-Related Injuries

I highly recommend <u>never</u> starting to use one.

If you feel you must use the one that great aunt Tammie gave you for a birth present, then do the following things: first, watch the child just as though you were at the swimming pool. Second, make whatever changes in the household structure that you must, such as stair and/or door gates, to ensure that falls won't occur. Third, try to get or exchange for a walker that is more than three feet wide and thus won't pass through standard three-foot wide doors. Or, with heavy duty strapping tape, tape a couple of lengths of cutoff broomstick handles to front and back of the walker. This, of course means that anything on the coffee table is at risk, but it does help keep the child in the same room with you -- perhaps.

> *Never sleep with your baby in your bed with you. There have been many cases where the infant somehow slipped down under the covers and suffocated. That happened to a baby that I personally delivered.*

Changing Diapers

If you use a bathinette, be sure to fasten the strap around your baby's tummy. And be sure the legs are firmly set to avoid tipping over. Have the clean diaper ready on the surface, with a container for the dirty one beside you. Never leave or take your eyes off your baby for even a second while changing it. If something that you need falls on the floor, keep one hand on the baby as you bend over to pick it up. And let the phone ring!

> *My wife made these mistakes with our second child. She left our eight-month old son lying on the bathinette in the care of our five year old daughter while she answered the phone. Our daughter carefully watched him and even played with him a little. But he kicked something off on the floor, and when she bent over to pick it up, he rolled off. Our daughter, bless her heart, reached out and caught his head, so that the only thing to hit the hard floor was his leg, which broke above the knee. But it wasn't a bad fracture, and in six weeks he was out of the cast and in eight weeks he was walking. It could have been lots worse! My wife, of course, was devastated.*

I have treated several little ones with variations of the same story. The stories are the same; only the characters have changed. One child rolled suddenly and the whole bathinette fell over. Another played with the strap until it came undone, and he rolled off. Most of the caregivers had slavishly gone to answer the phone.

Do not be a slave to your phone. It <u>rarely</u> rings when you want it to. It is almost always an intrusion upon what you are doing, though often a welcome one, as in kids or other loved-ones calling home. If you <u>must</u> break to answer the phone, then grab up the diaper, put it over the dangerous part of the baby's anatomy, and grab up the baby before going to the phone.

Pets

These can be a source of great joy for kids, or a source of great danger. Dogs left alone with a newborn have killed and eaten part of the child before being found. Cats have curled up over the baby's mouth and nose, suffocating it. Cats have scratched the eyes. Dogs have chewed on the ears and hands and feet. Pets are unpredictable, especially one whose territory is being invaded by a new baby who is now getting all the attention. Don't think for a minute that pets don't get jealous.

I grew up with a female German Shepherd who came when I was three months old and was my (and later my sister's) faithful companion in every possible respect, no matter how many indignities we heaped upon her. We have had dozens of cats and dogs all my life. So please be aware that I am not an animal hater. Quite the contrary, I love animals, and they reciprocate my affection almost always. My problem is that I have had to repair the wounds inflicted on little ones by a family pet (or a neighbor's), usually a dog, more than two hundred times in my long career. And a dog that I thought was my friend bit me suddenly on the forearm as I was stroking his neck and back last summer, only the second time I have ever been bitten.

So if you have a pet and decide to keep it, be sure it is <u>never</u> alone with your baby. Better yet, give it to Uncle Greg before the baby comes.

Many kids become allergic to animal dander. There has recently been a controversial study that seems to indicate that kids who have furry pets are less likely to develop asthma as they grow older. I doubt it, but it was presented in a well-respected medical journal. One thing for sure is that the pets have to go if the child actually becomes asthmatic.

Sleeping

For most of my medical career I advised new mothers to lay their new babies on their stomachs so that they wouldn't spit up and suck it down their windpipes. Very well-done studies in the past ten years, however, have conclusively indicated that there is a much lower rate of sudden infant deaths (SIDS) in those who sleep on their backs. No one can explain any reason for it, but the numbers are almost overwhelming. So, lay your little ones on their backs to sleep. And be sure there is no bed bumper or loose blanket around to tangle around the head or neck, and no pillow to press the nose and mouth into.

Tobacco

One other thing. There is a huge increase in Sudden Infant Death Syndrome (SIDS) in infants soon after exposure to second hand tobacco smoke. One study indicated that at least 40% of these deaths occurred after exposure to second hand tobacco smoke. Other studies have recently shown that exposure to second hand smoke increases the risk of SIDS by 50% to 500%, depending on the study.

So, be sure to never allow anyone to smoke in the house or car even when the baby isn't there. Stay out of restaurants and country clubs where they still allow smoking. And change your clothes before handling your baby after smoking yourself or being around someone who smokes. The child will inhale it from the fabric of your clothes as you hold it in your arms.

More about bad tobacco stuff in the **Tobacco** chapter.

Many country clubs, including my own Arizona Country Club, in spite of the efforts of some of my colleagues and me to persuade the Board of Directors otherwise, allow smoking either in the dining room or in a bar adjacent to the dining room that is not physically separated from the diners. Both situations mean that everyone in the dining room will be exposed to second hand smoke, including any little babies brought to the club of grandfather or parents. All of these private clubs have a rule requiring that all members spend at least a certain amount, typically $500 to $1,000, per year in the dining room. So even those who know as I do about the dangerous effects on little babies and kids can either leave their babies with a baby-sitter when they have a family dinner or pay the club the $500 or more per year and stay home.

I was horror-stricken last year when a grandfather in my club was allowed to smoke right beside his newborn little grandchild, presumably ignorant of the fact that he could be conferring a death sentence on the baby. I hope this book will prevent such ignorant behavior in your family!

CHAPTER 15 -- BACK INJURIES

Bed rest is no longer felt to be effective in helping people with back pain to recover. Many studies have shown that bed rest for as little as two days slows down full recovery by at least several days. Those who do best are those who continue their normal activities as tolerated. That is why the most enlightened employers now offer a wide variety of modified duty to those who have been injured on the job.

The one thing that consistently both improves the quality of recovery and shortens it is exercise within the limits of the injured person's capability, ideally starting the day of the injury. The sooner those with back pain go back to their jobs, the sooner their symptoms improve.

Exercise

Back injuries occur 10 times less frequently in those who are physically fit than in those who aren't. <u>All forms of exercise are helpful for people with chronic low back pain.</u> Exercise helps weight loss, particularly in the abdominal area, where a big belly causes the lower back to change contour. Instead of bearing the weight of the upper body, and anything lifted, on the flat surfaces of the vertebrae as a person with a normal flat abdominal wall does, the abdominally obese person is overbalanced and the weight is thrown onto the front corners of the vertebrae. This causes strain on the rearmost supporting ligaments of the vertebral bodies, as well as causing increased wear and tear on the front bone surfaces, with resulting arthritis at an early age.

Tightening the abdominal wall through weight loss and abdominal muscle strengthening not only helps to favorably change the weight-bearing load distribution on the vertebrae but also pushes the contents of the interior of the abdomen against the front of the backbone to provide support by direct hydrostatic pressure.

Exercise improves endurance and allows for more tolerance of activity. It improves the strength and flexibility of the lumbar muscles and ligaments. The endorphins produced in aerobic activities lasting over 30 minutes at a time provide actual pain relief by direct chemical action, with positive psychological effects also.

A positive motivation to exercise is a very strong indicator of a successful result in lower back pain patients.

Prevention of Back Injuries

Follow these few simple rules, and you will prevent 90% or more of possible back injuries.

1) Never lift anything that you think is too heavy.

2) Have the object you are going to lift as close to your body as possible. Do not reach out to lift anything more than a foot in front of you. Use some alternative method.

3) Pretend that it weighs 500 lbs (remember that you are lifting at least 100 lbs of your upper body weight plus whatever you are lifting.)

4) Tighten your stomach muscles and let your breath out (exhale) as you lift.

5) Always bend your knees and keep your back as straight as possible.

6) Never twist your body with a load. Move your feet as you pivot like a basketball player with your load (or ball).

Spinal manipulation must not be done in people with fractures, osteoporosis, osteomyelitis, malignancies, ankylosing conditions, and nerve root disorders. The consequences of manipulation can be devastating in someone who has not been properly evaluated before manipulation. These include paralysis in arms or legs or both (I have seen two such low back cases requiring emergency neurosurgery after manipulation), damage to the vertebral arteries in the neck, with possible stroke and death, and fractures of the spinal structures.

Approximately 12% of neck manipulations produce bad results, most of which, thankfully, are mild. I have seen two of these also, however, that required emergency surgical decompression of the spinal nerve. Massage therapy is as useful as manipulation without the risks, and generally provides considerable short-term relief.

These are good generalizations of care. For a much more extensive discussion of these and other injuries, see the chapter on **Muscle, Bone, and Joint injuries.**

CHAPTER 16 -- BAD BREATH

Bad breath (Halitosis) is a big problem in our society. A whole industry, it seems, is devoted to controlling it enough to make your mouth "kissing sweet."

The causes are many, but by far the most common one is food left in the mouth in which germs begin to grow within a few hours. Some of them produce a sulfur compound that is pretty rank. Places the bacteria can grow include between the teeth (where they can also cause gum disease and cavities), in the spaces between the cheeks and gums if you don't swish your mouth with water after eating, in the tiny cracks between the taste buds on the tongue (which is noticeable when you have a coated tongue), in your tonsils, particularly if they are somewhat large and have holes in them, and in the mucous fluid that drips from the nose down the back of the throat in most people at least occasionally.

Poor cleansing of the teeth and gums, often accompanied by gum disease, in my experience, causes the most offensive bad breath.

Certain foods can cause changes in your breath that can last up to 72 hours after you eat them. Smoking is a very common cause of bad breath.

Certain drugs, the medication DMSO for arthritis or bladder problems, and many chronic diseases, such as diabetes, kidney or liver conditions, along with respiratory tract infections, especially sinus infections, from the nose to the lungs all cause this problem.

GERD, with regurgitation of food from the stomach at night, is another common cause. Read the **GERD** chapter for how to deal with that.

Some people I have seen thought they had bad breath, but they actually didn't. This can be a terrible phobia for some. They brush their teeth six times a day and constantly use all different kinds of mouthwash.

How can you tell whether you have bad breath? Your best friends won't tell you. Once in awhile someone will give you a delicate hint, but you will have to be sharp to pick up on it. Perhaps your spouse will, but your significant other may just drop you instead of telling you.

One way to tell for yourself is to take a small breath and puff out your cheeks to fill your mouth with air. Then put your hand over your mouth and nose. Then inhale through your nose as you open your mouth and let the trapped air out, thus forcing the air in your mouth out through your lips and up into your nose. If it doesn't smell good, then you have a problem.

How do you cure or control bad breath? That depends, of course, on the cause, but I will give you some ideas here, hopefully even one or two you haven't already thought of. Some cases are easily cured by just stopping use of the offending substance.

First, if you smoke or chew tobacco, stop. Here we go again about tobacco. There is hardly any part of your body that isn't affected badly by tobacco! So here is still another reason to stop. Your non-smoking lover(s) will give you a lot more passionate kisses if you do, I promise.

Second, if you have gum disease already, treatment begins with totally clean teeth and gums, which are hard to obtain without a trip to a dental hygienist for a thorough cleaning. After that you can do the following and be pretty successful in keeping your breath "kissing sweet."

Swish some water around in your mouth after you finish eating anything, and then just swallow it. That will get rid of most food particles between your teeth and your gums.

Brush your teeth at least after breakfast and dinner, using an up-and-down motion while rolling the soft bristles a little to get most of the food particles out from between the teeth. Start on the gums and brush away from them over the teeth, both inside and out. This won't replace flossing, but it helps keep the food particles low until the next time you can floss.

To help prevent cavities always use a fluoridated toothpaste. In addition there are a number of preparations that add "tartar protection," "whitening," and others. Be careful of some of these. They may be using chemicals too strong for your teeth. I can't begin to list here the ones which have been approved by the American Dental Association, but if so approved, it will say so on the label. Do not use one that is not so approved. I feel confident with Crest and Ultrabrite formulations and haven't personally tried any others. (I have not received a fee or other consideration from them for mentioning their products or any others in this book.)

For those with large tonsils with holes that collect food particles in them, try gargling some water daily. You may not be able to get them all out this way, so I highly recommend a Water Pik, which is a pressurized water device used by most kids with orthodontic appliances on their teeth to clean food out of the cracks. Use it once a day, and direct the stream on the spots where you can see white stuff. You may gag a little the first few times, but you will soon get used to it.

Use the Water Pik also on your gums between the teeth every night before you go to bed, especially if you don't floss as often as you perhaps should. That will clean out the old food and improve your breath. It won't, however, replace the need to floss to prevent plaque buildup on the teeth, along with prevention of gum disease.

Sometimes the tongue gets tiny particles of partially digested food or tobacco stuck between the taste buds. You can easily tell by looking to see if your tongue is coated or discolored. If your tongue isn't nice and pink with no white or other stuff on it, then gently brush your tongue also. Smokers and chronically sick people are more likely to get the coated tongue problems.

Third, if you have a chronic post-nasal drip, see the chapter on **Allergy** for suggestions for improving it. Saline nose spray, 8-10 sprays in each nostril once or twice a day, may provide enough cleansing to greatly reduce the problem. A Neti pot (see the index for more about this) is even better. Also a Chlortrimeton tablet, which you can buy over-the-counter, 12 mg twice a day, is a pretty good antihistamine. It isn't as likely to make you sleepy as Benadryl and may actually be a slightly better medicine.

Fourth, avoid foods that you know cause bad breath. Onions, garlic and strong cheeses (especially limburger) come to mind immediately because my wife won't let me eat them when I am going to be seeing patients or otherwise out in public. Also she won't let me eat them unless she eats them too.

Fifth, there are numerous mouthwashes on the market. Some claim to kill offending bacteria, but mostly they just cover up the odor for a short time. It's OK to use them, but just be aware that they are not solving the underlying problem.

CHAPTER 17 -- BEHAVIOR PROBLEMS IN YOUNG CHILDREN

Dr. Tom Irons, a renowned pediatrician, has Seven Simple Principles, which make the most sense to me of anything I have encountered.

1. Threatening is harmful.

2. Guilt is destructive. Making laws is a most important parental duty. Parents must see themselves as enforcers of the law, like a policeman. Unreasonable laws are at best unenforceable, and at worst, just plain mean. Parents shouldn't feel guilty about discipline.

Tell the kids, "you have to do this. It's the law." Don't get into the "why game."

3. Parents must be teachers.

4. Limits are required, but they must be reasonable.

> *A woman I was once close to was scarred for life by her mother's threatening to "give her away" if she wasn't good. I don't think she has ever felt secure in her whole life.*

5. Actions, not words, are effective. <u>Actively</u> ignoring a child who is misbehaving is a <u>very</u> effective approach. Basically what you say is "I don't have anything to do with you when you do that." Then you turn your back to the child and keep turning if necessary.

6. Regular regrouping is essential.

7. Everybody backslides.

Remember that, if there are two parents in the picture, even if divorced, both of you are in it together.

CHAPTER 18 -- BIOLOGICAL WARFARE THREATS

There are a couple of problems that terrorists have to surmount in order to make an attack of bioterrorism: producing the chosen agent in a laboratory, one that is a pretty good one, while protecting the workers who are producing the bad stuff; and finding a way to deliver that agent to a large number of people in a short period of time. Some agents are transmissible from human to human, but most are not. In the case of Botulinus toxin enough could be carried in a carry-on bag to wipe out a large city if properly delivered.

Some of these are the germs themselves, while others, like botulinus, are the toxin (i.e., poison) produced when the germ is incubated or allowed to sit out on food at room temperature for too long before putting it away in the refrigerator.

One thing is certain, no matter what the agent employed by a terrorist group: there will be panic and hysteria which will overwhelm our emergency medical systems, and that will accomplish almost as much as a truly deadly killing agent because it will upset our way of life.

Below is a list of the most likely bioterrorism agents. There is not a lot of information about some of these in this country.

ANTHRAX

We have already had a dose of terrorism by anthrax, primarily in the eastern states, although the scare penetrated all the way to Phoenix, Arizona, where a post office received a broken shipment from the contaminated one in Washington, D.C., with possible white powder spilling out.

Anthrax has been called "wool-sorter's disease" because it has been common in that occupation, with spores getting into the wool. One spore can potentially produce disease, so it is a pretty good bet for terrorism. The terrorists are potentially at risk too; so a fairly sophisticated laboratory facility has to be set up in order to produce serious quantities.

Distribution can be very easy through the mail, as we already know, to our regret. The governor of Arizona recommended that no one should ever open mail from someone we don't know. That certainly would put the third class mail solicitations out of business.

Air ducts can be very easily contaminated, witness the Legionnaire's Disease epidemic in Philadelphia in the 1970s.

Water reservoirs are a major concern, but not as bad as you might think. The water we drink that originates from surface water is all contaminated with all kinds of germs and other organisms, some pretty bad ones. So our water has to be purified by filtration, aeration, chlorination, and I don't know what all else, before we can safely drink it. Sometimes one of the steps breaks down, as it did in part of Peoria, Arizona, in 2002, and people get sick and perhaps die. But mostly our water supplies are safe from bad germs. Toxic chemicals are another story.

I personally saw two of those postal workers, took cultures, and started them on Cipro, which the CDC was recommending to treat the anthrax cases. None of our patients developed the disease and no cultures turned up positive, but there was considerable anxiety among all of us for a couple of weeks.

I did find a very unusual sore on one man's hand two weeks later and spent thirty minutes on the phone with a very helpful person at the CDC who had no idea what the skin signs of anthrax look like. I followed his instructions though, and arranged for it to be drained and cultured, while prescribing Cipro until the culture report came back as a common staph aureus.

Well water in the mountains is pretty pure as it is. But well water around a big industrial city has to be suspect because all too many industrial plants have not been good citizens for years and dumped their waste fluids into the ground where toxic chemicals can leech into the well water layer of the ground.

What I'm leading up to is that we watch and test our drinking water supplies on a daily or weekly basis in most communities, thus providing a substantial bulwark against most massive chemical and biological weapons. Cyanide and others of the extremely toxic variety would take a little while to spread out in a reservoir. During that time we hope that the periodic testing would give us some warning.

Some people will die with any bioterrorist act, but we already have procedures in place in many areas to limit or contain the contamination and thus protect most of us.

That is scant reassurance to those involved, but it's the best we can do, at least right now.

BLACK LOCUST BEANS

I don't know much about this one except its symptoms. These include severe weakness, irregular pulse, severe shortness of breath, and diarrhea leading to dehydration if the other symptoms are not fatal. There is no antidote, but careful nursing in a hospital ICU can save a lot of people. I don't know what the dispersal method would likely be.

BOTULISM

The probable method of transmission: aerosol. Not spread from human to human because it is the toxin produced by the germ that is the killer. The germ itself usually just causes some diarrhea for a day or two. It is part of the same family as tetanus. It can live for weeks in non-moving water and food. The toxin is found naturally in spoiled or canned food, e.g. cans that bulge at the ends. This is a really bad chemical!

Botulinum antitoxin is lifesaving, but it must be given early in order to prevent damage to the respiratory nerves. The CDC and some state health departments stock the antitoxin. We don't have enough at this time to save very many people in an attack.

Isolated cases will usually get well if placed on a ventilator for several weeks until new nerves grow in to replace those damaged by the toxin. Unfortunately in a terrorist attack no such treatment will be available for hundreds or thousands of those exposed.

CHOLERA

The probable method of transmission would be water contamination. But it is unstable in fresh water and aerosols, though stable in salt water. It is transmitted from human to human by fecal-oral route. In other words, wash your hands before you handle anything you are going to put in your mouth and always after going to the toilet.

GLANDERS

The probable method of transmission would be by aerosol, with only a low dose needed to kill a lot of people. Very stable. Deadly. Little transmission from human to human. I have never seen or heard of an actual case in this country.

OLEANDER

This poison is used as for killing rats. Symptoms include vertigo, heart irregularities, convulsions and coma. I'm not sure at this time what is the most likely method of dispersal.

PLAGUE

This Black Death of the middle ages has three main types: the bubonic, which is spread by fleas mainly from rats; the pneumonic, which is very contagious, spreads from human to human and can be cured with antibiotics if diagnosed in time (within 24 hours after the first appearance of <u>any</u> symptoms); and the septicemic, which can be spread both ways and is always fatal (you go to bed feeling fine and wake up dead).

Plague is found in the Four Corners area of the Western U. S., particularly in the fleas of rats and prairie dogs. We have a case in our hospital in Flagstaff every three or four years. They are of the bubonic (swollen glands or bubos) variety, so they all get well on antibiotics. The disease moves so fast in the pneumonic, and especially the septicemic forms that asking your overwhelmed doctor's nurse to phone in a prescription at the first symptoms (after local health care providers become aware of what we have been attacked with) might be the only thing that will save you. You sure won't have time to go to an ER or Urgent Care facility and wait several hours.

RICIN

This is made to order for biologic terrorism. Types A and B are made from castor beans. Ricin is used commercially for killing moles. The probable method of transmission would be by aerosol. The incubation period is less than one day, and it is highly lethal. It causes nausea, vomiting, severe GI bleeding, and rapid dehydration. I know very little else about this one.

SMALLPOX

Before Jenner discovered that vaccinating people with the fluid from cowpox sores would prevent them from getting smallpox, we humans had to become infected with a disease, let our bodies produce enough antibodies to kill the germs, and then, if we survived, we would forever be immune. Jenner changed all that. Viruses had not been discovered at that time, and no one knew what an antibody was, but it didn't take the equivalent of a rocket scientist in those days to figure out that it is better to get a mild case of something, so as to be immune afterwards, than to get the full-blown disease. In the case of smallpox, a deadly disease was conquered.

Let's talk about smallpox a little more. It was declared in 1980 by the World Health Organization that smallpox was no longer present in our world and that vaccinations for it could be stopped. The only problem with such a declaration was, in the light of present day fears of biological warfare, that some incredibly stupid people in two countries, Russia and the United States Centers for Disease Control and Prevention (CDC), decided to keep some cultures around. If <u>all</u> smallpox virus in <u>all</u> laboratories in the whole world had been destroyed at that time, then we truly would now be rid of it. Instead there is now the very well-founded fear that a terrorist country or group could spread smallpox around the world again because the Russian lab was found in 1996 to be "a half-empty facility protected by a handful of guards who had not been paid for months." The scientists who previously were known to be at the Koltsovo facility had disappeared. This authority went on to say that there is now no confidence that there are not other sites where the smallpox virus is being stored or stockpiled.

It has been variously estimated that perhaps as many as half of our country's people have no resistance to smallpox. Further, most of us who are old enough to have had the vaccinations probably need badly outdated boosters.

There are two strains of the smallpox virus, and five types of cases. The overall fatality rate in the last big epidemic in Madras, India, in unvaccinated people was 35%! The variola minor strain generally causes a very mild illness, with less than 1% fatalities. Variola major causes the rest: ordinary smallpox and hemorrhagic smallpox are the serious types, while the modified type occurs in those who have been previously vaccinated, and the so-called flat type has a considerably different rash and, with mild symptoms, may not even be diagnosed as smallpox without cultures. Hemorrhagic is always fatal, while perhaps as many as 70% of those with ordinary smallpox will survive and recover completely.

The politicians in Washington are having a field day dithering about what to do with our small supply of smallpox vaccine. Should they vaccinate healthcare workers? That is probably a good thing because we will be caring for people with a very contagious disease. Unfortunately we have nothing that will cure this disease. Antibiotics don't work. But we can and have been able to prevent it from Jenner's time to the early 1980s.

Should they additionally vaccinate this group or that group, or this part of the country or that part of the country? Or should they hold the vaccine until cases appear and then try to vaccinate just a circle around the land area where the first cases appear? What about possible lawsuits from the inevitable scattered bad reactions?

This thinking is so fuzzy that it doesn't bear thinking about! Do you have any idea of how many people fly from one place to another just in our country every single day, even with the reduction after 9-11? The good news is that, unlike chickenpox, smallpox is usually not very contagious before the sores break out; airborne transmission, as with a ventilating system (remember the first outbreak of Legionnaires' Disease?), is possible but not the usual method.

The bad news is that not very many respiratory droplets from coughing and sneezing are required to contaminate a whole planeload of passengers and cabin crew as the infected person passes up and down the aisle to the restroom a few times. These people become contagious in 3-4 days and contaminate their friends, co-workers, co-passengers in buses and other airplanes, as well as the movie theaters they attend, and everyone in the waiting rooms of the doctors' offices, Urgent Cares, and ERs they go to for care when they finally realize that they are sick enough to need help.

The spread is exponential (which means like a forest fire in the dry country of the western United States -- remember the 480,000 acres burned in just one fire in eastern Arizona in the summer of 2002 and the almost one million acres burned in California in 2003?).

There is one very simple solution. But only one! Just declare smallpox undestroyed and start producing the vaccine again as soon as possible. And vaccinate everybody in the world again.

This will take several years. Hopefully the terrorists will give us that much time because they will experience some production and distribution problems with the virus. Our Rangers and other Special Forces heroes may see to that.

So there will need to be some prioritizing of who gets the first doses. I think police and firemen and military people should be right up there with healthcare personnel. Don't give the vaccine to anyone who has ever been vaccinated until vaccine supplies are adequate. That means anyone over about age 35-40 because we may not have full immunity but we are also not likely to die if we come down with the disease.

Allow no one to enter our country (as we and other countries used to do -- remember the little yellow immunization records we used to have to carry along with our passports?) who has not had a smallpox vaccination.

Aggressively seek out the illegal aliens in our country for vaccination. They could, for example, come to free vaccination stations and have the vaccine without having to give their names or any ID. I know this flies in the face of current "picture ID" and all kinds of documentation requirements, but our goal would be to protect our country from what those illegals might inadvertently bring into our country first and foremost. I once had an illegal from Rumania who brought in a case of tuberculosis and died from it, after infecting at least seven other people.

Our Kosciusko County Medical Society, in 1965, immunized every unvaccinated person who allowed it in our county during one three month period, free of charge, against polio. Doctors, nurses, teachers, medical assistants, and who knows who else, volunteered our services to man vaccination centers in the schools around our county. Afterwards we knew how many thousand doses we distributed, but kept no other records of our activities. No one sued any of us. We may even have given some poor wetback a dose or two.

The risk of really serious complications from smallpox vaccinations is 1.5 cases per million doses for progressive vaccinia, 12 cases per million doses of postvaccinial encephalitis, and **only one case per million doses of death from the vaccination.** 242 people will get cowpox all over their bodies but get well OK. 38 little kids with eczema who shouldn't have been given the vaccine in the first place (we never gave smallpox vaccine to children with eczema) will get bad cases of eczema vaccinatum and be pretty sick. **That's about as good and safe as a vaccination program can possibly be.**

But Congress might have to pass a special law that prevents anyone from being able to sue for anything involved with the national vaccination program.

The point is, there is still smallpox in the world. As long as it is present in a single cow, or a single laboratory, everyone in the world should continue to be vaccinated against it. It is ultimately much more deadly than Ebola and the other hemorrhagic fever viruses because it is more easily passed from person to person. It is far more dangerous than the Black Death of the Middle Ages because we have antibiotics now that kill plague like penicillin kills a strep throat. We see a case or two of plague in Flagstaff every year or two. It lives in rodents, such as rats and mice, but also in prairie dogs. I don't believe we have lost a patient to plague since I moved to Arizona in 1966. So the terrorists can't throw that at us. But we have nothing except our immune systems to help us throw smallpox off.

I strongly suggest that you contact your representatives in Washington and tell them how you feel about this.

How can you tell you have smallpox? Good question. Since I have never seen a case, I just hope I make the right diagnosis when the first case comes my way.

The incubation period is about two weeks (chickenpox is about three weeks) but can vary from seven to eighteen days, depending upon the amount of exposure and your immunity. The first symptoms are much like many other infections: fever, lack of energy, back and other muscle aches, but the headache is one of the worst you have ever had. Half the people vomit, and some become delirious and may convulse just like an epileptic. The outlook is more grim with such a severe onset. On the second or third day the rash appears, the fever falls, and the person feels better.

The rash usually appears all at once, with all spots in the same stage of development, instead of in "crops" over a couple or three days like chickenpox. First it may be small flat red spots, then the red spots become little bumps, and then suddenly, by the fourth day, they all turn into blisters that soon become yellow with pus. Most of these are on the face, arms and legs, with much fewer on the body. They may also be on the palms of the hands and the soles of the feet, much different from chickenpox.

The sores are <u>teeming</u> with the virus, and any contact with one will spread the infection until the scabs dry and drop off in three to four weeks, if the person survives. Also unlike chickenpox, the sores leave really bad scars in the survivors. Smallpox is not spread by animals or insects, but only from person to person.

When I was young, there were still occasional cases of smallpox. When that diagnosis had been made, the county health department came around and put a red "Quarantine" sign on your door. No one in that family was allowed to leave the house until released by a doctor. Neighbors and friends brought and bought food for the family, and the wage earner was usually given (at least in *our* town) paid time off from work. That was a pretty effective way of controlling the spread, and it would be the best way to limit the spread again if terrorists use it to attack us.

The CDC, under one plan, would fly in vaccine to a place where a smallpox case has been confirmed. They would do what they refer to as "ring" vaccination, where they vaccinate and the monitor a ring of people around the case, such as family members, other close contacts and their family members, medical personnel involved in care of the case, as well as lab workers who processed specimens from suspected cases. They would also try to vaccinate anyone who had possibly been exposed to the same viral release as the first case.

This is all well and good, and I think <u>very</u> highly of our CDC. They have helped me on some tough cases, and they are always there, on the other end of the phone, 24 hours a day, 365 days a year. But realistically there will be some, perhaps a lot, of deaths with this approach. With universal vaccination re-instituted no one needs to die (that is, if terrorists give us enough time).

We need to resume the worldwide smallpox immunization program as soon as possible. Then, at least, there will be one less biological weapon to worry about. And right now, I'm worrying!

STAPHYLOCOCCUS TYPE B ENTEROTOXIN

The probable method of transmission would be aerosol or food. People will get very sick with this, but a normally healthy person won't die. Think of it as a bad case of food poisoning. See the chapter on **Vomiting** for home care, because there won't be many IV fluids left for you after the rest of your city becomes ill.

TULAREMIA (Rabbit Fever, Deer Fly Fever)

It normally comes from contact with infected animals or from bites from carriers such as deer flies, mosquitoes, and ticks. By these routes the infection is usually a skin ulcer, with a swollen and tender lymph gland toward the heart from the ulcer.

Other routes of infection with different symptoms include taking in contaminated food or water (this results in severe abdominal symptoms of cramps, vomiting and diarrhea, along with chills and fever, aching, and headache) or inhaling contaminated air, which produces pneumonia.

The probable method of transmission would be by aerosol. It is not transmitted from human to human except through blood exposure. It may come in the form of a skin ulcer when contracted in nature, but would be pneumonic in the event of a terrorist attack.

> *My father got the pneumonic form from rabbit blood that got on his gloves, which he used to wipe his runny nose on a cold day in Indiana, No one had seen that form before, so the initial diagnosis was influenza. As his condition deteriorated, he was sent to the Indiana University Medical Center in Indianapolis, where the correct diagnosis was soon made, an experimental antibiotic given, and he got well.*

There is a vaccine for this, and it responds well to certain antibiotics.

T-2 MYCOTOXINS

The probable method of transmission would be by aerosol, with a one or two day maximum incubation time and 30-40% mortality. These are designed for biological warfare, and I know of no cases in everyday life.

VIRAL HEMORRHAGIC FEVERS (e.g., EBOLA)

Ebola is the worst, but this group also includes Marburg (after the town in Germany where it accidentally got out of the lab), Lassa fever, Bolivian hemorrhagic fever, Hanta viral fever (from exposure to the urine of deer mice in the Four Corners area of our Southwestern United States in the past ten years), Congo-Crimean hemorrhagic fever, and Rift Valley fever.

These viruses truly strike terror into our hearts, with good reason. The death rates are <u>extremely</u> high. Incubation periods vary from 4 to 21 days, with the shortest incubation carrying the highest mortality.

Symptoms begin usually with the usual viral fever and muscle aches and prostration. The eyeballs may be red, the face flushed, the blood pressure low, and there may be scattered little black or purple spots on the skin (called petechiae). (If you see these during <u>any</u> illness, they are an ominous sign and the person needs very rapid medical evaluation.) The liver is soon affected, then in a matter of hours or a day or two there is a sudden deterioration, with hemorrhage into the mucous membranes, shock, bleeding into the lungs, and death.

The drug Ribavirin may be effective in all but Ebola and Marburg if given early enough. The CDC provided us with it in Flagstaff within a few days after the Hantavirus was identified in our Four Corners epidemic, and that soon cut the mortality rate by about 90%. But it took awhile to isolate the organism, and a number of deaths occurred during that time. I think the total was less than 50, however. Four Corners is among the most sparsely populated areas of our country; so we were lucky the epidemic struck there instead of in an urban area.

The probable method of transmission in a terrorist attack would be by aerosol initially, then human to human by contact with feces, saliva, or urine. The Belgian nurse who was one of the only two persons who survived the first outbreak in Zaire (Congo) also was the only one who washed her hands after touching every patient when the gowns and gloves ran out. The other survivor was an African medical assistant who had symptoms for three days, then awoke on the fourth day without a fever and quickly got well. I hope someone analyzed his blood for the antibodies; but if so, I've never seen a report.

Any terrorist attack with a virulent germ will probably not be apparent for at least several days after the attack unless they are caught in the act. The incubation period has to progress to the symptomatic phase before any germs can be identified. The first hours or two or three days produce symptoms exactly like most other infectious diseases. Local laboratories will not be up to speed in testing for exotic stuff, and they will have to overnight specimens to the CDC for evaluation. But that can occur only after health care providers see the patient and order lab tests. It will be at least two or three days before it is apparent to the various physicians in their offices and to those in Urgent Care and emergency facilities that something different is going on. Then one or more will make some phone calls to other physicians or talk at lunch, call other ERs, or whatever. Then things will move very fast.

Each branch of the armed forces has a unit specially trained to respond to biological attacks on constant standby. They can be mobilized at a moment's notice. So massive help will soon be on the way once enough evidence to arouse the suspicions of us in the medical community appears. But that will take too long to help most of those infected in the first wave, and they will die.

If you think you may have exposed to a biological attack, decontamination is essential as soon as possible. Fortunately that is fairly easy in most cases. Just remove all of your clothes and bathe thoroughly with soap and water. Dispose of your clothes in the trash, and wash your hands again. The DOD would prefer that everyone bathe with a 0.5% (dilute) bleach solution, but soap and water will work almost as well and is much more readily available.

This is scary. But, to put this into perspective, even the most successful bioterrorism attack will probably not kill as many people as die from the use of tobacco in our country every year! We die at the rate of at least 500,000 per year from tobacco. Think about that the next time you light up.

Isolation of all people with respiratory illnesses will be very important to prevent spread from person to person, so wear a surgical mask if you have to be near anyone so afflicted. And stay out of crowds. If you yourself are so afflicted let someone check you into whatever medical facility waiting room you are going to while you personally wait out in the car. That will minimize your exposing others there.

CHAPTER 19 -- BLACK MOLD

There is a toxic mold called Stachybotrys atra that can invade a home when there is a flood or leaking water system. Sudden catastrophes, as occurred when a valve in our washing machine malfunctioned several years ago while my wife and I were on our honeymoon, are common.

A couple of things to remember: 1) turn off your washing machine at the wall before you go on a trip, 2) insure with a reliable company for homeowners insurance, and 3) expect to have your insurance refuse to renew your insurance if you incur too high a cost on a single claim, or if you incur as many as three claims in a two year period of time. If you have any reason to expect that you may be refused renewal, then apply for other insurance before you are actually canceled. That way you can truthfully answer no when asked if you have ever been refused insurance.

The reason we are here is to talk about black mold, believe it or not. I mentioned our story because it was handled properly, quickly, and thoroughly. The story of the Ballard family, which was on the cover of USA WEEKEND magazine in 1998, is about the bad things that can happen when the insurance company *doesn't* handle things properly. The Ballards apparently had leaky pipes which the insurance company took so long to cover that the black mold began to grow in their large home. They had many problems, and ultimately obtained a jury verdict against the insurance company for $32 million.

Molds play a major role in the allergy symptoms of many people. Asthma and other respiratory complaints can be traced to mold and mildew. It can be found almost anywhere, but is particularly common in the wet states of the oceans, the Gulf coast, and in the lake country areas of the northern tier of states.

At least one type of mold, Stachybotrys atra, can cause severe nerve problems, particularly memory loss. According to Mrs. Ballard, she had in her computer a list of almost 11,000 people who have or have had mild to severe mental problems from living in places where that mold contaminates the air of the building. It can also cause breathing trouble and even bleeding in the lungs. Dizziness, fatigue, and headaches also have been reported. So far it seems to be the most toxic one in this country, partly because it produces an airborne toxin. But there are thousands, if not millions, of strains of mold, so others may well appear.

The only successful treatment is prevention. <u>That means keeping your house dry</u>. To begin with, don't put carpet on a cement floor, nor anyplace else that might get damp. Use tile and throw rugs instead. Firmly wring out your washcloths when you finish bathing. Have an exhaust fan turned on during bathing and for a few minutes after with the door to the shower stall open. Wipe down the glass portions of your shower stall with a squeegee (like you use on your car windows at the gas station). Paint your bathrooms with semi-gloss paint for better moisture resistance.

When you find any hint of mold, clean it up <u>immediately</u> and eliminate the source of moisture. In the case of condensation, e.g., from air-conditioning ducts or cold water pipes, add insulation around the ducts or pipes. Use detergent and water to clean the mold off of hard surfaces. Dry any wet building materials within 24 hours.

When we drove into our driveway that night, there was water running out under the garage door and down the driveway. When we opened the kitchen door from the garage, a veritable flood of water came gushing out, soaking our feet instantly. The source was easy to find. The water was pouring from the top of the washing machine, even though it had been off when we left ten days before, and the switch was still in the "off" position.

There are companies that specialize in cleanup and drying out your house in such an event. We were fortunate that our insurance company immediately, that very night, retained the services of such a company. They came instantly and began the process of drying us out and salvaging our furniture and anything that had been sitting on the floor. All furniture was removed, dried and cleaned, and, where appropriate, sent to a refinisher.

We were not allowed to return to live in our house for almost two months, during which time the insurance company paid for our living at a nice hotel. New dry wall had to be installed in most of the rooms because black mold had already started to grow behind the walls. The house had to be dried out with heat and fans going 24 hours a day. They replaced the carpets, rugs, and hardwood floors. The insurance adjuster was a jewel; he had encountered this problem many times before.

In short, this was an ideal solution and result for us because the insurance company and adjuster retained experienced cleanup and repair people who were really good at what they did, and did not try to cut corners to save on costs. We had no sign of mold or any other problem related to our personal flood at any time in the ten additional years we lived in the house. The cost of all the services, we were told, was about $50,000. The company had an engineer come in to check out the cause of the washing machine malfunction. He found and removed for a later lawsuit against the washer maker the malfunctioning valve that apparently flipped to "on" during a thunderstorm a few days before. We certainly would recommend that company, which was State Farm, except that they then canceled our insurance even though all agreed that we were not at fault. The insurance adjuster had warned us that this happens with many companies after claims exceed a certain level for that company. So it was no surprise. I probably don't blame them much, but they did recover their costs from the maker of the washing machine.

People who live in moist climates need to use dehumidifiers to reduce mold and mildew prevalence, even if they don't presently have any medical symptoms related to molds. Aim for indoor relative humidity of 30 to 50%. Our respiratory passages need at least 30% humidity in order to function best, while most molds don't grow unless the moisture in the air around them exceeds 60%. It is not unusual for just a small dehumidifier unit to take as much as three <u>gallons</u> of water out of the air in one 24 hour period.

If you get leaks or indoor floods, be sure that everything is <u>thoroughly</u> dried out before any repairs are begun. Be sure there is no mold behind the drywall. If your insurance company doesn't want to do everything to make it right, get to a lawyer immediately. Don't wait until mold gets a foothold in your house, or the only recourse may be to burn the house down and start over. Most insurance companies probably wouldn't stand still for that, but I read of a couple who did that on their own because they had a great location and wanted to live there. This is mentioned just to illustrate that once a house is infested with black mold, it has what we call the "sick building syndrome," for which there is no cure.

One company that my employer handled worker's compensation claims for two or three years ago had such a building, and had well over one hundred employees with complaints that we had to evaluate. We also led the investigation of the building, bringing in specialists from New York, among others. I was transferred to another clinic before all reports were back, so I can't accurately report anything except that the building was finally cured, without burning it down, and all employees got well.

Careful scientific studies are under way in an attempt to pin down the many symptoms described in the many stories about these organisms. So far there is little scientific evidence of actual damage to organ systems. But the jury is still out. Tune in next edition.

CHAPTER 20 -- BLEEDING

A bleeding wound is a scary thing for most people. Unless someone has seen at least one before, it is easy to panic. The first thing to do is to immediately put pressure directly on the bleeding spot with as clean a piece of cloth as you can find. If you have a handkerchief, open it up and use the inside of it, or tear off a piece of a shirt tail that has been inside the pants. Ideally, of course, you will have a first aid kit with sterile (or at least clean) gauze pads and cloth wrap to apply. If the wound is relatively small and the bleeding is easily controlled, then washing it out vigorously with soap and water (and elbow grease, as one of my close relatives used to say) is a good thing to do before applying the bandage. The sooner a wound is cleaned out the less the likelihood of its getting infected.

A bleeding wound is almost always one that should be sewed up. And the sooner it is sewed up the less likely it is to get infected.

When do you need to have a wound repaired?

I see enough people who wait till the next day, when it is usually too late for a primary repair, that I think a few words are in order about that situation.

Probably most of the time this is obvious, because you are actively bleeding from an open wound and little globules of fat stick out. But sometimes the blood is just on the surface and the cut doesn't penetrate the deep layers of the skin, as with a barbed wire scratch, which I've seen a lot of. Here the edges of the wound are slightly separated and usually a little ragged. This is a tough call for a doctor, and most will just clean those out, trim them if necessary, and put a dressing on until the bleeding stops. That approach will result in a noticeable scar, but not a big wide one.

A few doctors (I'm one, because I <u>hate</u> any kind of a scar) will clean, trim, and put in tiny little stitches to bring the outer edges together and thus reduce the amount of scarring. An alternative to that approach is to do the cleaning and trimming and then pull the edges together with Steri-strips, or possibly butterfly bandaids until the wounds heal in 10 days or so.

If you aren't concerned about scarring, you can just scrub out the wound with soap and water with a clean washcloth, gauze, or whatever, as long as it is clean. If you don't have any clean cloth material handy, then use your hands to thoroughly work the soap into the wound, and use your clean fingers to pick out as much visible dirt or other foreign material as possible. Then pour water over the wound, for several minutes if your water supply will allow it. This will probably hold it until you can get home and use a really clean washcloth or gauze. It is OK to cover the wound after thoroughly washing it out, but if you do cover it, be sure to use something clean. Cleaning out the wound right away also extends the time when it is safe to do what we call a primary repair, one in which we sew it up as soon as possible rather than waiting a few days to control any possible low grade infection and then doing a secondary closure. Secondary closures tend to leave larger scars; so get to the doctor as soon as you can.

When you get home after you are wounded, you can clean out the wound one more time (it will hurt a little more because the shock will have worn off by then). Then you must decide whether to go to the doctor. If you haven't had a tetanus booster for over five years, that pretty much makes the decision for you, because you definitely will need one. If you are up to date with the shots, and don't care much about a scar in that particular place (somewhere besides the face, for sure), feel free to clean the skin for two or three inches on each side of it with alcohol to get rid of the skin oils and leftover soap. Then attach one end of a Steri-strip or butterfly bandaid to one side of the wound, and stretch it straight across to the other side, thus pulling the cut edges snugly against each other. Put several of them close together up and down the wound. Then put some tape parallel to the wound on each side to help hold the Steri-strips or butterflies in place for the next ten days.

It is _very_ important not to get the wound wet until it is fully healed. If you do, it increases the risk of infection, as well as allowing the closure strips to come unstuck. In that case the wound will split open. So pretend you are out camping and wash yourself with a washcloth. Also, under no circumstances use an antibiotic ointment on any wound once it has been closed by any method. Ointments slow down the healing, and a wound that has had the stitches removed will just flat come apart in all too many cases if you put on ointment. Once a wound has been cleaned out, the best treatment is to let it dry in the air as much as possible and keep it dry.

To Control Bleeding

Do not use a tourniquet. 99% of the time it will actually cause the bleeding to _increase_ rather than slow down and stop because it will close the veins so that blood can't flow back to the heart and must thus come out of the wound, following the least resistance. That said, if someone has an arm or a leg with the major artery only partially severed, then a tourniquet that is tightened until all bleeding stops may be life-saving. I say partially severed because the blood vessels all have muscles in their walls, the arteries more than the veins, and none in the capillaries. If a major artery is completely cut through, then its muscles will constrict it closed. On the other hand, if a part of the vessel is still attached, the muscles can't completely close the opening.

> *I had a very personal example of this when I was covering the Emergency Room in the little town of Warsaw, Indiana. I was coming down the hospital hall toward the ER entrance when my office receptionist/bookkeeper came around the corner with a man I recognized as her father walking beside her. I quickly noted the he was missing his right arm below his shoulder. There was nothing covering the stump except a few shreds of shirt. But there was no blood. Because all the vessels had been severed when his arm was caught in a cornpicker, the muscles in their walls had been able to contract powerfully and stop even the high pressure in the Brachial Artery.*

**WARNING TO FARMERS! Always turn off your cornpicker before clearing a jam! I know it's a pain to do so a dozen times per field, but I helped to treat three men who ignored that advice and lost their arms in the eight years I practiced in Warsaw. Even in these days of fabulous microsurgery the tissues are usually too badly damaged to successfully reattach. But bring your arm with you if you can get it out of the machine, just in case.

If you do use a tourniquet in a really desperate situation and the bleeding stops, you must be able to personally make sure that it is totally loosened at least every thirty minutes, or the tissue on the far side of the tourniquet from the heart may die from lack of oxygen before you can get to the doctor or hospital. It's a good idea to write down the time it was applied on the person's body part beside the tourniquet and call that to the attention of anyone who takes responsibility for the injured person from you.

> *Farmers and cowboys are the toughest people on Earth! In addition to my employee's father, I had another farmer who crawled across an eighty-acre field to the highway with a broken hip. The horse of a cowboy patient of mine took him under a low tree as they chased a cow. A sharp branch caught his scalp just at the top of the forehead and ripped it 90% off his skull. This man rode back to the ranch house and drove himself 50 miles in a pickup to the ER, where I spent three hours putting 200 stitches in it. (It healed just fine.)*
> *These people are so often out far from other people by themselves that no one misses them until they are late for supper. Then a desperate spouse has to look for the injured loved one, often in the dark.*

> *The elderly mother of one of my best Native American friends was involved in a motor vehicle accident far out on the Navajo Reservation. She had several injuries, but none were really serious if she could get prompt medical attention. She was, however, slowly but steadily bleeding internally from a wound to her spleen. As we discussed it later, her husband had heard somewhere that an injured person shouldn't be moved until the ambulance came. So he sent the only car that came along on the small dirt back road 60 miles to the nearest hospital at Tuba City, Arizona, for an ambulance. That took almost three hours while she slowly bled to death. She was beyond resuscitation when the ambulance finally arrived.*

** ***Forget the old lessons that said not to move an injured person.*** Use common sense. If the person is bleeding and you can't readily stop it or you suspect internal injury, pick him up, put him in a vehicle, and transport him to the nearest place where a medical professional can be found. Don't wait out in the middle of nowhere for an ambulance to come to you. In this era of cell phones and CB radios, call for help or have someone at the scene call for help and tell them you will meet them along the way.

CHAPTER 21 -- BREAST CANCER

Risk Factors

First and foremost is a history of breast cancer in a woman on your mother's side of the family. Then, in no particular order are: never having a baby, never breast feeding. Smoking and drinking alcohol while taking female replacement hormones almost doubles the risk in older women. There is much controversy right now over some recent reports that taking hormone replacement medications (progesterone compounds) after menopause *may* increase breast cancer risk.

I'm not totally sure about this. My personal impression is that taking continuous progesterone products is not a good thing. I believe that taking estrogen by itself is not a risk factor for cancer. I also believe that simply taking progesterone (or provera) for ten to twelve days once a month or once every three months to bring on a period is probably not a significant risk factor. I feel that if you have a uterus, then taking the estrogen-progesterone cyclically so that you will have a period several times a year is necessary to protect against uterine cancer. With the current information I am recommending using the provera for twelve days only once every three months, so that one will have a period four times a year and be exposed to progesterone only 48 days a year, rather than the 365 days in the initial study. **If you don't have a uterus, there is no reason under the sun to ever take any progesterone.** For more on this, see the chapter on **Hormone Therapy.**

Breast Self-Examination (also see the chapter on Staying Well Physically)

On one of our exams in medical school was the following question: "Who finds the most breast cancers? (a) husband (b) boyfriend (c) doctor (d) the patient herself?" To these today we would have to add (e) girlfriend, and (f) mammography. The answer was and still is (d) the patient herself.

Every woman should start examining her breasts once a month at the conclusion of her menstrual period from about the age 21 for the rest of her life. These instructions will give you an idea how do this accurately, but you should also ask your doctor to give you some instruction when you go in for a Pap smear. Most women's breasts have some small lumps or nodules in them. It's best to become acquainted with those that are present normally in your breasts long before you need to worry about cancer. Then if you notice something new or different, you can watch carefully and call it to the attention of your doctor.

This should be done by every woman after about age 21 on about the day after her period is over. The reason for that particular time is that the woman's hormone effect on the breasts is at its lowest at that time and the fluid retention that often occurs in relation to her periods has gone away. Thus there are less likely to be hormone-related lumps or cysts that might be confusing. Also it is easy to remember.

Approach the self-examination in a methodical way. I suggest that you first sit or stand in front of a mirror with a good light and look at how your breasts are supported and how they hang. It is unusual for both to be totally identical and symmetrical, but they

Whether to use hormone replacement therapy is a scary decision for women right now. On the one hand is hot flashes in many women, along with increased risk of osteoporosis if you don't take estrogen. Also, a patient of mine this week had talked with her gynecologist last month about this very thing and decided to quit taking the estrogen she had already been taking for twenty years without a problem. So here we were, a month later, and she had burning on urination, as well as irritation of the opening of the vagina. She also was totally dry when she made love for the first time in her life. After a urinalysis was normal, a pelvic exam revealed what we call atrophic vaginitis, in which the vaginal mucous membranes become thin, dry, and irritated. Estrogen keeps those tissues normal when you take it, but the effect wears off quickly when you stop, as my patient discovered.

We discussed at length the pros and cons. Included was the fact that estrogen patches do not follow the same metabolic pathway through the liver that the pills do. Also estrogen cream is available for local use in the vagina. It doesn't help prevent osteoporosis, but it will make the vaginal tissues healthy again. And the risk of its causing breast cancer should be as close to nil as possible. She elected Vivelle patches, which at present are the smallest and easiest to stay on of all the patches, and we started her on a low-medium dose.

should look the same every time. Look for **dimples in the skin**. Look for *irregularities in the skin surface*. These are possible danger signals.

Clasp your hands in front of you without blocking your view, and first push the hands together. That causes contraction of the underlying pectoral muscles and may cause a **dimple to appear that wasn't there before** if there is a lump or other tissue in the breast that is attached to the muscle. That is another danger signal. Then clench your fingers together as you try to pull your hands apart to contract slightly different muscles to produce the same result.

Lie down. Place a small pillow under your right shoulder blade. Put your right arm over your head on the bed. That position will flatten your breast as much as possible on your chest wall, making it easier to feel any lumps. First with the palm of your opposite hand, push firmly down on all parts of the breast, and notice any lumps or unusual sensation of fullness down deep in the breast. Now mentally divide your breast into four parts (as north, south, east, and west). Next with the flats of your fingers start out at the very farthest edge of your breast, which is out at your armpit in the northwest quarter, and push first lightly and then firmly as you go like the spokes of a wheel from the rim to the nipple area (we call it the areola) all around that quarter. Then move to the southwest quarter and do the same. Repeat for the northeast and southeast quarters, and you are done.

<u>Expect</u> to find lumps and nodules (maybe lots) that are perfectly normal. Get acquainted with where they are and how they feel. **What you are looking for is a lump that wasn't there last month.** That needs to be checked by your doctor. Also:

**Anything that feels hard like a rock should be checked by your doctor right away.

In spite of mammography, which is hugely important in picking up early breast cancers, breast self-examination still finds a significant percentage of these tumors. If you are sure that a lump is new (and you will be when you become acquainted with the contents of each breast after a few months of self-examination), see your doctor immediately for a biopsy or aspiration. If your doctor doesn't do these, then he will refer you to someone who does. Don't waste time. **Breast cancer is curable if it is found early enough.**

A patient herself cannot really be sure of feeling a lump until it is about 1/2 inch in diameter. Her doctor probably can't find it any better than she can, but he or she can <u>sometimes</u> have a better idea about whether it could dangerous. Mammography can pick up spots as tiny as 2 millimeters in diameter that may be cancer. Ultrasound can tell whether a lump is solid or cystic. Your doctor can put a small needle into a lump that doesn't feel solid to him and draw out fluid to send to the lab for cytology (if you get fluid, the odds are overwhelming that you have benign fibrocystic disease, a very common condition). Your doctor may suggest doing a fine needle biopsy of a lump, sucking out a few cells to be examined under the microscope. But the only absolute way to make the diagnosis of cancer is to take a biopsy.

A biopsy involves removing all or a portion of the lump and sending it to the pathologist, a doctor who specializes in laboratory medicine. His technicians will fix it in formalin, put it into a block of paraffin, cut it into ultra thin sections, which are then stained and attached to slides for examination under the microscope by the pathologist. This normally takes three working days but can be speeded up under certain favorable or emergency circumstances. The biopsy is usually done in the hospital, but can be done easily in the doctor's office under local anesthetic if the lump is fairly close to the surface of the breast.

We used to (and probably quite a few doctors still do) tell the patient that we would take the biopsy in the operating room, send it to the lab and have the pathologist freeze and stain a "frozen section" for immediate examination under the microscope. This takes only about 20 minutes if he has been alerted ahead of time as is usual. The problem with the frozen section is that it is thicker than a normal fully processed section, and the staining characteristics aren't as good. Therefore, the vast majority of us don't feel completely secure with a diagnosis until we see the report of the final sections. Sometimes our local pathologist finds something rare that he hasn't seen before. In such a case he will send representative slides to a reference lab, such as at the University of Arizona School of Medicine here in Arizona (they are particularly famous for their work with malignant melanoma). They may in turn send it somewhere else before a final determination is made. That can take awhile.

We would tell the patient that if the lump was cancer she would wake up without a breast, and with a lymph node dissection and whatever her surgeon felt was best to help cure the cancer. If she woke up with her breast still securely in place, then it was benign. We did this because we felt that cutting into a cancerous tumor would almost always spread some cells and increase the risk of metastases.

I quit letting that approach be used on my patients when a good surgeon, with me assisting, did a breast biopsy on a lady who was a good friend of both of us. We both felt that the lump looked benign, but eyeballing it isn't the final word, not ever. On frozen section the pathologist wasn't absolutely sure but thought it was cancer. The surgeon turned to me and said, "Carl, I'm not going to remove this lady's breast without a lot better diagnostic certainty than that!" I felt the same way, and we quickly closed the small biopsy wound. I notified the pathologist of our decision and heard his sigh of relief on the other end of the line. He expedited the processing, so that two days later he called with the news that the lump was, indeed, benign! If the frozen section diagnosis isn't absolutely certain, one should always wait for the permanent sections to be reported in writing.

Treatments

A yearly consensus statement by the National Institutes of Health (NIH) gives guidance for the most successful current treatments of breast cancer. I haven't seen the latest one.

Treatment with a combination of chemotherapy drugs, especially combinations that include anthracyclines (such as doxorubicin and cyclophosphamide) and tamoxifen, currently provides the best chance for survival. This approach is especially good for women with localized breast cancer (the "lumpectomy" patients).

Women whose tumors have estrogen receptors should receive female hormones.

Women who have undergone mastectomies and who are at high risk for recurrence should receive radiation therapy.

While these are generally thought to be best, patient input and other characteristics, such as age, tumor size and cell type, hormone receptor status, and cell turnover rate must be taken into account when planning the attack on the cancer. The quality of life issue may be a factor, especially in older women in whom chemo is being considered.

So women now usually have the input for what should be done (lumpectomy, radical mastectomy, etc.) after a certain diagnosis is made and before the major surgical procedure is done. Further discussion about cancer of the breast is beyond the present scope of this book.

It is essential to consult an oncologist (a doctor who specializes in the treatment of cancer), who will have the latest information, and will be aware of unpublished treatments with promising drugs not yet approved by the FDA for use outside of clinical trials.

CHAPTER 22 -- CHOOSING A DOCTOR

Your doctor should be, and given a chance will be, your confidante, your healer, your confessor, and most of all, your friend. He or she will deliver your children, sit up with them late at night when they are sick, help you talk to them about the birds and the bees, stitch up your and their wounds, advise you in all things secular, make you well and pray for you when he can't, find you a good specialist when you need one, give you drug samples when ordering a new and undoubtedly expensive medication, and give you literature on everything from unusual coital positions to caring for pinworms. (I'm not sure yet whether I'll include coital positions in this edition, but I will tell you about pinworms.)

People choose a doctor by recommendations from their friends, neighbors, or coworkers, out of the yellow pages, a name from a waitress, from the list provided by their HMO, whatever. Ask a nurse friend who works at the hospital which doctors he or she thinks are the best and nicest. If you don't know a nurse, then find one of your friends who does.

Try to choose someone who is Board-certified in his or her specialty because that usually means that the doctor has had at least a certain minimum training after medical school, then has done a certain minimum number of procedures, and/or cared for a certain minimum number of various types of cases, then passed an examination.

Board certification by itself doesn't guarantee a good doctor. But it's a start. In my own specialty of Family Practice an even better indication of a doctor who keeps up his training after medical school and residency is one who is a member of the American Academy of Family Practice (AAFP). The chief requirement of continuing membership is that a member must complete at least an average of 50 hours of continuing medical education (CME) every year. These hours have to be documented and turned into the AAFP. This is by far the most stringent CME requirement of any specialty, but it is necessary if a family doctor is to be able to keep up with so many different aspects of medicine.

Practically every vacation I have taken for almost 45 years has been sandwiched around a medical meeting! Fortunately some of them have been in pretty exotic places. So my wife goes sight-seeing during the day, and we get together for dinner and maybe an evening lecture. Plus we get to sleep in a bed together with no kids down the hall.

Ask to see the doctor's CV. I had mine on my receptionist's desk and each new patient was given one. That way you know more about your prospective doctor than just his or her degree. Note the way you are treated when you walk into the office for the first time. Also pay attention to the way the doctor treats his employees. Are there lots of smiles -- or just harried looks?

Ask to meet a prospective doctor before you choose him from your panel, because once you have signed on with one, it is less easy to change to another. He probably won't have time for much more than a handshake, but that often is enough.

One problem is that every year many employers change insurance companies, thus making you and all other employees change to new doctors. This is equally difficult for doctors, and the influx of many new patients makes it tough to have time for new patient interviews. But reading your prospective doctor's history plus a short 5-minute meeting is the best possible thing for both of you. So try to arrange it.

When you have your first patient visit, note whether your doctor washes his or her hands after examining you. This is the single most important thing a health professional can do to prevent spread of infection from patient to patient. Your doctor's hands should be scrupulously clean at all times, and he will usually wash them after any contact with you if you have an infection of any kind. It is not necessary to wash the hands after doing a blood pressure check or other clean encounter, but don't stay with a doctor who has dirty hands.

If you don't like your assigned or chosen doctor after one or two visits, by all means switch to someone else. You will be doing both yourself and the doctor a favor!

One more thing -- the most expensive doctor is not likely to be the best doctor.

CHAPTER 23 -- CIRCUMCISION

The pros and cons of having your baby boy circumcised are many and varied. Certain religions practice it as a ritual, perhaps, in some cases, not being aware of why their religion began the practice hundreds or thousands of years ago.

What, actually, is circumcision? The answer depends considerably on the person performing it. A Jewish rabbi may perform it himself, during a short religious ceremony, with a clamp that allows only 1/8 to 1/4 inch of skin to be removed, barely exposing the tip of the head of the penis. Then everyone present has a ritual glass of wine plus other celebratory aspects.

Similar results are obtained by doctors who haven't been trained adequately in the procedure and don't feel competent to remove more than just the end of the skin. Or they don't believe in the procedure in the first place.

The plastibel technique, in which a tiny plastic cup is tied in place on the penis inside the protruding foreskin until the skin dies and it falls off, takes more foreskin, but still leaves a lot behind, along with bits of skin that may be stuck to the head of the penis.

The above techniques all have the disadvantage of requiring the complete retraction of the foreskin daily for washing for the rest of the person's life, not a very difficult thing to do. The chief advantage is that the remaining foreskin produces some lubrication during lovemaking, and that can be helpful if the partner does not produce quite enough vaginal secretion on her own.

Gay men, even uncircumcised, need extra lubrication such as K-Y jelly anyway, so this doesn't really apply to them.

A doctor who is well-trained in doing these, using a Gomco clamp, will remove most of the foreskin, leaving behind just enough of a fold around the shaft below the head to allow for expansion when an erection occurs. Most of us who do these now use a little local non-epinephrine-containing anesthetic. But the pain of the procedure lasts such a short time that the little guys I performed it on, before we had locals that we felt were safe, would go to sleep as soon as the clamp was tightened and wouldn't even feel the knife.

Possible complications include bleeding, taking off too much skin, cutting into the urine tube (which is especially risky when the tube opening is out of the usual location -- a situation I have seen about once per thousand circumcisions that I have performed), and infection (I've never seen a case in a newborn, but this becomes more likely as the boy gets older).

In the uncircumcised boy adhesions often develop between the foreskin and the head of the penis, and this, if not corrected, will produce the condition called phimosis, which gets worse as one gets older. In this the foreskin cannot be retracted for cleansing, and interferes with erection and lovemaking. This is another reason that men have a circumcision done as adults.

Possible immediate advantages of circumcision include:

1. Prevention of phimosis adhesions

2. Probably less chance of urinary tract infections (which are more likely to occur in little girls, by the way)

3. Much easier to cleanse lifelong

4. Prevention of infections that may occur under the foreskin

Studies have shown that the wives of men who have been circumcised are less likely to develop cancer of the cervix. The explanation for that is pretty simple. Cancer of the cervix is caused by a virus. This virus, as well as other disease-producing micro-organisms, is more likely to be carried under the possibly somewhat unclean foreskin of an uncircumcised penis than on a circumcised penis, which is easier to clean and is mostly exposed to the air all the time.

A recent study indicates that AIDS is less likely to be transmitted to a man who has been circumcised.

The reverse of the man infecting the woman occurs when the woman has a vaginal yeast infection. If not always using a condom, the man gets the yeast under the foreskin, where it is warm and moist, ideal growing conditions for yeast. Many previously uncircumcised men whose partners have the yeast problem come in for an adult circumcision. In those cases they have all the foreskin removed, and their part of the yeast problem goes away.

Another advantage of circumcision is in quite a few men who have premature ejaculation that hasn't responded to any of the techniques taught by sex therapists and most urologists. The head of the penis is slightly desensitized by being in contact with the air and clothing, thus allowing the man to wait longer before firing off. His partner is then more likely to achieve her full satisfaction also.

I have yet to have a man complain to me about having been circumcised, but I'm aware that some men have little clubs or chat rooms where they share dissatisfaction with others who have undergone the procedure. I think those men might also be benefited by some psychological counseling directed toward other possible areas of problems in their lives.

Some insurances will pay for a newborn circumcision, while others won't. In my opinion, paying extra on your own will be well worth the expense and will save your child a lot of unwanted problems later in life.

If you elect not to have your child circumcised, then it is <u>absolutely essential</u> that you retract the foreskin completely back and away from the head of the penis, as well as away from the rim of the head, where little white patches are often found, every day during the bath, starting as soon as one week old. Then as the child gets older, teach him to wash it properly himself under your supervision. This is very important because the time will come when he becomes very shy about your seeing his private areas and won't allow your care anymore.

How do you retract the foreskin? In the newborn this is pretty easy. Just gently pull the foreskin back as far as you can every day when you bathe him. Each day pull it back a little farther. Within two or three weeks you will have it pulled back beyond the little depression that is back of the purplish rim of the head of the penis, where the shaft is attached. That allows you to remove with each washing the smelly whitish stuff, called smegma, that collects there. Thus no adhesions are likely to develop.

If you have trouble with this, ask your doctor to do the initial pulling of the foreskin membrane off the head at one of the first well-baby visits. He or she or you can just use some wet or dry gauze in each hand to steady the penis on one side while peeling from the other. Some doctors aren't aware of the adhesion problem, which <u>must</u> be taken care of in the first month or two of life, when it is easy for you or the doctor, as well as for your little guy. In those few cases seek another doctor's help.

In conclusion, as you may have guessed, I firmly believe in and highly recommend circumcision in the newborn by an experienced doctor, within the first two to four weeks of life, when the procedure is relatively easy, and risks are very low.

CHAPTER 24 -- CONSTIPATION

This chapter is pretty gross. Please feel free to skip over it if you don't have this problem.

I firmly believe that more people are caused discomfort by some of the treatments for supposed constipation than by true constipation itself. I still cringe when I think of having to endure what happened when my beloved grandmother told me periodically, when we lived with my grandparents during the Depression, "Carl Jr., you need a good cleaning out." That meant a dose of castor oil and some prunes usually, with the associated cramping stomach until I was thoroughly "cleaned out." Maybe I really was constipated, but I kind of suspect that she was as preoccupied as many others of her generation with keeping the bowels as empty as possible.

This condition has conflicting definitions, depending upon who is defining it. A lot of older people feel that not having a bowel movement at least once every day means that they are constipated. I'm more concerned with what their normal bowel pattern has been all their lives. To me, a change in the previous bowel habit that lasts more than about two weeks without an apparent cause may mean a medical problem has developed.

"An apparent cause" can mean being on a long journey with inability to keep up enough fluid intake to keep the stools from getting hard. It can mean eating too many prunes "because they were so good" and getting loose stools for awhile. It can mean getting food poisoning and taking a little while to get the stools settled down again. It can mean taking an antibiotic that kills the normal bacteria or germs in the digestive tract, with upset digestion until the normal bacteria return (taking acidophilus or lactobacillus pills or capsules during or after taking antibiotics often helps a quick return to normal). It can mean falling in a ski accident and breaking five ribs, thus paralyzing the GI tract (what we call an ileus, if you are interested) for three days.

Any definite change in the bowel habit that lasts more than two weeks can be a **danger signal** and you should consult your doctor. Parasites, bowel malfunctions, medication problems, even early cancers, can present this way. For the moment, we are just going to talk about the constipation change in the bowel function. Please remember that diarrhea is also a change in the bowel habit, and one that is likely to bring you to the attention of medical authorities sooner than constipation.

First, let's see just how the bowel plays a part in this problem. As digestion progresses from the mouth downward, a lot of digestive fluids are secreted rapidly into the GI tract. Normally it takes about three days for food to travel from the mouth to its ultimate destination in the rectum and out the anus.

Each area of the tract plays its own part in the digestive process, some areas absorbing one or more types of nutrients and others being absorbed into the bloodstream elsewhere. By the time the food has passed through 25 or 30 feet of small intestine, it is almost all liquid, the same as we see with diarrhea. Then it enters the large intestine, over in the lower right side of the abdomen where the appendix is located. Some further food is absorbed into the blood in the 10 or 12 feet of large intestine, but most of what is absorbed is water, especially in the descending colon and rectum. The longer the stool stays in those areas, the more water is absorbed from it back into the blood. If a person is a little dehydrated (as who isn't in Phoenix in the summertime), then the bowel works harder at sucking away the water.

Normally the smooth muscle action of the GI tract is like a wave, starting at the top and progressing all the way down in what we call peristalsis. After a meal this is particularly active. And, by no coincidence, that is the best time to have a bowel movement so it doesn't have to be forced. Warm fluids also stimulate peristalsis, and they can be hot water just as well as coffee or tea. So for someone who has a constipation problem, here are the first two suggestions:

1. Try to go soon after a meal.

2. Drink plenty of non-caffeine-containing fluids so that there is still some water in the stool by the time it gets to the anus. What is enough water? A good rule of thumb is that if you have to pee about every two hours, you are probably drinking enough. Another is that your urine should be very light in color. Deep yellow means it is too concentrated and thus you aren't drinking enough.

3. Next is to go when you first feel that you might be able to. If you decide to wait and finish a project, then you have "lost the wave," and another may not come along that day.

Stools that contain a lot of cellulose or other fibers, which are indigestible, tend to hold back more water from absorption and thus are quite a bit softer. This is especially important in people with diverticulosis and diverticulitis of the colon (see that chapter).

4. So eat a lot of fiber every day, some for every meal. Raw uncooked fruits and vegetables have a lot of cellulose-type fiber. Whole grain breads and cereals, particularly bran cereals, are also rich in fiber. Popcorn has the most of all, but the shell can be another problem.

Artificial fiber products, such as Metamucil (the oldest and probably still the cheapest one) and a bunch of others are a good way to treat constipation.

5. Exercise for at least 30 minutes without stopping every day.

A stool that follows the normal pattern will be somewhat firm when passed, but also somewhat compressible so that it won't overstretch and hurt the muscles and mucous membrane of the anus.

In someone with a bad case of diarrhea, what you put in your mouth can pass all the way through and out the other end in 30 minutes. Once the diarrhea stops, the tract may take two or three days to start you going to the bathroom again. This is not constipation. Food normally takes about three days to pass from the mouth to the toilet.

> *Some people have what we call a megacolon, where the nerve-to-smooth muscle tone relationship which most people have, just isn't there in the colon, and thus stool isn't moved along once the descending colon begins to withdraw water from the stool material. These people may have a stool only once a week, and when they do, it is huge. I had friend in college who had this problem. We used to tell him to go do his duty somewhere else besides our housing unit because he always plugged up the toilet so that it overflowed.*

So let's just talk about plain old uncomplicated constipation and what you can do about it. To me that kind of constipation means that at least the first part of your stools are hard, perhaps painfully so. It may also mean that you are now having stools every three or four days instead of once every day or two. It also means a change from your usual or lifelong pattern.

Certain medications slow down peristalsis (the intestinal wave), draw excess fluid out of the stool, or whatever, and thus cause constipation. Your pharmacist should give you a list of possible side effects whenever he or she fills your prescriptions. Be sure to always read that list. If constipation is on it and you are affected, short of stopping the drugs, especially if they are working, try the suggestions below.

Chronic laxative users have a problem that severely tests the ingenuity of their physicians. The laxatives they have used over the years have eventually caused the loss of nerve-smooth muscle function and thus proper peristalsis in the GI tract no longer occurs. In other words, the nerves don't stimulate the muscles, and the muscles may have gotten so over-stretched over the years that they can't move the stool along properly, particularly in the large intestine. This may have resulted in a sort of self-induced megacolon. So the bowels have gotten to the place where they don't move without some kind of help.

The program I had my elderly lady patient on (see page 99), and which I recommend to each of you with real honest-to-goodness constipation includes the five suggestions above, plus the following:

6. Never take a laxative. Metamucil is not actually a laxative, and you can take a lot of it (I almost wrote "all you want," but my experience has been that there probably is an

upper limit to how much Metamucil you can safely take. I just don't know what that limit is.) This substance is pretty mild, gentle, and safe.

7. Do all the stuff above, and if you haven't had a BM (bowel movement) after three days but feel there is something in your rectum, put about four ounces of mineral oil into the rectum at night before you go to bed and leave it there.

8. If you then don't have a BM by lunchtime or so the next day, take a warm tap water enema. Or use a disposable Fleet's enema.

The best way to take an enema is to lie on your left side with the bag hung by a bent wire clothes hanger from the shower stall rod with the warm water in it. Lubricate the nozzle with Vaseline petroleum jelly, and point it toward your navel in the front of your abdomen, because that is the direction that the anal canal runs as it passes from the rectum. Then gently work the nozzle into the canal and on into the rectum. It helps if you pretend that you are having a bowel movement as you do that, because the anal muscle then relaxes somewhat. (When a doctor is going to do a rectal exam on you, remember this little tip also. It will definitely make the exam much more comfortable -- really!)

Hold the fluid in the bowel for up to 30 minutes, if you can. Then sit on the toilet and expel it.

9. You can repeat the enema the next day if no results. If still no results, then you must consider the possibility of a fecal impaction.

> *My elderly lady patient with congestive heart failure for twenty years that I tell about in the chapter on **Heart Failure** again is a perfect but extreme example of this kind of problem. (Bless her heart; we could fill up this book with all her medical problems! But she lived to eighty-four and still loved to watch basketball games on TV.) She had already been using Ex-lax, castor oil, cascara sagrada, milk of magnesia, and I don't remember what else, for twenty or thirty years before I first met her. She hadn't had a normal, unassisted bowel movement in all that time. X-rays of her large intestine showed that it was dilated to about three times its normal size, much as a megacolon would be. But she wasn't born with this as those with megacolons are. She acquired this by taking laxatives. Every now and then she would develop a fecal impaction if she didn't follow my program faithfully. And sometimes, even when she followed my program, it didn't work and we had to use dynamite in the form of cascara sagrada. Sometimes we used dulcolax, which is almost as strong and is used often as a bowel prep when we order a barium enema, colonoscopy, or sigmoidoscopy.*

Fecal Impaction

In the elderly, lack of strength in the abdominal and other muscles may make it difficult to push out the stool. Poor fluid intake may make the rectum work harder to reabsorb moisture in the stool. Sometimes the elderly go days or even weeks with no stool, then a little diarrhea appears, to the point where they soil themselves. So nobody thinks that someone with diarrhea is constipated. Until they develop abdominal pain and go to the doctor.

The doctor right away will do a rectal exam, and guess what? The patient is so constipated that he has a fecal impaction, which has to be literally dug out with the (preferably) double-gloved finger of the nurse or doctor. Enemas won't do it. If you ever have to do this unpleasant chore, be assured that the person you are doing it for will be very grateful. The technique is simple. Use some K-Y jelly if you have it, or Vaseline petroleum jelly and lubricate the rectum and your finger thoroughly with it. Keep it handy, as it will wear off and need to be renewed many times.

When you insert your finger into the rectum, you will feel something smooth, rounded, and pretty hard. The way to break it up is to push through it from the front toward the bony area just above the tailbone, and then pull out whatever breaks off with your finger. Have lots of Kleenex tissues or toilet paper handy, and a paper sack to put them in. Keep plugging away until you can't feel any more. I have taken as much as 45 minutes to an hour before the rectum was completely empty, and I have pretty long fingers. Then put about four ounces of mineral oil into the rectum to sit overnight. Then check the person again the next day.

When you are all through you can then gradually empty the contents of the paper sack into the toilet, flushing frequently enough that the toilet won't get backed up. Your rubber gloves can't go down the toilet. Just wrap them up in the paper sack and put them in the garbage. Then wash your hands several times. The odor may hang on it for awhile, but it will actually be clean. Just ignore it. You've done a good thing, probably for someone you love, which you could never have done if you had allowed yourself to be overly fastidious. Just think of those dirty diapers you used to have to clean up when you had a baby (if you were a mommy once -- and forever).

CHAPTER 25 -- CONSULTATIONS

Most of us, at least after a few years, recognize our limitations and seek consultations when we're getting in over our heads or just to be sure we're not missing something in diagnosis or treatment. A physician extender, such as a PA or CPN, should be quick to discuss your case with his or her supervising physician and can and should send you to a specialist for consultation under the same circumstances a physician would.

When you're being sent for consultation or referral to another physician your doctor should offer you a choice of at least two or three physicians in that field, or choose a doctor you yourself suggest. Most of us usually think that one consultant may be a little better than another in the list we give you, and we will usually put that name first in the list. You should always be given a choice. You may not want to make a choice yourself, but you should always have that right. Ask your doctor for a little information about each of them. After your doctor or his extender gives you the list, go home and talk to your spouse. Talk to your friends. Talk to your boss. Talk to your spouse's boss.

At night or on weekends you pretty much have to take someone who is on call and willing to see you. So the choice in emergencies is likely to be much more limited. This is also true in small towns. But most consultations are not emergencies, so don't hesitate to seek someone in a distant city if you aren't satisfied that you will get as good care in your own community. Here in Arizona I had to send people 150 miles from Flagstaff to Phoenix often, until we had that particular specialty in our own town. The big problem with this is that you would miss a day of work.

Always bear in mind that a doctor is more likely to recommend a course of treatment that he is personally trained in and comfortable with. Expect a surgeon to recommend surgery, an internist to recommend drug therapy, a sports medicine doctor to suggest exercise, etc. If your condition warrants, try to see a doctor in several different specialties to evaluate if there are different approaches to your illness or condition. Consider combining them, and always think about trying the most conservative, least invasive treatment first. This will often save you big bucks, because the more conservative treatments are usually a lot less expensive than surgery, with less risk of complications.

CHAPTER 26 -- CONTRACEPTION

There are two types, permanent, and temporary. Permanent includes only three categories: Hysterectomy (removal of the uterus in the woman), vasectomy in the man, and tubal ligation in women. All the main temporary methods are discussed below. Abortion is <u>not</u> contraception. It is termination of the pregnancy after implantation of the egg into the wall of the uterus. Contraception is prevention from implantation of a fertilized egg, or prevention of ovulation, or barrier means to prevent sperm from reaching the egg if ovulation does occur.

Vasectomy

There are two tubes called the vas deferens, which carry the sperm from each testicle (your balls) to the seminal vesicles (think of them as storage tanks for sperm) in the prostate area, where they are stored until ejaculation during intercourse, masturbation, or wet dreams. At those times they are squeezed out by the millions and mixed with the semen fluid to pass out of the opening of the penis.

In a vasectomy the doctor injects the area in the sack with local anesthetic, using a tiny needle. Then a small cut is made in the upper scrotum (sack that holds the testicles or balls) on each side over the underlying vas. This tube can be felt as a very firm string about 1/16 inch in diameter running in the softer tissue of the spermatic cord and muscle that makes your balls go up and down when someone strokes your thighs. <u>Nothing touches the testicles.</u>

A small instrument is used to grasp the tube and pull it up into the opening. After some further dissection, a small piece of the tube, from 1/4 to 1 inch long, is removed and usually either saved or sent away to the lab for identification, to be sure that the doctor did, indeed, get the right tube. The ends of the tubes are usually tied or lightly cauterized, or both. Then the wound is closed with a couple of stitches. The same thing is repeated on the other side. A dressing is then usually applied that will soak up the expected few drops of blood that appear in the first hour after the surgery. These dressings tend to be somewhat bulky and somewhat loose because the testicles are almost constantly in motion.

There is also the single incision approach where the only incision is made in the midline of the sack and the tubes are brought over to that opening, then cut and tied. Also there is the so-called no-scalpel approach where a special instrument with a sharp point on it is used to penetrate the skin on each side and then opened to split the skin so that the tubes can be brought out to be cut and tied or cauterized. I have done all types and will do whatever you, my patient, wants. However, the single incision often causes more interior bruising than two small separate ones. And it seems to me that the no-scalpel approach might slightly increase the low failure rate because not as big a segment of the tubes can be removed.

The Pre-Vasectomy Conference

This will be a meeting among the man undergoing the procedure, his spouse, and the doctor who will do the surgery usually. Sometimes an assistant will do the explanations and the doctor will wind it up. You will probably be given a printed explanation of the procedure, which will include much of what you are reading here (or more!). He will explain the possible complications, which include particularly post-op bleeding, infection (only 3% of all clean surgical procedures nationally become infected), life-threatening allergic reaction to the local anesthetic, development of a spermatocele, a sack in the scrotum which contains sperm that can't go anywhere. (I've seen just one of these, in a man who had not had a vasectomy. Treatment is usually just putting a small needle into it and sucking out the fluid), and failure of the spouse to enjoy sex as much afterwards because there is no longer an element of risk in it! If you had a good sex life before the surgery, then it will probable be even better afterwards. If you had a bad sex life, then the vas probably won't make it better.

You are just as much of a man after a vas as before. You have the same hormones; you still get erections (hard-ons); you still ejaculate; you still grow hair on your face. Nothing has changed except the removal of small segments of tubes. Think of a highway over a river. If the bridge is removed, there is no change in any of the countryside except that cars no longer can cross the river. That is what happens with a vasectomy. The sperm are still formed, but they live their lives and are recycled by the body locally instead of being expelled with the semen fluid when you ejaculate. If you are still worried about what might happen to you mentally, then wait. Talk to other guys who have had it. Talk to a psychologist. Whatever. Don't have it until you feel comfortable.

Two contradictory studies have been mentioned in the literature. One suggested that a man who had had a vasectomy is more likely to get cancer of the prostate. The other study suggested that someone who had this surgery would be more likely to live longer than those who didn't have it. I can easily believe that we can live an extra two minutes for every minute we exercise, as discussed under Benefits of Exercise elsewhere in this book, but as far as I'm concerned, both of these studies fly in the face of reason.

If your marriage is a good one, and you are sure that you will not ever want any more kids, even if one or more were killed in an accident, then go ahead with the vas. If there is a chance that your marriage will not survive, then don't have it. A new wife in the future might want to have kids.

Go into the procedure with the expectation that it will be permanent. The operation to repair the tubes after a vasectomy is delicate, very expensive, not covered by insurance, but about 90% successful with a skillful surgeon in the first year (dropping drastically in subsequent years). However, if either of you have any doubts about whether you might want more kids, use other contraception until those doubts are resolved. That's why the doctor wants your spouse also to sign the sterilization consent form before agreeing to do the case. I have turned down a small number of these when it was obvious that one spouse had serious doubts.

> *I performed one case when the wife had already had a hysterectomy and couldn't have more children. The man persuaded me that he didn't want his multiple girlfriends to get pregnant. That was in pre-AIDS years. I'm not sure how I would react now. I hope he might feel that he didn't now need the vas because he was already using condoms. It's probably too much to hope that he would come to his senses and seek psychological help.*

> *I've had a number of patients whose "friends" have scared them to death before the day arrived, in spite of my reassuring pre-vas conference. One closed his eyes and gripped the sides of the operating table with white knuckles throughout the procedure. When I was through 30 minutes or so later, he asked, "When are you going to start?" When I told him it was over, his response was, "I'll kill them!" The poor man was literally petrified by his co-workers' stories.*

Vasectomy Pre-Op Care

Take a bath and then shave or clip very closely all the hair on the sack from the top of the penis down to the lower third of the sack. This should be done within thirty minutes before you are due in the doctor's office, because shaving more than thirty minutes before surgery has been shown to increase the risk of infection. It's OK to eat your regular meals as usual, but probably best not to eat for at least an hour before coming to the office.

Vasectomy Post-Op Care

Every doctor will have different instructions. These have worked very well for me. First and foremost, keep the wound dry until the stitches are removed, or for at least five days. This means <u>no bathing in the tub or shower</u>. My feeling is that bacteria have to swim to get into a wound, and if you keep it dry the bacteria can't get in. I don't recommend the use of antibiotic ointment because a) it does <u>not</u> prevent infection, b) it causes maceration of the wound by keeping it moist and unable to get oxygen, and c) it slows down healing.

A couple of spots of blood on the bandage are normal. If the bandage becomes soaked with blood, then a stitch has probably come loose and you must call your doctor so that he can go back and stop the bleeder. That happens rarely, I'm happy to say. To help prevent post-op bleeding, plan on going home and lying down for the rest of the day until the blood in the tied-off vessels has a chance to clot. Take it easy as to physical activity for the next couple of days. There won't usually be much discomfort, so you really have to watch yourself not to overdo it. Try to schedule your surgery for a time when you will have the next day off. I've had guys get up off the table and go right back to work, but they were pretty tough customers, right up there with cowboys and farmers.

> *One couple decided after the husband's vas to try one more time for another child (or just ignored what I said). The wife did, indeed, get pregnant. So, no unprotected sex until you get a negative sperm count. Some doctors have yet another sperm count done in three or six months. I haven't done this, and I don't know what percentage show up with sperm later after a negative one. I've never had anyone get pregnant after a negative test.*

A study that I read about the results of vasectomies in a big medical center on the west coast indicated that they had had a failure rate of 5 out of 1,600 cases. Two of the five were due to the inexperience of the young doctors in training doing the cases. They got the wrong tubes! The possible causes of the other three failures were not found. Therefore, after the wound is all healed, I recommend that the couple not make love for three more weeks to give the tissues a chance to heal and some scar tissue to develop between the cut ends. That may help to make it more difficult for the sperm to find a channel from the end of one tube to the end of the other after the sutures eventually dissolve. Then four weeks from the surgery, start making love as often as possible for the next two weeks, <u>still using contraception</u>. That will usually flush out the remaining sperm from the seminal vesicles (remember? -- the storage tanks). At six weeks from the surgery, get a lab slip and a specimen container from your doctor, and go have a sperm count. This may be in the doctor's office or a lab. Someone has to look at the fluid under a microscope and see whether there are any sperm left. If there are, then continue to use contraception for another month and get another test. I've had only one man who still had sperm at the end of the second try. He was a traveling salesman who wasn't home very often but was true to his wife, bless his heart!

** Remember, you still have millions of sperm stored in your seminal vesicles (storage tanks) at the time of your surgery. After the vas no new sperm can get there, but the only way those stored sperm can get out is by repeated ejaculations. That is why you must continue to use contraception until the microscope says there are no more sperm.

Be aware, men, that having a vasectomy is one of the best possible presents you can give your wife if the two of you have decided that you don't ever want more children. The procedure is much easier for you than a tubal ligation for your wife, also cheaper, if your health insurance doesn't cover sterilization. Your wife had your babies. While the risk is low for tubal ligations, it is still significantly higher than vasectomies. I attended a vas conference three or four years ago where the speaker estimated that those in the room had personally performed or had had performed in clinics under their supervision about one million cases. Then he asked if anyone knew of a single death. Not one! So the vas is a <u>very</u> safe method.

Tubal Ligation

As done today in the hospital or outpatient operating suite under general anesthetic (you are asleep) through a laparoscope at least two tubes are inserted into the lower abdomen, one into the umbilical depression (belly button), and the other elsewhere. The abdomen is inflated, usually with carbon dioxide, and the operating table tipped so that the bowel falls toward the head so that the pelvic organs can be easily seen.

There is the uterus in the middle, with one fallopian tube coming off of each side to curve the short distance over to the ovary, the organs from which each egg (ovum) comes, and which produce the female hormones. As you may know the open end of each tube has little hair-like cilia that wave to produce a slight current that entices the egg to come to its opening and travel down its length to the uterine cavity. This current is strong enough to bring the egg from the opposite ovary to it.

The metal operating tube is used to grasp the fallopian tube on first one side and then the other, while the light and magnifying lens is on the other instrument. The cautery wire is passed through the fallopian tube, both cutting it and sealing the ends so that an egg can't pass anymore. The procedure is repeated on the other side and the wounds are closed with a stitch or two. The lady almost always

> *I had a young patient with endometriosis who first had a ruptured tubal pregnancy on the left side and thus lost that tube. A year later she had a large chocolate cyst containing old blood that pretty well destroyed the right ovary, which had to be removed. The good news was that she had no other signs of the endometriosis. She then had a normal left ovary and an unharmed right fallopian tube. Within six months she was pregnant and I delivered a beautiful healthy baby for her. She later had another child.*

goes home the same day. After effects are few, some nausea, perhaps, and some shoulder pain from irritation of the diaphragm possibly. She is up and around the same day, but hopefully her husband won't expect her to do dishes for a day or two! The risks are low, but there are some that the surgeon should go over. Bleeding that requires making a large incision to control is one. Infection is always a risk in a surgical operation. Inadvertent cautery of something other than the fallopian tubes is another. Adverse reaction to the general anesthesia yet another. Death from complications is extremely rare.

The Pill

This is very effective and is the most commonly used contraceptive method at the present time. There are many different brands and formulas. All are designed to prevent you from ovulating (producing an egg) that month. Some have undesirable side effects, nausea one of the most frequent. If you can't tolerate the one first chosen for you, call your doctor before the end of the cycle in the pill pack and get a prescription for a different type. It may take as much as two or three trials before you get it right, but almost certainly there is one out there that will work well for you.

Basically you take your first pill when your doctor tells you to start, then one daily until you want to again become fertile, perhaps months or years later. In order to be sure you don't have a period on weekends, plan the initial dose so that your last pill always comes on a Saturday. In the combination packs there are usually two colors of pills. There may also be three colors. You can just ignore the colors and take the pills in their proper order. Normally the last seven pills are inactive.

Do not miss any pills. If you do, you cannot count on not ovulating that month and must use another form of contraception for the rest of the month, and/or the morning-after pill.

Be sure you are not pregnant when you start the pill. This can best be done by starting your pack on the 3rd to 7th day after your period starts. (Day no.1 is the first day you see any blood. Count from there.)

You will become much less likely to become pregnant by the fifth pill of your first pack, but you can't absolutely *count* on ovulation stopping until you have gone through a complete menstrual cycle and had your period.

You may experience some breakthrough bleeding in mid-month the first two or three cycles. This is nothing to worry about, and it does not mean that you are not protected that month. Some girls find it continuing longer or excessively, and they need to be changed to another pill at the beginning of the next cycle.

You can safely regulate your cycles to prevent having your period while on vacation, during a sports tournament or game, while your husband (or you) is home on leave, or any other inconvenient time. Check with your doctor, but usually extending your cycle involves just borrowing enough of the active pills (the first 1/4 of the cycle usually has these, no matter what the brand) to extend it the number of days you want to. Then just add them to the first 1/4 of the pills in your current pack, and finish your cycle when you get to where you want to be. You can't use the pack you borrowed them from for a regular cycle though. You will need a new pack with the full number. (Or just skip the last seven pills and start a new pack if you are taking pills that are all the same except the last seven, and go as far as you want to in the new pack before taking the last seven inactive pills.)

There is a movement toward totally eliminating your periods for many months at a time. In October 2003 the FDA approved Seasonale, a 91-day oral pill designed to reduce your periods to just four per year. According to the reports I have seen so far, they are effective, but there is a lot more breakthrough bleeding with them. The most reliable method, probably, is to follow the same program as in the last paragraph, but do it for months at a time, never stopping the active pills and just throwing away the seven sugar pills in each pack. There is probably nothing at all wrong with this as long as the pills you are using contain estrogen (which is necessary to prevent osteoporosis) and contain the same amount of hormone in all of the first 21 pills. The progesterone-dominant pills won't give this protection, while such multi-phasic pills as Ortho Tri-cyclen (which has 3 hormone levels) won't stop the bleeding. This approach costs about $180 more per year because you have to buy 18 packs of the pills per year instead of 13.

It is probably a good idea to go off the pill for two or three months about every five years just to let your normal hormone cycle click in for a little while. Be sure to use other contraception during that time. There is nothing magic about five years. You can probably go considerably longer without any problems developing.

Don't use them after age 35 if you are a smoker. Bad complications can ensue. There is some evidence that some formulations may provide some protection against either breast cancer or ovarian cancer, but there is still a lot of discussion about these areas. There are many different formulas involving various estrogen and progesterone formulas and combinations. Almost everybody now can find one that will agree with her.

Women at high risk for blood clots must avoid all formulas that contain estrogen. In addition, take a baby aspirin every day.

Injections of Depo Provera (every three months)

This long-acting method has many advantages that are obvious. And you don't have to be exact on the 90 days either. If you forget or are out of town, as much as ten days late usually won't hurt. You may have irregular bleeding for up to one year.

Implants (Norplant and a new one soon)

These are little hollow plastic tubes about the size of a large pencil lead, which are inserted under local anesthesia under the skin of the upper arm. Usually there is one stitch. The tubes contain a chemical that prevents ovulation for 5 years or more. Then they need to be replaced. Unfortunately they also have side effects in many people. To find out whether you may have a side effect with them, ask your doctor to give you five 10-mg. size tablets of Provera to take from the 21st to 25th days of your menstrual cycle. If you don't know you are taking them, then you may be an ideal candidate for the Norplant. If, however, you have *any* symptoms, then don't even consider the Norplant. Choose a doctor who does some surgery for the insertion and removal. It is a very easy procedure for someone versed in surgery.

IUDs

These are the real sleeper in the contraception list as far as cost effectiveness and ease of use is concerned.

Advantages are that they don't have to be inserted when you want to make love, cost the least of all methods of contraception when spread over the effective life of the device, and fertility returns rapidly when the device is removed.

Complicating side effects include involuntary expulsion of the device in up to 5% of cases in the first year, increased severity of menstrual cramps for at least the first two or three months, increased blood flow during menstruation, and spotting of blood sometimes between periods.

Problems that require removal are severe menstrual cramps that don't improve after the first couple of periods, severe menstrual bleeding, and uterine infection. They should not be removed if pregnancy occurs unless you want the pregnancy to be terminated. I have delivered two normal babies after uneventful pregnancies where I found an IUD imbedded in the placentas. These situations are quite rare however.

Originally the IUDs were made of a somewhat flexible material in various forms, which worked mainly by causing enough irritation in the uterus to prevent a fertilized egg from successfully implanting itself in the womb. These were the type I found in the placentas. Then compounds, such as copper and various hormones began to be added to the devices to make them more reliable at preventing pregnancy. Today the Paragard and Progestasert devices are effective for up to ten years after insertion. The new Mirena IUD releases a hormone and reduces menstrual bleeding by almost 90%. It completely stops the period in 1 out of 5 women who use it.

The IUD consistently ranks highest among contraceptive methods in patient satisfaction surveys.

Note: IUDs will not prevent any venereal disease. Condoms must still be worn for disease prevention. There is some evidence that IUDs may actually prevent ectopic pregnancies.

IUDs got a bad reputation during the late 1970s when the Dalkon Shield lawsuits were being filed virtually every day. They were a radical design, which was removed from the market soon after the first lawsuit. Then doctors, patients, and the IUD makers over-reacted to the point that we seldom used them, and those we did insert into a patient were made in Canada and imported. Inaccuracies, omissions, outdated information, and outright falsehoods were commonplace in nine widely used OB-GYN textbooks and manuals during the 1990s between 1992 and 1998, according to a recent literature review by an expert in the field.

As a result of this mostly misinformation many physicians, including some OB-GYN medical faculty have never put in an IUD -- 41% of the faculty members and 65% of the residents in training at one medical school surveyed.

So if you decide on an IUD, ask your doctor whether she has put any in before and if she has had any complications. The procedure is pretty simple and straightforward and easy to learn. I have done dozens with no complications. The risk of uterine perforation is only one in a thousand, but some physicians are less skilled at the insertion than others.

The latest one is **Mirena**, and it is the only one currently that may be appropriate for use in older teens who are at low risk for sexually transmitted diseases (STDs).

Barrier Methods

Be aware that no barrier method except a condom will give you <u>any</u> protection against sexually transmitted diseases.

Condoms

These may be rubber-based (that's where the term "rubbers" comes from) or synthetic. Some are thin, some have reservoirs at the tip, some are lubricated. And so on. The latex ones afford the best protection against AIDS. While being pretty inexpensive in supermarkets, especially, and drugstores, they aren't quite as cheap as they used to be, perhaps because of lawsuits if they break. And break they do, especially if they are not properly put on, or if the two of you do not have enough lubrication. One caution, lubricating with Vaseline may weaken the rubber material chemically. So if you need lubrication, use K-Y Jelly. Better yet, get the lubricated ones to start with. They may well be a lot cheaper at the supermarket than at a pharmacy. But use an old reliable brand, such as Trojans. <u>This is not the time to buy something made in China</u>. And they should cost less than $0.75 apiece.

Their use requires a little care. Wait until you get hard before putting it on. You may not want to stop when you get well into making love, so decide ahead of time when you will put it on. Always put it on before any serious foreplay, and especially before your penis gets anywhere near any body opening.

Girls often love to put it on for you and usually find that activity sexually stimulating to them. Be sure the rolled-up ring is on the outside. Always leave some room for expansion at the end, even if it has a reservoir tip, and squeeze the end with your thumb and finger to get the air out of the end before putting it on. Roll the condom all the way down to your hair. If the condom doesn't unroll, it is on wrong. Take it off and put on a new one. Don't <u>ever</u> try to reuse a condom.

The head of your organ will always grow a little more after insertion into the girl's vagina, so leaving extra room will help prevent breakage (which is often a disaster if one of you has a sexually transmitted disease like AIDS, or you aren't using backup contraception).

If the condom breaks and some backup contraception isn't being used, then the girl must use the emergency contraception described below to prevent pregnancy, wash with soap and water quickly, and douche with three or four quarts of vinegar water (two tablespoons of white vinegar to a quart of warm water) to try to flush out as much possible bacteria as possible. This isn't a very effective thing to do (and absolutely won't help at all in preventing pregnancy), but perhaps it's better than nothing.

After sex, pull your penis out slowly while it is still hard. Hold the ring end in place to keep from spilling your semen. Turn and move completely away before removing the condom so it can't spill even a drop on your partner. Dispose of the rubber by wrapping it in Kleenex or toilet paper and placing in the garbage, not in the toilet. Then wipe yourself off and return to bed, if you wish, for some pillow talk, which is often as much fun as the sex act itself.

Condoms must be kept in their sealed packets, in a cool, dry place, not in your wallet, although a pocket with nothing else in it is usually OK. Never use one after the expiration date because rubber deteriorates with age. Never use Vaseline or any kind of petroleum jelly for lubrication because it makes the rubber rot in minutes. K-Y and H-R jellies are only lubricants I consider safe.

If the man is using medication on his penis or the woman is using any kind of vaginal medication, they may also damage the condom.

Cervical Cap

These are fitted over the cervix up inside the vagina. I have had no personal experience with them. You will probably have to see an OB-GYN specialist for the fitting of one. They will not protect you against sexually transmitted diseases.

Spermicidal Jelly

These kill sperm. Any sperm unlucky enough to find itself in the jelly is a dead one. Spermicidal jelly will not protect you against sexually transmitted diseases.

The use of these jellies along with a diaphragm is a very effective method of contraception. Using the jelly by itself is better than nothing -- but not much. The reason is that sperm are often ejaculated directly from the opening in the penis into the opening in the cervix, which leads right up into the womb. So they just squirt through the jelly and aren't inactivated.

Diaphragm

Adding a diaphragm to the spermicidal jelly, however, keeps the sperm from being able to squirt directly into the cervical canal, and this means that the sperm must swim through the jelly on the inside of the diaphragm. They tend to not be successful in that attempt.

A diaphragm is a dome of a thin rubber surrounded by a circle of springy metal. A glob of spermicidal jelly about the size of a quarter is placed on what will be the upper surface of the dome. When properly positioned in the vagina, the front of the circle will be up under your pubic bone, and the back of the circle will be behind the cervix, which feels about like a warm wet nose when you check it with your finger. The rubber dome will completely cover the cervix. You must always check to be sure the cervix is covered, even after you have used it a hundred times or more. Otherwise you may be in too much of a hurry and wind up pregnant.

They come in several sizes and different types of spring to fit various sizes and shapes of vaginas. You have to have a doctor examine and measure you and then prescribe the proper one for you. You will use that same size until something occurs that changes the size of your vagina. Then you must be measured and fitted again. Having a baby usually leaves some permanent increase in vaginal size, thus have a new fitting at your six-week checkup after your baby is born.

Anyone can wear a diaphragm before a pregnancy, but sometimes the vaginal support tissues weaken too much with delivery of the baby for a diaphragm to fit adequately afterwards. Your doctor will be able to tell you at your six-week checkup.

Your doctor or assistant will teach you how to use it. You will have a chance to try to insert it properly in the examining room under supervision. Then you will take it home, practice with it without using it for real, and wear it back into the doctor's office to be sure you are doing it right. Only then is it safe to abandon other methods of contraception.

Let me suggest an easy way to properly insert your diaphragm. It can be put into its place while you are sitting, lying down, or standing with one foot up on a step. Before you try to put it in the first time, reach into your vagina with your middle or index finger and feel what your cervix feels like, where it is located, and which way it is pointing. Remember, it feels a lot like your nose, only warm and wet.

Be aware that the rubber is slippery with the jelly on it. Squeeze the spring together in the middle, using both hands if necessary, then insert it into the opening. As it passes into the vagina, try to direct it toward your tailbone.

Carefully push it the rest of the way in as far as it will go. Right now is the time to put your finger way up into the top of the vagina and feel your cervix. Is it covered by the thin rubber membrane? If so, then push the front of the spring up under your pubic bone, and you are ready for love. If the cervix isn't covered, take it out and try again. You may have to add some more jelly.

While we are on that subject, let me suggest that you put your diaphragm in before you become sexually excited. That may mean that sometimes you have the diaphragm in unnecessarily (either your seductive capabilities were slipping, or you changed your mind). But needing it when it is home in the drawer is not a good plan.

A diaphragm will <u>not</u> protect you against sexually transmitted diseases.

Rhythm Method

The safest time is during your period. This is not acceptable for some couples, but there is no medical reason to not make love during your period. Those who have menstrual cramps may find that they worsen somewhat the first day or two but are OK a little later. If the two of you are comfortable with a little mess, you can have great sex during menstruation. Soaking any soiled cloth overnight in cold water, and maybe some BIZ will remove blood pretty well.

A study in which the hormone cycles of 221 women were tested daily by the hormones excreted in the urine to see exactly when they ovulated was published in May 2001. The study attempted to aid in the timing of "the fertile window" of women to make the Rhythm Method more accurate for contraception, as well as to aid couples who were having trouble getting pregnant.

That study found that current Rhythm Method guidelines were reliable for only about 30% of healthy women. On each day between days 6 to 21 (day 1 is the first day of your period) there is at least a 10% probability of being in the fertile window, and late ovulation cannot be predicted. The conclusion was what we all already know, that timing intercourse to achieve or avoid pregnancy cannot be done with precision. That's why this little joke is no joke for a lot of Catholic couples: **[Question: Do you know what they call people who use the rhythm method for contraception? Answer: Parents!]**

New Contraceptive Methods

These are new in 2003.

The Today Sponge

This was offered in the U. S. and discontinued. It is about to be started in Canada and will probably be available over the Internet. It contains a chemical that inactivates sperm, is inserted like a tampon, and is available without a prescription. Its effectiveness is about the same as diaphragm or condom, but does not protect against sexually transmitted diseases. It is an option for women who are not in a long-term relationship or don't want to take hormones, or as backup protection when using condoms.

The Weekly Patch

This is called Ortho-Evra. You stick it on a smooth area of your skin, and it releases hormones through your skin that prevent ovulation for a week. It is resistant to getting wet, even swimming, but is visible when you are in your bikini. It was 99% effective in the trials but we won't know how it really works for probably a year or more. One thing for sure, it is cheaper than a lot of other options. Three patches will cost about $30.

The Vaginal Ring

This is called NuvaRing. It is flexible, relatively small, and much easier to insert than a diaphragm. Also it doesn't require a pelvic exam for fitting, although a pelvic exam is really important at least once a year, especially if you are young and sexually active. It is particularly good for teenage girls who don't want to take the pill or the shots. If you are comfortable using tampons, then you will have no problem using NuvaRing. There is no wrong way to put it into your vagina, and it can't get lost or get pushed too far up into the vagina.

You insert it while in a squatting, standing with one foot up on a step, or lying down with legs-apart position. Very explicit directions with good picture diagrams come in the box with the ring. It does not safely protect against pregnancy until it has been in for 7 days the first time. If it comes out (as when you remove a tampon or in moving the bowels, especially if constipated), it may be washed off with cool water and reinserted within 3 hours. If it has been out for more than 3 hours, you must use some additional form of birth control until the same or a new ring has been in place for at least 7 days again.

Insert it the first time any day from day 1 (the first day of your period) to day 5. You must insert it by day 5 even if you have not yet stopped bleeding. If possible, time it so that you put it in on a Saturday or Sunday, because you will then remove it 3 weeks later and begin your period three days after removal, after your weekend social activities are over. (If you forget to remove it on time, no problem. It is good for another 5-7 days of protection. But you are not protected if you go past 4 weeks.) Then 7 days later put in a new one. You should mark your calendar when you put it in and take it out so that you will be sure to stay on schedule.

There are some possible side effects, as with all hormonal products: vaginal discharge or even infections, headache, weight gain if you don't watch your eating, nausea, and irregular bleeding for the first two or three cycles. Other less common ones are listed in the package.

You can get one sample ring, good for a month's protection, by calling 1-877-NUVARING, or at the company's website, www.nuvaring.com.

The Monthly Shot

This is called Lunelle. It is as effective as the Pills, and you have to think about it only once a month. It is injected into your arm. BUT it requires a visit to a doctor or nurse once a month, which may be a pain for those not in a healthcare field (or who don't have a nurse handy at work). It also costs somewhat more than the Pills because there is a professional's fee in addition to the cost of medication, about $45 to $50. As I write this it is not available due to some kind of manufacturing problem, but may again be available by the time you read this.

Emergency Contraception: The Morning After Pill

<u>Always</u> use this as backup protection for all other contraceptive methods to avoid pregnancy after accidental exposure to sperm (as in a rubber or condom breaking, or in a rape. By the way, the most common reason for a condom breaking is inadequate lubrication. Best to use a lubricated condom and perhaps some K-Y jelly).

1. "**PLAN B**": Take the first dose as soon as possible and the second 12 hours later. You may become nauseated with this. A few people vomit. So it is a good idea to swallow one of the following over-the-counter medicines 1 to 1 1/2 hours before taking the pill: Meclizine, 25 mg. Dramamine II, or Bonine, 2 tablets.

Also it is a good idea to have a little food in your stomach when you take it, a piece of bread and some milk, for example. If you vomit within one to two hours after the dose in spite of the anti-vomiting pills, then you need another dose of the emergency pill. Call your doctor for a medicated suppository called Tigan, 200 mg, which you put into your rectum about 1 to 1 1/2 hours before you take the pill again. And get another 2 pills when you get the suppository at the drugstore. Headache can occur. Just take some Tylenol for it.

Plan B may soon be available over the counter without a prescription.

2. "**PREVEN**" Take the first dose as soon as possible and the second 12 hours later. Nausea and vomiting are much more common with this one, so just get some anti-vomiting medicine when you get the Emergency Pill, and take the anti-vomiting medicine 1 to 1 1/2 hours before the Emergency Pill.

If you are sexually active, ask your doctor to prescribe the Emergency Pill for you when he or she helps you with some regular contraceptive method. It is a good idea to have these on hand in case a rubber breaks, for example, or if you missed one or more of your regular birth control pills during the cycle.

The Emergency Pill is <u>not</u> a substitute for other, more reliable contraception methods. There is a movement afoot to have them sold over-the-counter. I hope it happens. BUT there is considerable concern that it will be used instead of other methods.

The Emergency Pill is 99.5% effective if the first one is taken within the first 12 hours after making love. It <u>may</u> still be up to 96% effective if the first pill is taken within 72 hours, and still has <u>some</u> protective effect even up to 4 days afterward. But we all agree that taking the first pill within the first 12 hours prevents probably ten times as many pregnancies as taking the first one in the last 12 of the 72-hour window.

Doctors are liable from a medical-legal standpoint if they don't order the Emergency Pill for a woman in need. So you should be able to obtain them if you don't already have them.

Emergency Contraception Hotline: 1-888-NOT-2-LATE (1-888-668-2528) or www.not-2-late.com

CHAPTER 27 -- COPD or EMPHYSEMA

Chronic Obstructive Pulmonary Disease, also known as **Emphysema** has become the fourth leading cause of death in the United States. About 20% of our adult population currently has this condition. By some estimates, it is involved in 14 *million* doctor visits every year. **You will save tens of thousands of dollars in medical bills by quitting smoking before it's too late for your lungs to heal, not to mention the enormous difference it will make in your quality of life.**

It is an almost totally preventable condition, with more than 90% of cases caused by smoking yourself or by inhaling someone else's smoke (second hand smoke) over a period of years, at home or at work. Asthmatics who smoke are absolutely guaranteed to develop COPD, and usually at a much younger age than other smokers. This is true even if the asthma cleared up before the teenage years. The next time the wheezing comes back it will be the harbinger of COPD.

The second hand smoke aspect has become a major source of friction between smokers and non-smokers. It has also become a major cause of workplace litigation since it was accepted as a workplace health hazard by the Environmental Protection Agency (EPA) in the early 1990s. That finding by the EPA led to legislation banning smoking in airline flights. It also played a part in the ongoing banning of smoking in the workplace, first in California, then in New York City, then elsewhere, to the point where smoking is now banned in areas affecting more than half the population of the U. S.

There is a story going around legal circles (my stepson is an attorney) about one recent lawsuit involving injury from an employee's long-time exposure to second hand smoke in a Las Vegas casino, which was settled out of court for $5,000,000 in favor of the employee. The non-smoking wife of an acquaintance of mine, who smoked more than three packs a day, died of COPD a few months after her husband finally quit smoking.

But second hand smoke is the cause of only 10-15% of the many problems caused by tobacco. 90% of all the really bad stuff is from what you do to yourself. See the chapter on **Tobacco** for the rest of the story.

What actually is going on in the body of one who has COPD?

COPD is the end stage of damage to the lungs that began with the first cigar or cigarette and has progressed, usually for at least twenty years, with destruction of lung tissue and loss of the tiny air sacs, increase in dead space in the lungs, where there is little or no air exchange, thus allowing carbon dioxide accumulation higher and higher there and in the bloodstream. Those dead spaces also allow sticky secretions to just lie there and fester, providing a great place for all kinds of nasty bacteria to grow.

One recent legal case I was called to review had a patient whose lung culture grew three of the most deadly and resistant germs that we ever see in the lungs. Any one could have killed her. The family wanted the doctor to pay them damages because he didn't save her to die a month or a year later when she got infected again. I had to testify that she had essentially committed suicide by deciding to continue smoking when her doctor had first told her to stop 12 or 15 years before.

Don't blame the doctor if he can't bail you out after years of ignoring his advice to stop smoking!

The other main problem is progressively worsening obstruction of the bronchial tubes, caused by years of inflammation and swelling of the membranes of the bronchial tubes. The little hair-like cilia that work to cleanse become paralyzed, and the thin mucus that constantly washes the surfaces of the membranes becomes thick and won't flow readily, so that the lungs lose more and more of their ability to get rid of air pollutants and germs. You develop a morning cough and have trouble coughing out the thick phlegm that has accumulated overnight. Then you begin to cough all day.

Shortness of breath becomes a daily part of life. You may have to start carrying around a small tank of oxygen. Your lungs don't transfer oxygen to the blood and remove the carbon dioxide properly. You develop pulmonary hypertension, which leads to right-sided heart failure (see the chapter on **Heart Failure**). Your red blood count builds up to very high levels, producing what we call "polycythemia." This very thick blood often leads to blood clots in the deep veins and some less severe conditions. I can often look at someone's red blood count and tell that they are smokers whose lungs are going bad even before ordering lung function tests.

When infections flare up there is more and thicker phlegm production, and it may become more yellow or yellow-green. Not pretty stuff. And shortness of breath gets worse. You may not have a fever to speak of.

Other things that may make the symptoms worse are cold air, exposure to something you are allergic to, exposure to air pollution (as in the ozone alerts so often seen in larger cities), and inhaling your own or someone else's tobacco smoke.

A COPD flare-up is much like an asthma attack. The problem here, however, is that in asthmatics, once the proper medications are administered and the spasm of the airways is controlled, the lung function returns to normal. In COPD the lung function never returns to normal. The airway spasm may improve, but your condition is permanent and can never, ever return to normal.

The good news, however, is that as soon as you eliminate all exposure to tobacco smoke, the situation quits getting worse so fast. The lungs will actually heal themselves to some degree for up to a couple of years, and the annual decline in lung function will slow down a lot.

How can you help yourself to a better quality of life?

First, and foremost, stop all exposure to tobacco smoke. (See the chapter on **Tobacco** and stopping smoking.) Second avoid all kinds of pollution. Stay indoors on ozone alert days. Live somewhere where there is no smog. But don't even think about moving or even visiting anyplace above about 3,000 feet altitude. At least not without a continuous oxygen supply. Because, if you have shortness of breath at your present altitude, there isn't enough oxygen as you go higher, and you can soon get to a critical level and die. Early in my medical career in Flagstaff (at 7,000 ft. altitude) I frequently was called out to pronounce someone dead in a motel who had had COPD. They didn't last even one night.

If you currently live at high altitude, and you are doing everything else right and not having much shortness of breath, then you may be able to continue there for a while. Eventually, though, you will find that moving to sea level will give you a lot more energy and exercise capability with your breathing.

Exercise daily as much as you can tolerate. You don't have to walk fast, just walk as long and as far as you can. If you get too tired, stop and sit down, on the curb, if necessary. Don't suddenly start, however. Start with perhaps one block and increase it by two or three steps every day, till one day you may even get up to a mile.

If you are overweight, then it is very important to take as much strain off the heart and lungs as possible by losing down to what your doctor and you feel is normal for you. If you are underweight, then consider adding a diet supplement, such as Ensure, or Ultra Slimfast, or even Ovaltine or an eggnog (non-alcoholic, of course) to what you are eating now.

You may need to do some daily breathing exercises, as well as postural drainage with someone gently pounding on your back to loosen the secretions in the lungs and help you to cough them up so you can breathe better. You will need a respiratory therapist to help train you in "pulmonary rehabilitation."

In postural drainage you lie over the edge of your bed so that your trunk is bent at the waist and your head and chest hang down at as much of an angle as you can tolerate for about ten minutes at least twice a day. If you take nebulizer treatments, or use a bronchodilator inhaler, then the time for postural drainage is right after you do one of those.

Turn your chest from side to side while you gently cough and try to loosen up the mucous plugs from deep in your lungs. This is where having someone pound on (gently) your back with a cupped hand is very helpful. When you feel something loosening up, then cough more forcefully to bring up as much as possible. Some folks have so much phlegm that they need to have a small pan for it on the floor. If a respiratory therapist is assisting you in the hospital, you will feel as though you've had a pretty good workout by the end of the ten minutes.

Getting rid of the mucous plugs morning and night gives a lot more breathing space. It also removes material for germs to grow in and slows down the downward trend of the disease.

Prevention of infections is extremely important. They tend to be more common in the colder months of the year. For this reason you absolutely must get a flu shot every September or early October. In addition you must get a pneumonia shot about every 5 years.

We give kids shots to prevent Hemophilus influenzae, a bacteria which is not related to the viral influenza that spreads around the world every year, some years worse than others. The Hemophilus (otherwise often called "H. flu") also affects adults, especially those with weakened lungs. So I'm not quite sure why we aren't using the vaccine for at-risk adults too. Currently the only place an adult can get such a shot is from a family doctor or a pediatrician. Watch for it in health news, and if it becomes generally available for adults, get it.

Avoiding exposure is very important for prevention. So stay out of crowds. Don't travel on long flights, where the air breathed by all on board a plane is re-circulated many times. Church is probably OK because it usually lasts only an hour or so. A movie may be all right if the crowd isn't large and the film doesn't last more than two hours. Other forms of entertainment may require you to use your own judgement.

Be aware, though, that even shopping for groceries can be a source of exposure. For shopping, try to go in the morning on a weekday, when there aren't many people there.

No one should go out among people when they are ill, but many do. So if you are seated near someone who is coughing or sneezing, get up and move right away if you possibly can.

If you are invited to someone's house, and you walk in and find someone who may be ill (usually a moist cough is a dead giveaway), make your excuses to the hostess and just leave. Same thing if someone is smoking.

Avoid little kids, even family, unless you have a surgical mask on. Especially avoid those who go to daycare centers because they are exposed to everything and literally bring everything home.

Take your vitamin C, at least 500 mg daily, and at least 1,000 mg daily when you feel something coming on.

How can you tell when you are headed for trouble? I highly recommend that you get a Peak Flow Meter just like those with asthma. Test yourself with it at least twice a day.

When it begins to deteriorate, then you need more oxygen, more bronchodilator inhaler, more inhaled corticosteroid, and whatever else your doctor has ordered for you.

If your phlegm changes in the amount you are coughing up, or the color, or the consistency or thickness, this usually means an infection is starting. We physicians like to wait a day or two or longer before prescribing antibiotics for normal people, but those with COPD need to start them right away, or at least get a sputum (phlegm) culture started while watching you, probably on a daily basis. Since mixed infections are common in those with chronic lung disease, you will often be given a combination of two or more antibiotics.

CHAPTER 28 -- DANGER SIGNALS

Significant change in bowel habit needs a GI work-up, especially if you have black tarry stools. Bright red blood in the stools is usually less likely to be immediately serious than black sticky stools that can be identified as blood only with a simple chemical test. The black tarry blood usually comes from up high in the GI tract, for example, the lower esophagus, or the stomach, or the duodenum, where ulcers bleed, and the blood has been partially digested before reaching the rectum. Bright red blood, however, usually comes from the left side of the colon, or the rectum, or the anus where bleeding hemorrhoids and fissures are common.

A small child who is coughing, short of breath, inconsolable, and unable to sleep must be <u>seen</u> by a doctor right away. It may have epiglottitis, where the windpipe swells shut. Don't settle for a phone call to a tired doctor in the middle of the night. Do call your doctor. But insist that he see your child if he tries to recommend a vaporizer, etc. (which <u>is</u> a good idea, by the way, and every household with young children should have one. I prefer a cool mist one if the child has a fever and a hot steam one if there is no fever.)

If, however, your child has a croupy cough but is able to go to sleep normally (or almost so), then the condition is much less likely to be really serious. But talk to your doctor anyway if you have the slightest doubt.

When you are taking a habit-forming drug, or mood-altering medicine, or <u>any</u> medicine, watch for signs that you are becoming dependent on that medication. The two main signs of dependence are: 1) the feeling that you "cannot live without it", and 2) you find that you need more and more of this medication to get the same relief.

A pressure pain in the chest that feels "like a gorilla sitting on you" anytime after about age 25 could be a heart attack. Especially if there is also the same type of pain going up into the neck and/or down the inside of one or both arms. Chest pain plus a cold sweat is especially ominous. Feeling faint in addition adds to the risk. **This set of symptoms requires immediate medical evaluation. Call 911.**

Anxiety sometimes produces a feeling that you can't get enough breath into you, and chest tightness may result from overbreathing (we call it hyperventilation). You may even pass out. But you won't have the pain into the arms and neck, nor the cold sweat in those cases. If you are older, the risk of it being a heart attack increases.

Sudden loss of use of one side of the body, inability to speak, loss of vision in one eye or one side of your visual fields may mean you are having a stroke. Strokes can be short-circuited if you get to the ER within an hour: so call 911.

CHAPTER 29 -- DEALING WITH HMOs

My advice is: if you have any other option, don't allow your company to put you in an HMO. Quite frankly, the reason that I have the time to write this book is because dealing with the five HMOs that I felt I had to belong to in order to keep my patients and continue to make a decent living made my quality of life deteriorate so much that I quit private practice much earlier than I had always planned.

I now work for someone else, get a paycheck every month, have no night calls, no hospital work, and most of all, no hassle with insurance companies. But I really miss my old patients!

You have all heard horror stories about denial of services and benefits, not paying for prescription drugs if they are not on the formulary (and no drug is <u>ever</u> on the formulary of any HMO until two years after the rest of the world is using it), taking forever to allow certain lab or x-ray tests. All those stories are true, and more.

When you are having a problem with an HMO, there are two avenues of help available short of taking them to court (which you can't do till the Patient's Bill Of Rights that hasn't been passed by Congress as of this moment) or calling an investigative reporter: 1) see if your doctor will intercede on your behalf (we do it all the time -- <u>hours</u> every day. See the next paragraph.) And 2) complain with the facts to your employer, who has, in effect, hired the HMO to care for you, his employee.

A recent poll indicated that 53 percent of all physicians over age 55 plan to quit practice within two years. The primary reason they gave for quitting so early was the HMO hassle factor. You are giving away much of your freedom of choice in the medical care of yourself and your family when you are under the care of an HMO, especially if your doctor, PCP, gate keeper, or whatever, is capitated.

For example, in order for you to have the HMO pay for a drug that isn't on the formulary, your physician has to make a request in writing to the formulary committee and/or speak directly to the company pharmacist. Of course the company pharmacist never answers the phone and doesn't return your doctor's calls for hours. These obstructions are deliberately designed to inhibit the busy doctor from seeking approval for newer, and often better, drugs.

For example E-mycin is an antibiotic that is relatively cheap, but still a few cents more expensive than its close generic cousin, erythrocin. E-mycin is never on any formulary, while erythrocin is on all of them. They both contain the same amount of antibiotic, but this antibiotic upsets a lot of people's stomachs. E-mycin has a special coating which greatly reduces or prevents the stomach upset. But no one from the HMO is interested in protecting your stomach. All they are interested in is their bottom line.

Another example: the drugs Claritin, Zyrtec and Allegra. They are excellent antihistamines which are used for hay fever and certain other allergies. While they are somewhat better than all previous antihistamines as far as allergy control is concerned, they are far superior in not making you sleepy. So you can safely drive and work around machinery without a stuffy nose while taking them. How long do you suppose it took to get these drugs on the formularies of the HMOs I was contracted with? At least three years! To respond to this foot dragging by HMOs, drug companies began direct consumer advertising about two years ago. They hoped that you, the consumer, would complain to your companies who provide your health insurance, to the HMOs, and to your physicians about this problem. It has succeeded to some degree, but not to the extent hoped for.

When your company offers a choice in health insurance plans, always take the **indemnity plan** if you possibly can. If you take the HMO, you will receive the same kind of discount care that Medicaid provides, in all respects. They will tell you that all "approved" tests, drugs, consultations, surgical procedures, etc., are covered. But there is a huge amount of stuff that isn't covered without a battle. My medical assistant and nurse spent many hours each week fighting that battle for our patients. After awhile many of us begin to take the line of least resistance, or quit the HMO rat race as I did.

> *My medical assistant who had to deal with the HMOs spent so much time on the phone that she looked as though she had a tumor in the shape of a telephone attached to her ear all day long. Doctors were supposed to have a private line, but very rarely did she complete a call without at least a 15-minute wait on hold. It was so bad she was able to spend only about ten percent of her time on patient care and the rest on HMO telephoning and paperwork.*

> *One of my colleagues told me last month that he had just had to borrow $60,000 to pay salaries and other unpaid debts of his practice. They were unpaid because the HMOs he had contracted with had cut his reimbursements while at the same time waiting a very long time to pay him for his work on their behalf. He is canceling all of his HMO contracts as soon as the contracts allow and switching to a cash basis. I'll be interested in seeing how it works for him and whether others in his situation join him.*

The federal government won't allow physicians to band together in a city or town to negotiate collectively with these giant multi-billion dollar companies. A group of dentists in Tucson, Arizona, tried it and were taken to court by the Feds, which resulted in large fines and the HMO then being able to impose its will on each dentist individually. Imagine how much negotiating power a single physician or dentist has in a situation like that. "Here's our deal. Take it or leave it!"

The HMOs call us the "product" they are selling. To our face at our hospital during a quarterly meeting of those physicians who had signed up with one of them. Let me tell you, it is a pretty poor product if the physicians are as unhappy as most of us are.

A doctor won't be as happy to care for an HMO member as for a regular patient. I wasn't. I'm sure my HMO patients were aware of my feelings at times, even though I always did my utmost to treat them like every other patient. And I particularly tried to treat my Medicaid (AHCCCS in Arizona) patients better than anyone else, because I figured that they needed all the help they could get.

Ideally most of us look upon and try to treat all of our patients as friends. In the days before HMOs I felt really complimented whenever a new patient came to see me for care. I figured that one of my patient friends had helped in the selection process, and I had better live up to that trust.

Nowadays more people come in to see the new doctor because their employer switched health plans. So they probably aren't happy about having to see their third or fourth doctor in the past two or three years. They would rather have stayed with their previous "product." They have to fill out their history forms again and remember to tell about allergies and possible genetic or hereditary problems. If they haven't been in an HMO before, then they may have a long grocery list of things that need to be done for their health. And inevitably the plan won't cover some of those items, even though someone on the HMO phone had told them that all the doctor has to do is order it. Then when that new patient has to be told by the doctor that something isn't covered, they become more unhappy, and, what for centuries has been the doctor-patient relationship that is highly valued by both sides, is off to a rocky start.

You will have to choose a doctor who has agreed to accept the reduced fees of the HMO in return for their promise of increased business. Many HMOs offer the doctors on their lists a bonus at the end of the year for staying below the HMO's budgeted expense per person. That often means that your doctor has an incentive to avoid new drugs, costly lab tests, MRIs, CT scans, etc. And fewer referrals to specialists. My own experience is that the better doctors often don't need as many tests and referrals because of their own experience and training. But, given a financial incentive to help pay off those humongous medical school loans, what would you do?! So find out (ask) if the doctors in a particular plan have such a bonus plan before you sign up.

Find out if your own doctor is in the new plan, if you want to keep him.

When Your HMO or Other Insurance Denies Coverage

A corporation of urgent care clinics in the Phoenix area is never able to pay the salaries of its employees on time because of slow pay by their contracted HMOs. The doctors never know when they can then pay their own bills, and many of them seek moonlighting jobs just to pay their most important bills, like mortgages. The president of this corporation has had to take out a second mortgage on his home to keep the clinics afloat. These clinics have a valuable place in medicine, especially so in a rapidly-growing urban environment. It would be a shame to see them go under because of the shoddy business practices of HMOs in particular, and health insurance companies in general.

First, be aware that most claim processors are in entry-level jobs with minimal and/or insufficient training.

The most important thing you can do in preparing for a dispute of any kind is to keep all your records, with notations of whom you spoke to at each level, with the dates and time of day. Also make copies of all correspondence. Send a letter to the person at the company to whom you spoke, stating your understanding of what was said. Keep a copy of that. If it involves a critical decision, send it certified mail with a return receipt requested.

Refer back to the records you have on file each time you get a new record or letter or statement. Get a copy of your policy and the policy booklet that many companies distribute to employees before they sign up for a plan. That particular document is very important because what it tells you will be held legally binding in Court even if the fine print in the policy you receive later says something else.

Search through the actual policy for the benefits it specifically offers first. Look for words and phrases, such as "medically necessary," "necessary tests," "necessary office visits," and "necessary medications," which may limit coverage somewhere down the line. Always to their benefit, of course!

Look especially under the section that describes basic facts about the plan for information about primary physicians and the use of specialists, along with other limits.

Whenever a person refuses to grant you something you are requesting, sweetly ask for her full name and write it down. Then ask to speak to her supervisor. If you get no satisfaction there, repeat the process. You may have to go through several layers of administration before you get to one who has the power to make a favorable decision. Be aware that all of the lower layers have the power to refuse you. But you inevitably will have to go higher before you find someone able to say "yes" and be able to make it stick. If you get a "yes," then that person will get one of your certified letters the next day.

The Fine Print

Throughout the policy you will find, almost hidden, various "services not covered," "conditions," and "exclusions," not all in one place. The exclusions list may be short, but the language can give them a lot of leeway for denying or reducing claims. "According to accepted standards" is a favorite one that basically means whatever they want it to. "Definitions" is another good place for concealing exclusions.

> One horror story of the patient of a colleague of mine involved the necessity of notifying the plan or getting a referral from your PCP (primary care physician) before going to the Emergency Room, so that the company won't deny your claim for not following the rules. **A man whose son had been stabbed in the liver carefully called the plan and his PCP to get permission to take the boy to the ER, all while his son bled to death!** Don't be that scared of your insurance plan's often-ridiculous rules. Even the worst plan couldn't deny such a claim. Well, probably not.

Certain conditions are required of the policyholder. Be aware of these hidden traps. All too often people discover them too late or don't fully understand them.

If your claim is denied, check with the insurance department of your state. Most states have their own rules about what insurance policies must cover if the company is allowed to operate in that state. These rules are in force no matter what the policy says.

For example, West Virginia requires coverage for cosmetic surgery if the condition was caused by violence in a family setting. Most states allow the exclusion of all cosmetic surgery coverage. Wisconsin allows coverage of grandchildren under age 18. New York and California, among ten other states, require coverage for infertility. Some states even require coverage for toupees in alopecia (total baldness) caused by cancer chemotherapy.

Some issues, as pointed out in John Grisham's excellent book, *The Rainmaker,* require an attorney or other patient advocate to get the insurance company on the straight and narrow path. Others may be resolved by a lot of persistence on your part.

Also in *The Rainmaker* an insurance company was portrayed as automatically denying all claims the first time around, and I suspect that there is more truth than fiction in that scenario. The longer insurance companies can wait to pay a claim, the longer your premium money can earn interest for the company. Also some insureds may get tired of the hassle and just give up. Both ways the company makes money with such a policy. That's why they routinely don't pay your doctor for three months, or six months -- or a year, in the case of my younger son one time.

I'm afraid that by now you may be suspecting that I'm not a friend of HMOs. You are right! To me, "HMO" is a four-letter word.

CHAPTER 30 -- DEATH AND DYING

The actual or impending death of a friend or loved family member creates severe stresses in our lives. The actual stress points, which are discussed in the chapter on **Staying Fit Mentally**, are 100, the most of any of our many life stresses. As those who read that chapter will recall, it takes only 150 stress points in a six-month period to cause emotional and/or physical impairment of some degree in many people. The more points accumulated, the more likely that you will have problems develop.

The physical breakdown includes our immune systems, our blood pressures, our endocrine systems, and several others. Virtually the entire body is at risk.

Mentally, depression is the most likely and most obvious problem, with all its many physical symptoms noted above.

Acceptance of the fact of death is tough for us. Sometimes it helps to realize that it is the person's time to go, regardless of your religious background. You may not like it, and the person may not either, but there it is. So try to help the person to make the best of it, along with other members of the family and close friends.

Family members should not fight to keep the person alive, as they often do, even long after the person has accepted his or her fate and made peace with the emotions. The family and friends should be supportive. Tell him he has fought a good fight, and it's OK to slip away. When the quality of life deteriorates to a certain point (different for each of us), most of us are not only ready, but actually often eager to move on. Many stay alive until they reach a goal, like a wedding, the birth of a child, a graduation, then say good-bye.

Prayer, for those who can use it, is very therapeutic. But be careful what you pray for.

Organ donations have a healing power of their own, when possible. The deceased one lives on in another's body. Consider giving "the gift of life."

Keep in mind that for those with children our DNA lives on. For those with no biological children, the positive effects and teachings of the deceased one on those around him will live on.

Choosing the place of the dying process can be a great comfort to the dying one, while enabling the loved ones to be closer. Medicare has a lot of stuff available for home care if the patient's physician certifies that he is terminal. For example, the person can stay in his or her own home, while using oxygen, a hospital bed, two shifts of licensed practical nurses daily, medications, a shower stool, walker, etc. paid for by Medicare.

Hospices are now in almost every town or city of any size. Use of the hospice people and/or facilities to assist the dying person in many ways is a much preferable alternative to spending the final days in the hospital if pain medications are necessary and the patient is pretty immobile.

Hospice caregivers provide wonderful support and use many spiritual or meditation techniques, along with physical therapy to help minimize the need for mind-clouding anti-pain drugs. I urge anyone facing death, especially from cancer, to go the Hospice route.

Every adult person should have a living will. Don't think that you don't need one until you are old. Bad things happen to young people every day. Right now in Florida there is a woman who has been brain dead for 13 years. She suffered the injury to her brain when she was only 37 years old. She had told her husband that she did not want to be kept alive by artificial means. But she didn't write it down. In Florida that means that her husband cannot carry out her wishes and must pay what must be over a million dollars so far to keep that poor vegetable alive. The story is that her children are hoping for a miracle and thus oppose taking her off life support.

Regardless of the merits of that case, you have the absolute right in all states to make sure that your wishes in such a case are carried out according to your desires. But the only way to be sure is to make a living will that expressly states your wishes. It must follow certain forms in various states and must be witnessed by two people who have no possible financial connection to you or your estate. Lawyers follow the state format. In some states you can get that format right off of the Internet. Do it now!

CHAPTER 31 -- DEPRESSION

This is something that happens to most of us from time to time, usually because of something sad or devastating, such as the loss of a friend, lover, family loved one, divorce, or the loss of your job, or a crash in the stock market brought on by Alan Greenspan that wipes out your life's savings.

How we react to these events and their resulting effects on our lives determines whether we need professional help in recovering. Some of us deal with disappointment better than others. These are more likely also to deal better with depression than others. Some let the obvious precipitating cause begin to take over their every waking moment. Others seek help from friends and acquaintances to work through the grief, or immediately look for constructive activities to help overcome misfortune without looking back. Most of us are somewhere in between.

About twenty million people in our country suffer from clinical depression each year, and about one out of every six people will have it sometime in their lives. About twice as many women suffer from this as men. It can affect any age and any race, rich or poor.

Recognizing depression is not easy. Many of the symptoms can fit other conditions, or just fatigue. You may have both physical and emotional symptoms. You may not be feeling like yourself. You may feel tired all the time for no apparent reason, with total lack of energy. You may have aches and pains that don't go away and don't respond to any treatment.

You may lose interest in things you once loved to do, including sex. You may not want to talk to or get together with family or friends. You may feel sad and hopeless, like you are carrying the world on your shoulders. You may want the world to stop so you can get off. You may just not feel right. You may feel helpless and unable to control your life.

Food may not taste as good as it used to, so you are not hungry. You may be losing weight. Oddly enough, you may also <u>gain</u> weight, perhaps because you mistake food for love. Your activities of everyday living may suffer. You may have trouble sleeping or may sleep all the time. You may cry a lot more than you ever have before. You may think about ending it all by committing suicide.

Each of us may experience a few or all of these symptoms at various times in our lives without being clinically depressed. But if they last for two weeks or more, then they become potentially serious.

A common working definition of depression then is a condition where you emotionally have **a constant sad mood or loss of interest or pleasure in activities which you used to enjoy, for at least two weeks, along with one or more physical symptoms, such as changes in appetite or weight (particularly loss of appetite or weight), changes in your normal sleep patterns, difficulty making decisions, difficulty concentrating, feelings of guilt, feeling that you are worthless, lack of energy or feeling tired all the time, restlessness or decreased activity that is noticeable to others, and, worst of all, repeated thoughts of death or suicide.**

Depression that has an identifiable event as the cause, if not repeatedly reinforced, loses its strength with the passage of time. The first year anniversary of the loss of a loved one, for example, usually marks the end of the severe grieving process and leaves just a dull ache behind that flares up less and less often as more time passes. If a person with this type of depression can just make it from day to day long enough, he or she will eventually snap back to normal.

Unfortunately some are so overcome by grief or guilt that they don't make it past the first shock. That is about the time when they decide whether they

> *The first two weeks can be critical, as it was with my mother in Indiana after my father died. I went home to Arizona a couple days after his funeral, and my sister had to go back to South Bend, 170 miles away, to care for her family. No friends were near either. When I called her the last time about two weeks after Dad's death, no one answered the phone. My sister called the police, who found her, with a suicide note beside her body.*
>
> *Needless to say the two of us felt considerable guilt for a long time. But ours is not an unusual story. Suicide, I know now, is very common by the initially surviving spouse in the first few weeks after the death of the loved one. Sometimes it occurs within minutes after the dead one is found.*

want to live or die. If some one is there for them, for example, in the week or month after the funeral, then they may decide to live. In the death of a family member most families come together as they haven't for years just for the funeral or memorial service. But after the funeral, hardly anyone has time to stay around for the surviving spouse unless they live in town.

> *One old patient and friend of mine was in his eighties and prided himself on the strength of his handshake each time he came to my office. His medical problems were few, and I thought he would probably live to be a hundred. Unfortunately he developed an eye problem that caused him to lose his driver's license. He thus had to rely on family and his few surviving friends who could still drive for everything he did. I instantly recognized that the will to live was gone from him. His grip strength became that of a child from one office visit to the next. His smile was gone. Recognizing the depression was easy. But neither I nor a psychiatric colleague nor his children and grandchildren could successfully treat it. He just quit eating and was dead in less than six months.*

I firmly believe that one should not be blamed for committing suicide. People just get to the end of their ropes and find nothing compelling to keep them fighting to stay alive. Life has been tough and is getting tougher, so why not move on? This is especially true of the elderly, who try to survive on a meager social security check while paying more and more money for medicines and doctor bills. Our life savings, in a great many cases right now, have been depleted by the government's forcing our money management company into receivership or by Alan Greenspan's Recession of 2000 and 2001 and 2002. Most of us don't want to be dependent on our kids, who usually can't afford to raise their families and take care of aging parents at the same time. Most of us want to be independent until the end and don't want to be warehoused in a nursing home for years. When our ability to be independent is lost or taken away, then the spark that keeps us going often is snuffed out.

The scout leader, with whose troop I hiked to Havasupai Canyon every spring for several years, was a very vigorous man who loved the outdoors. When he had a stroke and was paralyzed on one side, he soon took his own life. Perhaps other factors also played a part. I understand and don't blame him. I hope God doesn't either.

This chapter is written for those of us whose loved ones may be at risk, and whom we don't want to lose just yet. It may be up to us to, possibly in collaboration with the person's doctor, to try to provide the sense that the person is still needed and do anything possible to enhance their feeling of self worth.

It has been well known for years that death occurs in a high percentage of men within one year after full retirement. Thus I suggest that when you or your spouse is near retirement, that person should develop other consuming interests that can be pursued vigorously starting immediately after retirement becomes a reality. Also be sure that exercise within the limits of your capability is an even larger part of your daily routine than it is now.

The depression that has no apparent cause may be part of a bipolar disorder, or an overt psychosis. Or it may be to the lack of enough of a certain chemical in the brain. Or something else. People who have a relative who has had depression are more likely to have it themselves.

If depression is left untreated, it may affect our lives in several undesirable ways. These include marked feelings of isolation and loneliness, loss of interest in life in general, as well as in personal hobbies or projects, difficulty with relationships with family, friends, and coworkers, poorer work performance, reduced self-esteem, possibly increased alcohol use.

We now have quite an arsenal against all types of mental disease, and especially depression. Counseling has come a long way. Medications include Prozac, Zoloft, Paxil, Effexor, Welbutrin, Lithium, the tricyclics such as Elavil and its cousins, and some newer ones in the pipeline.

So we need to get people with depression diagnosed, which you can do now that you have read this chapter, and then get them to a doctor who can help them as soon as possible. There are mental health clinics available in almost every county in every state in our country now, most of which have at least some public funding. Public funding means that they are cheaper than private doctors on a sliding scale, or may even be free. Most colleges and universities have counseling centers with well-trained psychologists and psychiatrists to treat students who need mental care, as well as physical medical care during their time in school. Many family and some other types of doctors treat milder types of depression all the time. We are trained to do this.

Depression is very treatable. **You can get well!** You can resume a normal life. You just need to get yourself or your friend or loved one to one of these options. Do it soon!

Treatment of depression has come a long way since I first started working as an extern in Central State Hospital, a mental hospital in Indianapolis, my last two years in medical school. In those days, and even today in many states, a person could be committed to the state hospital if a judge determined that you were a danger to yourself or to others. Treatment of really bad depression often included electroshock treatments, and I assisted at quite a few of those while I worked there. Mostly, though, I worked as a doctor. Even though I hadn't completed my training, there were a lot of conditions I could treat, much as the physician extenders of today do.

I well recall, since I lived on the campus of about ten buildings, that when I first began working there in the summer, with no air conditioning and all windows open, the patients in the locked violent wards would yell and scream all night. But during my first year a new medication called Thorazine was discovered and came into general use for especially the more violent of the mentally ill. So by the time my two years were up, and I was ready to move on to my internship, we were able to sleep all night with all windows open (we had Thorazine but still no air conditioning) without hearing a single yell or scream. And all but one of the locked wards had become open wards, with patients able to come and go at will (although they still had to stay on the campus, as well as observe a ten o'clock curfew).

CHAPTER 32 -- DIABETES

How do you know when you have diabetes? Often the first knowledge occurs when you take a pre-employment or DOT physical exam and your urine turns up positive for sugar. Symptoms may include unusual thirst, urinary frequency, and weight loss, along with lack of energy and perhaps some other general feelings of something just not right. Your vision may deteriorate. Or you may have no symptoms at all if the disease is in its early stages. Those who are obese, and those who have a family history of diabetes should have a fasting blood sugar done at least once a year just to be on the safe side.

*I can't stress too much how important the family history is. Studies have confirmed what many of us physicians have been pretty sure of for years.

If you have a family history of diabetes and you want to keep from getting it yourself, then is particularly important for you to get your weight down to normal and keep it there, along with exercising daily for at least 30 minutes for the rest of your life.

To help you with these, please see the chapters on **Obesity** and **Exercise**.

Rapid weight gain predicts impending Type II diabetes. The sudden increase or rapid gain of more than 11 pounds greatly increases the risk of developing diabetes in those individuals who are at risk already. Diabetes is likely to develop within the following 3-6 months after the sudden weight gain.

The patient's weight at age 18 is a big issue. A body mass index greater than 27 correlates with an increased risk of Type II diabetes. (See the chapter on **Obesity** for an explanation of the new body mass index, which you will hear a lot more about in the future.) Another marker is a belt size of 40 inches or more. As discussed elsewhere fat in the belly is a _huge_ risk factor for diabetes.

Insulin resistance, which is the cause of Type II diabetes, is associated with the amount of fat in the abdominal cavity; increased fat in the areas under the skin has little influence on glucose metabolism (which is abnormal in diabetes).

Treatment of diabetes should not be limited to simply controlling the blood sugar. It must also include <u>prevention of or control of already existing high blood pressure, along with control of the blood fats, cholesterol and triglycerides.</u>

A study from Finland in the Internal Medicine News of August 2000 reported a 57 percent reduction in the incidence of Type II diabetes among adults with impaired glucose tolerance who participated in an intense diet and exercise program. The average age was 55 years. The average body mass index was 31 kg per square meter (see the chapter on **Obesity** *if you want that explained). 1) The diet portion of the program involved reduction of total weight, reduction of total and saturated fats, reduction of total calories, and increased consumption of dietary fiber. 2) The exercise program focused more on exercise strengthening by resistance training and weight lifting than on aerobic activity. The controls were given general advice about healthy diet and activity.*

The most obvious complications of diabetes are associated with blood sugars that are too high for long enough to produce ketoacidosis, or too low, even to the point where the person loses consciousness. Ketoacidosis to more than a mild degree requires a trip to the ER at least, and often admission to the hospital if the consciousness is affected at all.

Those are the obvious extremes of diabetes and its treatment; but bad things are going on in your blood vessels, and your eyes, and your kidneys, and these are silently accelerated by inadequate control of your blood sugar.

Ideally your blood sugar will always be below 110. Most diabetics who get it that low have to contend with occasional spells of too low blood sugar (hypoglycemia). Too low a blood sugar can lead to falls when you feel faint or unsteady on your feet, in addition to just plain passing out. You can die a whole lot faster from low blood sugar (minutes to a few hours) than from blood sugars that are too high (days to weeks, or even years in milder cases). If a diabetic is on the verge of passing out or has passed out, you won't do any harm by giving sugar-containing fluids (<u>not</u> a <u>Diet</u> Coke) right after you call 911. If the blood sugar is too low, the sweet fluid drink will help quickly. If the blood sugar is too high, that won't cause any additional problem. Also dextrose or glucose in some form are ideal if available, and all diabetics should carry some of these with them at all times

Since 110 is hard to attain without side effects, we often aim for 130 or better in the fasting blood sugar and a hemoglobin A1c of 6.5 or better. The hemoglobin A1c measures how well you control your blood sugar over time -- the past 30 days or so, and I rely more on that than the blood sugar. If you are a brittle diabetic, that is, very hard to control, then you will be testing your blood up to four times a day. You must keep that record and bring it to your doctor at each visit. Try never to exceed a blood sugar of 200. You should also test your urine with a dipstick periodically. First, it is very important to know whether you have acetone (a ketone) in the urine because that means you are getting into trouble with acidosis. That takes just one test on the dipstick and is pretty cheap. Second, the dipsticks now have gotten very complete, and we can test for bacteria, pus cells, nitrites, and a lot of other stuff that can indicate the early presence of urinary tract infections. These are much more common in diabetics than other people, probably due to the sugar in the urine providing more food for the bacteria. A really good insurance policy is to do one of the infection-detecting dipsticks the first thing in the morning once a month. Do this especially if you don't see your doctor very often. He can order a bottle of the sticks for you. The dipstick doesn't adequately replace looking at the specimen under the microscope, though, so your doctor should check a urine specimen at each office visit too.

Diabetics get hardening of the arteries (arteriosclerosis) very early in life, with reduced blood flow to all organs.

Cataracts of the lenses of the eyes develop much earlier and more often.

High blood pressure is much more common; almost all will eventually get it.

The kidneys fail and need dialysis in most diabetics if they live long enough. The blood pressure pills called ACE inhibitors have been a recent big help in protecting the kidneys (e.g., enalapril, lisinopril, Accupril, Monopril, and others). I believe that all diabetics should take one of them, even if their blood pressure hasn't become high yet. The dose will have to be lower, of course, if the BP is normal.

The nerves to the feet lose their sensitivity and may actually become very painful (neuropathy), while their blood supply fails. Diabetics therefore may not notice something rubbing a raw spot, or a toenail that is ingrowing. Shoes need to be wide and soft.

Diabetics must carefully inspect their feet at least once a week, and keep them clean and free from blisters, ingrown toenails, corns and calluses. Wash them daily. With the reduced blood supply little scrapes don't heal well and often something that would be trivial to a non-diabetic leads to an amputation of toe, foot, or leg. So be sure you <u>always</u> wear comfortable well-fitting shoes. Never buy a shoe that feels tight when you first try it on. The sales person may try to tell you that it will soon stretch and get broken in. Don't you believe him. It's your feet that will be "broken in," often to your sorrow when you are a diabetic. It's better to try the shoes on in the afternoon because your feet expand a little (sometimes a lot) after you walk around awhile during the day. And always have your foot measured while standing up on the measuring device. You will always measure a half to a full size larger when standing. And you are buying shoes mostly for standing and walking, aren't you?

The use of tobacco is an absolute no-no in diabetics because tobacco in any form causes the blood vessels to shrink even more in size. No blood means gangrene and amputation if even the slightest thing goes wrong with the feet.

Treatment

The treatment of diabetes comes down to a few simple things that are extremely important: <u>Exercise daily. Control your weight. Avoid simple or refined sugars and carbohydrates. Avoid alcohol, which is also a refined carbohydrate with the same bad effects as sugar.</u> (See the chapter on **Weight Loss** for some excellent diets that diabetics can use for both weight and sugar control.) <u>Take your injectable insulin or oral medication</u>, and <u>carefully watch your blood sugars and hemoglobin A1c tests</u> to be sure you are keeping them under control. <u>Watch your blood pressure.</u> <u>Take an ACE inhibitor</u> for its kidney protecting effect if possible even if you don't have high blood pressure. If you do have hypertension, then insist that you be put on an ACE inhibitor, to as high a dose as you can tolerate, as one of the medications used for your blood pressure control. <u>Don't use tobacco.</u> <u>Keep your cholesterol and triglycerides down in their normal ranges</u>.

Many people with diabetes can "cure" it. By "cure" I mean that they can keep their blood sugars down in the normal range and avoid all of the diabetic complications through the simple measures of weight loss until you have a lean body, and daily aerobic exercise of at least 30 minutes. I have had several dozen highly motivated patients who have been successful in doing just that. Perhaps you can too. It's worth a try!!

CHAPTER 33 -- DOCTOR'S FEES

The fees charged by most physicians are related to several things:

1. The most obvious is the amount of time spent with the patient. If that were all that was involved, then you would feel even more short-changed then you already do when a doctor spends about two minutes with you then charges you $60-80 plus lab, shots, etc. I am embarrassed for some of my colleagues who have to do that to make a living.

2. How hard it is to make the diagnosis (the "complexity" of the decision-making process). In other words how many possible diagnoses have to be considered? When the complexity is high, a specialist may be necessary. They, rightfully, can charge more and be paid more by Medicare and the insurance companies.

Not all doctors charge the same, no matter whether in general practice or a specialty. So it may pay to call a couple of the offices of doctors you are considering and ask what they charge for "99203" and "99213" office visits.

3. Is the diagnosis straightforward or convoluted? (Easy or difficult?) Again, the specialist will usually have a higher fee. If your condition is difficult to diagnose, then your dollars are better spent in seeing a specialist in that field. If, on the other hand, the diagnosis is relatively easy, then you will have a much better bargain by going to a family or general practitioner.

Medical fees of all kinds rise, in part, because constantly changing state and federal regulations, such as those requiring new record-keeping methods to protect privacy, are adding billions of dollars of new expenses for doctors and hospitals in the U.S. A very expensive example is the new requirement that all patient records be computerized so they can be "portable" and thus instantly accessible to doctors and hospitals far away from your home. *But these entities never provide any additional funding for us to implement those new regulations.* So we have to hire more people, and buy more computers and computer programs. Who pays for all of those regulations? You do!

I was just as embarrassed by having to hurry my patients out occasionally myself on a Friday afternoon, as I was trying to get through with office hours in time to make the team bus for an away game, when I was team doctor for the Warsaw Tigers in a little town in northern Indiana. (My high school English teacher must be turning over in her grave after that sentence!) Of course in those days I charged only four dollars. And I sometimes had a patient come back for free during Saturday morning office hours if I really had to short change him. And they all knew I was the doctor for the Tigers. So not a soul ever complained. Boy, that was fun!!

The new privacy laws to the contrary notwithstanding, the scary thing about these totally computerized records is that any hacker hired by an insurance company, a prospective employer, a vengeful ex-spouse, and who knows who else, can access them. All they need is your social security number -- or the last four digits of it. I know a little bit about computers. At one time I was president of a computer club. In our club were some girls and guys who could make a computer do <u>anything</u>. I don't know about you, but I really don't want any of those entities I mentioned above to know whether I have an active sex life (my wife and my urologist know, and that's enough), or whether I had Tsutsugamushi fever when I was in the U. S. Air Force, or whether I have ever been treated by a psychiatrist -- I haven't but you get the point).

But doctors and hospitals are now being pressured to produce these "portable records." And it's going to cost them <u>Big Bucks</u>. Medicare and the HMOs are not going to pay for all the new computers and the software and especially the salaries of the new employees needed to input all this information. So we physicians are going to take yet another hit in the pocketbook and the quality of life as we are pushed to spend more time on the records than we spend with our patients. Currently, in one of my urgent care settings I have to make some notation on a total of five pages of paper for each non-work-related medical patient I see. For work-related injuries I have to do seven pages. It <u>often</u> takes longer to treat the chart than it does the patient! I have frequently wondered how many trees are cut down each year for each page.

Below is a list of doctors and facilities providing medical services, from least to most expensive. Consider this list when you are about to seek medical help. Keep in mind that even though you may be paying only a small co-pay for all of these, if you always use the most expensive, then your medical insurance premium will inevitably go up next year.

1. Least expensive: Teaching hospital's outpatient clinics
2. Family doctor's office, during the day on weekdays. And if you are having a temporary financial problem, you may often be able request and receive a reduced price.

3. Specialist's office, during the day on weekdays. I suspect they also may reduce their fees under special circumstances.
4. Family doctor or his on-call doctor, at night or weekends
5. Specialist or his on-call doctor, at night or weekends
6. I'm constantly amazed by how many people just go directly to an urgent care facility or an ER, even on a weekday, without even calling their doctors first. Also, many specialists are available 24 hours per day, even if you are a new patient. (You probably will have to pay in cash or have good insurance in that case however.)
7. More expensive: Urgent Care. These are great for a person who has a relatively minor semi-emergency and who can't reach a doctor. Also very good for someone from out of town. (See the chapter on **Emergency Rooms** and Urgent Cares for more complete information.)
8. Even more expensive: Hospital Emergency Rooms, where only true emergencies really belong.
9. The most expensive of all: certain high profile clinics who over charge, over test, and over treat.

For those patients on Medicare, many doctors now limit their practices to people under 65. The reason is that Medicare fees are set by the federal government, based on federal budgetary restrictions, which generally bear little or no relationship to office costs and other factors and are considerably lower than our actual costs in many cases. Also we are required to charge the same reduced prices to millionaires as to the truly indigent person. When I was in private practice, I had three really rich people whose office fees were required to be drastically reduced when they turned 65 and went on Medicare. They each offered to continue to pay my regular fees, but I was required by law to charge them the same as the truly poor widow lady.

There are some <u>very</u> good things about Medicare. When I began practice more than forty years ago, Medicare was a socialist idea whose time had not yet come. When I had a retired patient, I automatically reduced my bill unless I knew that he was well off. And I treated <u>many</u> elderly patients free of charge. I saved medication samples for those who had trouble getting their medicines (most of us still do). And I often made house calls instead of putting people in the hospital.

Now I definitely take in more money than before Medicare, even with their reducing my charges. The problem comes in the fact that Medicare has caused my costs to rise <u>a lot</u> because of all the paperwork and documentation that they require, and because they literally change the rules every month! They send out a monthly newsletter with the latest changes, and we must read it carefully and then either program our computers ourselves (which I did, but can't anymore) or pay someone to modify the software. Or buy all new software, which is happening with the new "portable records" requirements. And all of us have to hire additional office personnel to do the paperwork. And more trees have to be cut down to make paper (the "Paperwork Reduction Act" to the contrary notwithstanding).

So a lot of us lose money, according to cost accounting, for each Medicare patient we see. But I will testify that it is a whole lot better than it used to be for those of us who have practiced on both sides of the street. And for all patients, except the very rich, the gain in available medical care is <u>huge</u>.

Medicine is by far not the only area where the government changes the rules but provides no funds to help pay for the costs of those changes. It just happens to be the area I know about from long personal experience. In my opinion the <u>very least</u> that Congress should do when they mandate something is to allow a tax <u>credit</u> instead of a deduction for costs incurred in implementing their laws.

CHAPTER 34 -- DRUGS IN THE ELDERLY

For a number of reasons, certain drugs should be avoided or given in very reduced doses in elderly people. One reason is that these older folks often have kidneys that don't function as well as they used to, thus not excreting the medications taken as they should. This often allows the levels of medication to build up to possibly toxic levels in the blood, thus causing undesirable and sometimes bizarre side effects. Another reason is that our brains become more sensitive to certain drugs as the circulation inevitably diminishes.

Another drug problem in our older friends is that they often have multiple little brush fires going on in their bodies, each of which needs its own medication to control or put out. By the time one reaches three or four (or <u>more</u>) medicines, there is a high risk of undesirable and perhaps unexpected drug interactions occurring. Usually if you use just one doctor and one pharmacist, they will be able to warn you about 90% of the time when such things may occur. But the elderly people I see often see a specialist for one thing, their family doctor for others, and an urgent care center for sore throats and acute stuff. And they may just use the pharmacy nearest each of these, so no one really has an idea just what all the patient is taking. Your best defense in those cases is to pay attention to the list below. Your second best defense is to keep an updated list of all your medicines in your wallet or purse and show it to every doctor you ever see.

If you or an elderly relative are on one or more of these listed medications, talk with the doctor about possible alternatives that are less likely to cause side effects.

Tri-cyclic antidepressants. Elavil (generic name is amitryptiline), Limbitrol (generic chlordiazepoxide- amitryptiline), and Triavil (generic perphenazine-amitryptiline) are used for depression in younger people. They cause too much sedation in the elderly, with falls and inability to think straight. They also cause dry mouth and constipation.

Barbiturates. These have more side effects than other sedatives and sleeping meds and are very addictive. Their only use in older people should be for seizure control.

Benzodiazepines. These include Librium (clordiazepoxide), Limbitrol (chlordiazepoxide-amitryptiline), Librax (chlordiazepoxide-clindium), Valium (diazepam), which for years has been one of the most-prescribed medicines in the world, and Dalmane (flurazepam), a long-acting sleeping pill that causes a hangover even in younger people. All of these last much longer in older people, with prolonged sleepiness and more falls and fractures.

A good idea at any age, but especially in older folks, is to throw away all drugs more than a year old in the medicine cabinet on New Year's Day or your birthday. This can be modified somewhat if you know what something is for, and you are pretty sure it isn't far out of date. Older people, however, tend to forget what meds are for what, and need some encouragement to throw them out.

To go on with the list:

Aldomet, Aldoril (Methyldopa, also with hydrochlorthiazide). These drugs for high blood pressure may cause slow heartbeat and aggravate depression. Also sometimes the liver is affected. We now have much better choices for blood pressure treatment in older folks.

Bentyl (dicyclomine), Levsin and Levsinex (hyoscyamine), Probanthine (propantheline), Donnatal and others (belladonna alkaloids), and Librax (chlordiazepoxide-clindium). These are intestinal anti-spasm meds and cause toxic effects of various types. They aren't very effective in the very small doses tolerated by the elderly. They are best totally avoided.

Demerol (meperidine). This is a pain med, usually given by shot, and has few benefits when given by mouth, with some bad side effects.

Diabinase (chlorpropamide) for diabetes, which is prone to cause severe low blood sugar in the elderly, along with some other bad hormonal stuff.

Lanoxin (digoxin). This is a very potent and good drug for congestive heart failure. Unfortunately, there isn't a very wide spread between therapeutic and poisonous. So it has to be watched closely to be sure it doesn't cause heart block, among other things. The dose in younger people is usually 0.25 mg daily, but older patients usually shouldn't exceed 0.125 mg daily -- especially those with some reduced kidney function. Kidney function plays a *huge* part in medication doses in people of *all* ages, but even more so in our grandparents and great grandparents.

Equanil and Miltown (meprobamate). We used these before Valium came along. They are very addicting, and habit-forming, with sedation a big problem.

Norpace and Norpace CR. This may cause heart failure, as well as constipation and dry mouth. Avoid it totally.

Sinequan (doxepin) is a drug for depression that affects the intestinal tract strongly, and makes one sleepy.

Talwin (pentazocine) is a narcotic that causes more effects on the brain than many other narcotics.

Ticlid (ticlopidine) is an anti-clotting drug that is probably no better than aspirin for clot prevention, but with quite a few more side effects.

One of the patients I was called to see at home for one of my physician colleagues when he was away was the 89-year-old grandmother of one of my own patients. She had been well and still fairly vigorous until about two weeks before. But now she was almost comatose, and the family was starting to make funeral preparations. She had a living will (something I highly recommend -- see that chapter), so no hospitalization was considered. I examined her and couldn't find anything in particular wrong with her except that she was very groggy and had trouble talking as though she was tongue-tied. I asked to see her medications because, first it's always a good idea, and, second, because the patient was very private and no one could give much of a medical history, least of all the patient. I thought that I might be able to tell something about her medical history by the medicines she was taking.

There were literally dozens of bottles of pills in her medicine cabinet, some dated as long as 20 years before. When I held out the bottles, my patient was able to show me which ones she had been taking recently. It turned out that she had consolidated some pills and was taking Valium, Dalmane, and Phenobarbital, none of which had been prescribed by my colleague for at least ten or fifteen years! No wonder she was sleepy. She thought one was for constipation and one was a vitamin. Well, I took the lady's daughter into the bathroom, and we flushed several hundred pills down the toilet. Then we just gave her plenty of fluids, with light food as tolerated for about three days. Bless her heart, she woke up and lived for another 5 or 6 years, doing her own housework every day. This is an extreme case (or else I probably wouldn't have included it here), but not unusual in lesser degrees.

As reported elsewhere in this book, I recently had an elderly lady from out of town who was taking an anticoagulant medication for stroke prevention in atrial fibrillation (a heart rhythm disturbance). She came to our urgent care clinic because she was getting a lot of bruises all over her body, but did not recall ever bumping herself. She said that her blood test just 2 weeks before at her new doctor's office was in the "good" range. After an otherwise normal physical exam I ordered a prothrombin time blood test to see how well her blood was clotting. It came back the next morning as 90 seconds! (The normal therapeutic and safe range for anticoagulants is generally 20-25 seconds.)

I called her right away and asked her to bring in all her medications. When she came in that afternoon, I found that she had a bottle of 5 mg Coumadin tablets, about half empty, and a bottle of 5 mg Warfarin tablets, nearly full. She said that she had recently had to switch doctors in a new HMO, and she was still taking the Coumadin from her former doctor. She had also had to switch pharmacies; so the new pharmacy had no record of what medications she was on.

Her new doctor had done the blood test, then gave her the new prescription for generic Coumadin, otherwise known as warfarin (also sometimes known as rat poison). The new bottle was labeled "Warfarin," and, in tiny letters I needed a magnifying glass for, "generic coumadin." So she had been taking a double dose of this powerful "blood thinner" for a little over two weeks. No wonder she had bruises all over her body. Another few days and she would have been bleeding into her brain, a frequently somewhat fatal situation!

Since we are no longer able to keep the same doctor and the same pharmacist for long periods of time, your only real defense against such potential catastrophes is to always bring every bottle of everything you are taking to your doctor at every visit. He or she may not look at all of them each time, but you have them if needed.

CHAPTER 35 -- EARS

Take good care of them early in life and they will repay you with good hearing when you are old. Well, within reason.

Never put anything smaller than your elbow into your ear! All right, nothing smaller than your finger. Certainly no Q-tips. I have personally seen several dozen eardrums damaged by the use of Q-tips for cleaning the ears. A few of those actually had holes in them. Quite a few ears had earwax that was packed down tightly by the Q-tips. Others had damage to the ear canals. Keep in mind that Q-tips are almost like sandpaper to the delicate membranes inside your ears.

Be aware that our ears are self-cleaning for most of us. Sometimes wax will build up when outdoors in the dust in dry weather, but even then most of us don't have a problem. For 98% of us all we need at most is a little soap from the washcloth on our finger when we wash our faces, then a little rinse with water from the cloth.

If you are one of the 2%, then it's a 100% situation for you to fix personally, and **save money**. You have some easy options before heading to a doctor's office for help. First, ask someone to pull your ear lobe back and peer into your ear canal in a good light. That may not be much help, but most of the really severe wax impactions I've treated have been visible with the naked eye. Then go to the drugstore and buy a rubber bulb syringe. It may even be called an ear syringe. Or it may be called a suction syringe (as for suctioning thick mucus out of a baby's nostrils). Whatever. Fill it with <u>warm</u> water (if you use cold, or sometimes even room temperature water, you will probably get very dizzy very soon. If this should happen to you anyway, just lie down for a few minutes. It will go away as soon as the inner ear warms up.)

Next, put your head over the sink and start squirting the water into the ear, directing it toward a slightly different part of the ear canal at each squirt. Be patient. It is rare that a big wax plug comes out with the first try. What usually happens with the first syringe full is that an ear that was only partially plugged up before now becomes completely closed. Stay with it. You will notice some little specks of wax coming out with each blast.

If you are ready to quit after 15 minutes or so, I don't blame you. You can then put two drops or so of olive oil or baby oil into the ear and let it soften overnight, or for two or three nights, coming back to irrigating it every day until the wax finally floats out or you give up and go to the doctor. You can use Cerumenex or Debrox instead of oil, but the oil works about as well as those two usually. If you do wind up at the doctor's, you will have made his job a lot easier. I don't mind telling you that I have spent as much as 45 minutes cleaning out a really tightly adherent plug of wax.

After your ears are clean, then for the rest of your life just put a drop of olive oil into each one once a week, and get a little soap into them when you wash your face. Your ears will keep themselves clean from then on -- probably.

For prevention of deafness you should prevent exposure to loud noises from birth on. I gave my kids shooters' ear plugs for use whenever they went to a concert. They told me later that they even used them … sometimes.

Loudness of noise is measured in decibels. Exposure to any noise that is 80 decibels in strength or more for a very long period of time -- eight hours at a time may be the minimum -- will cause damage to the ears, slight but definite. Exposure to 90 decibels for a much shorter amount of time will produce even more damage in a shorter time period. (Audio tests done in a small single engine airplane produced a noise level of 92 decibels. The sound at the muzzle of a .45 caliber pistol is 140 decibels.) The higher the noise level, the more likelihood of loss. So protect your ears with earplugs and ear muffs (both together in higher noise levels like shooting, running a chain saw, or working in a truck factory like I did when I was working my way through school). Loud noise exposure leads to loss in the high frequency ranges but spares, relatively speaking, the lower tones. Thus we may hear men's voices better than soprano women's speech if we have such high frequency loss.

As we grow older a high percentage of us fall prey to hearing loss in all ranges. This tendency is very much accentuated by previous noise exposure, as well as repeated or severe ear infections.

When infections cause the eardrums to rupture, obviously, if they do heal, a scar is left on the delicate membrane that affects all the frequencies.

Preventing rupture of the eardrums in infection is therefore a major consideration when you have an ear infection. What happens in those cases is that the tube that leads from the back of the nose above the back of the throat up to the middle ear (the eustacean tube) gets swollen. Usually that is because the nasal membranes are swollen, which closes the nose end of the tube. This tube is important in equalizing the pressure in the middle ear. When you change altitude that tube has to open for your ears to "pop."

When you have an infection in the nose, the tube may be unable to open. If bacteria are trapped in there, a middle ear infection may result. <u>It is very important to not change altitude if you have an ear infection. You may rupture your eardrum</u>. That means don't leave town if you live in the mountains, and don't fly in an airplane. I have written probably a couple hundred excuses for people who needed to get their airline tickets changed. I have also had three or four patients who left Flagstaff, at 7,000 feet, heading for Phoenix, whose eardrums ruptured as they went down the steep grade of the Mogollon Rim on I-17 at about the Stoneman Lake exit.

How can you deal with a plugged up ear yourself and save money? When it first feels plugged up, have someone look as far into the ear as he or she can see. If no wax can be seen, spray your nose three times with Afrin while sniffing the spray back, perhaps even lying down for five minutes and looking at the ceiling while you sniff. Then repeat three sprays and the rest of the procedure again. Remember, the tube opening to the middle ear is clear at the back of the nose; so the spray has to get all the way back there to do any good. Gargling with hot salt water is also sometimes helpful because the tube opening is behind the soft palate just above the throat. Then, after the nose is as clear as you can get it, pinch your nose tightly and blow, and try to make your ears pop. This is more likely to be successful if you are staying at the same altitude or dropping in altitude than when you are going up.

Nasal decongestants, which are available in massive quantities over the counter -- pick your favorite -- may be helpful over time, but not as quickly as the spray.

If there is a bug in your ear, use a rubber bulb syringe with <u>warm</u> water and just squirt it into the ear repeatedly until the bug comes out. If it is a tick, you may not be able to remove it yourself because they often sink their little pincers right into your eardrum then suck your blood until they are as large as a pea. For a tick you will

A bead in the ear (or nose) of a little kid can be a challenge, even for doctors with our special instruments. One thing that I have personally found effective is to put a drop of Super Glue on the plastic end of a cotton swab, and then quickly but carefully touch it to the bead for about 15 seconds. Then gently pull out on the stick. And there it is! I had read about using some kind of rapid dental adhesive not long before this cute little three year old girl came in with a bead in her left ear a few months ago. Unfortunately the clinic at which I was working that day did not have a dentist nearby. So I thought maybe Super Glue would work as well. I sent her father to the pharmacy two blocks away, and when he returned, we tried it. This little sweetheart was as still and good as she could be. It took two tries. The first time I used a wooden applicator, and the glue just soaked into the wooden tip. The second time I used one made with plastic and dislodged it right away. Then all my PA student had to do was gently put the end of a paper clip behind it and push it the rest of the way out.

almost always need to see a doctor. But try flooding the ear canal with rubbing alcohol (water won't work with ticks). Often that makes them pull right out. For a tick in a more exposed location, you can strike a match, then blow it out and quickly apply the still-hot end to the tick's body. It will immediately do its best to get the heck out of Dodge! Vigorously wash the spot where the tick was attached to try to prevent infection. (See the chapter on **Tick-Borne Diseases**.)

Ringing in the Ears (Tinnitus)

This is caused most of the time by exposure to enough noise to produce permanent damage to the hearing mechanism. This can be 80 decibels or more without hearing protection on an almost daily basis for a long time. Or it can be from personally firing, or standing beside someone who is firing a .357 magnum revolver, which produces a muzzle blast of 150 decibels, without ear protection just once. I've seen both situations, the first more than the second, but I live in the huge Coconino National Forest, where hunting every year without ear protection is a way of life.

Sadly, once tinnitus appears, there is no cure. All one can do is to prevent it from getting worse by wearing double ear protection (ear plugs plus ear muffs) from now on whenever personally doing or being around anything noisy. The obvious noisy activities include running a chain saw (another favorite pastime in our forest), shooting, running a lawn mower, running some vacuum cleaners, and blow-drying your hair. Others include flying behind the engines in a lot of airplanes, attending concerts, working in factories with lots of punch presses, or just driving in a car with the speakers turned up to max. Some electric razors seem a little loud. Think of loud things in your own life.

Some people have trouble sleeping because of ringing in the ears. There are some machines that produce a low background noise, which you can turn on when you go to bed. Options include rain, waves on a beach, wind in the trees, and others. These machines are also useful for relaxation purposes. They cost $50 or $60, I believe.

Hearing Aids

These are many and expensive. $5,000 for a set of two digital aids. Medicare, the last I heard, would pay up to $300 for a set. A little more for the examination and fitting.

Most fit in the ear. Some fit behind the ear, and some are in the form of earmuffs with directional microphones, very high tech for people with little usable hearing.

The complaint of the vast majority of people with hearing aids is that they amplify every little sound to the point where meaningful conversation is drowned out. So they are no better than they were before and often abandon the aid within a month or two. The aids that are advertised most are the ones most likely to be discarded, with a feeling that you were gypped. You probably were.

Once you pay your money, you are usually stuck with what you have.

Save Money

Go to a certified audiologist, preferably one that will not profit from the sale of a particular brand. An ear exam by an Ear, Nose and Throat (ENT) specialist will be necessary. Many ENT doctors have audiologists working right in the same office. Others will refer you to one they feel comfortable with.

Audiologists have multiple types of aids for you to try out right in the office. They can order aids that amplify only the frequencies in which you are deficient. **A good audiologist will save you big bucks!** And he or she will help you choose a hearing aid that you won't throw away.

CHAPTER 36 -- EMERGENCY ROOMS

These are where everything that is really or potentially serious belongs, and as soon as possible once you have reached that decision. Your doctor may be prepared for almost anything (and as a small town doctor I had to be), but he cannot properly cope with massive bleeding or a heart attack or stroke in his office. Same for an Urgent Care facility. If, however you are a long way from a hospital and you happen to know of a nearby doctor's office, by all means stop there first. The doctor will almost certainly be able to do something you couldn't know how to do that may make the situation better.

You have all heard of and probably have experienced many hours of waiting in one or more ERs. This is inevitable at times, and be assured the doctors and nurses working there feel almost as badly about the wait as you do.

A nurse (not a nurse's aide) will do triage, a term that originated in the military where there were a lot of casualties suddenly being brought to the field hospital or M*A*S*H unit all at once (remember the movie and the TV series?) This means that a trained person briefly checks every person who comes to the ER to determine the severity of the condition. The worst problems go first (i.e., get top priority), then the next worse, etc. So when you entered the ER has little relation to when you are seen if your condition does not *seem* relatively urgent to the triage nurse.

If you or your friend or family member you are accompanying begins to feel faint, especially when standing up, **get help** from the ER staff any way you have to. Try everything you can without making them call Security because you made someone angry. Just say that you know of someone who died in the ER waiting room and that you or your friend or family member is having almost the same symptoms. Ask for a new triage evaluation. Go to a phone and call your family doctor. Stop a paramedic as he or she passes by. **Call 911 from the phone outside the ER.** Stop a doctor who comes out to the waiting room to talk to the family of a patient he has just taken care of. Say that you are very worried.

The one almost unfailing symptom that should cause concern for possible internal bleeding is a feeling of faintness upon standing up and not having it go away in a few seconds as that feeling does when we have been sitting or lying down for awhile and suddenly stand up. And the face may be pale. And the pulse, if you can find it, will be rapid -- over a hundred beats per minute almost always.

*If you think you are worse than the nurse thinks you are, **you must be your own advocate in the ER**. Don't just sit there and let yourself bleed to death internally as my step-cousin did from a ruptured spleen during "only" a four-hour wait in the ER after triage. She was a beautiful and gentle lady who had been in a relatively minor auto accident that jammed her left lower rib cage against the door handle protrusion. She didn't want to complain and just gradually bled to death without making a fuss.*

Going to the ER for a cold is a terrible waste of medical resources. Same for a lot of other routine medical problems. A really good alternative medical source between your family doctor and the ER is an **Urgent Care** facility. These are facilities which provide the general practice of medicine for <u>acute</u> care. In other words go there for problems that are not serious enough for the ER (which is also a lot more expensive), for which you can't get in to see your doctor as soon as you need to. Or go there if you are on vacation. Or if your doctor is not on your new insurance plan. Or for whatever reason. For best results don't wait until almost closing time. The staff in most cases has been there for a long time, up to 12 hours, under stressful conditions and is getting tired and looking forward to going home.

Be aware that there is a great variation among Urgent Care facilities. Most have at least limited X-ray capability, chest and extremity x-rays, while some can do much more. Some have small office labs on the premises, with microscopes and machines for doing at least a complete blood count (something that is very important in deciding how to treat infections in little kids). Others have to send out everything except a urine dipstick, a rapid strep screen, and a pregnancy test.

Some have considerable minor surgical capability, depending on the training of the doctor working the shift when you appear there, and the surgical equipment provided by the company which owns the facility. All can repair minor skin wounds that just take four or five stitches but no deep layers.

All can administer oxygen or give a small volume nebulizer treatment when needed. All can put a splint on a minor fracture until you can see a bone doctor the next day. All can provide pain medication if needed; but don't go there if you are hooked on legal drugs -- you won't get any more sympathy there than anywhere else. The federal Drug Enforcement Administration (DEA) regulates Urgent Care doctors and PAs just as strictly as those physicians who practice individually.

All can treat non-emergency conditions of everyday life. But they aren't cheap. *<u>The most economical use of your medical dollar continues to be your own family doctor</u>. (See the chapter on **Choosing a Doctor.**)

CHAPTER 37 -- ENERGY FIELDS

Our bodies have an invisible but measurable energy field, often called an aura. The Department of Kinesthesiology at UCLA Medical School at one time had a $500,000 machine that could actually measure auras. The Russians developed a technique called Kirlian Photography that could take pictures of auras. They could be compared from year-to-year and would show undesirable changes in the aura several weeks to months before illness in the person's body actually showed up. What a great technique to use at each annual physical exam! So I looked for and found such an apparatus in a catalog for sale in this country. When I tried to order one, however, I was told that it had been "discontinued. There were some problems with it." Since it used high voltage electricity, I've always suspected that "some problems" meant that someone had been electrocuted. It still sounds like a great idea.

Some researchers have found people who can actually see auras. They estimate about 1 in 10,000 people have that ability. I know one. She played first violin for a symphony orchestra for many years before she finally retired about ten years ago. Her husband was a schoolteacher. He told me that they had been married for 43 years before she let him know that she could see auras. She was afraid he would think she was crazy! Unfortunately I lost touch with her before I could learn more.

I do plan to investigate the body energy field and other aspects of so-called psychic energy that have been studied for years at the Rhine Institute at Duke University. You may have heard of Duke. They also have a basketball team (coached by a man whose last name makes one wish he had never studied phonetics). That will be in future editions of this book.

CHAPTER 38 -- EXERCISE

Exercise is the keystone for good health throughout your life. Our bodies are strange and wondrous things. The more we use (but not abuse) them the better they function.

My great grandmother died in her sleep at age 105. She was still tending her yard and, according to family lore, cleaning her house the day before she died. Her quality of life was excellent to the end, partly, no doubt from heredity, but mainly because she exercised every day of her life. Her philosophy was, "if I don't use my mind and body, they will rust."

The Harvard Medical School study of their graduates, which I believe began in 1929 and is updated every year with a long questionnaire about all kinds of activities of living and health, told us a couple of years ago that we live almost an additional two minutes for every minute we engage in some kind of active aerobic exercise. The doctors who participate in this study are highly motivated to provide accurate information each year, and there is a very high response rate. Therefore those of us in the medical profession have always valued reports from that study very much. This report, for the first time, actually proved what many of us had long suspected. We've known for years that regular exercise enhances the quality of life. Now we are being told that it also increases the length of life.

Realizing that there were fatal accidents, homicides, and suicides that shortened some of the lives in the study, exercise may play an even greater role in the aspects of our lives that we have more control over than the report implied.

I suggest that even these three causes of death may be favorably affected by regular aerobic exercise. Suicide, for example, is usually a result of untreated depression. We now have wonderful medications for depression called SSRIs (the full name doesn't mean a whole lot more to me than it would to you). But 20 years ago a psychiatrist in Minnesota found that his patients recovered from depression much faster than those of any other physician or psychologist in the country because he demanded that they exercise for an hour each day in addition to whatever medication and psychotherapy he was also using.

There was a running track next door to his office; and when the snow wasn't too deep, the therapeutic session was carried out as both doctor and patient walked or jogged around the track for 45 minutes.

We know from other studies that endorphins, chemicals produced in the brain which have anti-pain and anti-depression effects on our bodies, begin to be produced after about 30 minutes of continuous exercise and produces the so-called runner's high. I have experienced that for years, as my custom is to exercise right after I get home from my always-stressful work. After 45 minutes to an hour I feel as though my brain has been run through a car wash and all the bad stuff of the day washed away. I feel human again! The same will happen to you. I guarantee it!

Aerobic exercise is sometimes referred to as cardiovascular (or cardio) exercise. It can be computed, on a treadmill for example, (remember videos of the astronauts on treadmills and bicycles with tubes in their mouths?) by measuring the amount of oxygen consumed by a person engaged in that activity for a given time.

I was privileged to attend medical school at Indiana University, where Dr. Sid Robinson pioneered these studies, which are used all over the world today. He used as his first famous guinea pig Don Lash, an I. U. track star who was the top miler in the country. Other famous athletes beat a path to his door from around the country to be tested. A more obscure athlete he tested was myself.

As a result of his innovations, eventually virtually every activity known to man has been checked out and the amount of oxygen consumed per hour measured. (The first Kinsey Report on sexual activities also came from Indiana in this same era.) The oxygen consumed is given as METS, and exercise prescriptions given by doctors, in particular after heart attacks, are based on what treadmill tests tell him or her about that patient's exercise capabilities.

Basically, without referring to the chart (at least not yet), aerobic exercise is any exercise that does not build up an oxygen debt (is not so demanding that lactic acid builds up in the body because the muscles aren't getting enough oxygen from lungs and blood). Ideally it should be an activity that causes an increase in your heart rate to about 2/3 of your VO max and keeps it there for at least 30 minutes. That probably means a heart rate of 120-140 beats per minute for most of us. If in doubt, go for the lower figure.

A lot of activities are aerobic. **Walking** at what <u>you</u> feel is a brisk pace for at least 30 minutes is aerobic. You should be able to talk to a walking partner without getting breathless while doing this and all aerobic activities. Riding a **stationary bike** at a resistance setting you feel comfortable with, using a **cross country ski machine**, **swimming**, **jogging**, actual **cross country skiing**, **jogging on a mini-trampoline**, which is reputed to exercise every cell in your body, and **working the pedals on an inverted bike with your hands** for those who have leg infirmities are all acceptable aerobic activities.

For your own personal exercise program, get some <u>comfortable</u> (see the chapter on **Foot Problems**) walking/jogging shoes and start slowly with whatever you can do easily right now. Do it every day for six days. If you have sore muscles anywhere by then, rest for a day. Then start gradually increasing the amount of time spent exercising each day. Just add one minute each day; don't ever increase your total activities for a week more than 10% per week. We are aiming for a <u>minimum</u> average of 30 minutes per day, or a total of 3 1/2 hours per week. I suggest that, if possible, you do a different activity on alternate days so as to train as many parts of your body as possible and give stressed muscles a day to recover. This will help you to avoid sore muscles that might interfere with continuing your program. If your feet become sore, read the chapter on **Foot Problems**. If you are starting to put in a lot of miles, it may be a good idea to get a second pair of athletic shoes and alternate which pair you wear each day.

As you begin to become enthusiastic about your workout program, you may find it difficult to avoid overdoing it. Prevention of injuries to muscles and ligaments will allow you to continue your program without the aches and pains that often develop to the point where you stop.

To keep that from happening, observe these suggestions from the American Academy of Orthopedic Surgeons:

Warm up and stretch: I know you're eager to get on with your workout. But take a few moments to warm up first. Studies show that cold muscles are more likely to be injured.

Spread out your workouts: Compressing all of your physical activity into two days a week on weekends sets you up for pain and doesn't increase your fitness level.

The rules for physical fitness are that your fitness level declines with less than 3 days of exercise per week. Your fitness level can be *maintained* by exercising three days per week, but it can't be *improved* with less than four workouts per week.

Take a lesson: It's better to spend an hour with your tennis or golf pro, or a personal trainer than to spend an hour in your doctor's waiting room. Experts can teach you how to improve your form and workout program to avoid injury.

Buy the best equipment you can afford: Especially your shoes, as described elsewhere here. This can apply to all manner of things that enhance our lives, such as musical instruments. I'll never forget how excited my younger son was when he finally was allowed to play his band leader's concert quality trombone instead of the one we got from the school when he started out. And my own improved golf scores with some Ping clubs. And my wife's improved groundstrokes after I gave her a new Sledgehammer tennis racquet for her birthday last year.

Listen to your body: Your ego may tell you that you're 28 while your body is telling you that you're 48. Listen to your body!

Take small steps: The AAOS says to use the 10% rule. That is, boost your level of physical activity by no more than 10% a week. As a sports medicine doctor for many years I have encountered dozens, perhaps hundreds, of athletes who violated this rule to their sorrow and wound up in my office with a musculoskeletal injury.

The most common of those are runners who want to run a marathon.

I recommend, particularly for those just starting out, the 5% rule. In other words don't increase your total activity more than 5% per week until you are very comfortable and set in your workouts.

In recent years, studies have been done on nursing home patients, ranging from 60 to over 90 years of age. In these studies physical therapists have gone into the facility as little as three times a week (with the permission of their physicians) to make every patient exercise within the limits of their capability. The results are startling. As many as 25 percent of patients who were totally bedridden were able to get out of bed and resume some caring for themselves. More than 30 percent of all patients were able to either go home or move into an assisted care facility where they mainly cared for themselves. Over 90 percent had some measurable improvement in their physical as well as mental conditions.

As a direct result of these studies, many of the higher quality nursing facilities now have an on-site physical therapy department.

An officer of the law for Coconino County, Arizona, for many years and a dedicated runner was not my patient but a good friend, so I won't betray a doctor-patient relationship with this revelation. The good officer desperately wanted to run the Fiesta Bowl Marathon, which used to be held on the first weekend in December every year in the Phoenix area. We who ran it would start our training the previous January and run at least 1000 miles in training for it. The better runners probably ran 2000 miles. He was, and is, very competitive; so if his times were not coming down enough by about Labor Day, he would drastically increase his weekly mileage far more than 10% per week for several weeks. Inevitably his body broke down year after year in the weeks leading up to the event. I finally asked him what his goal was, to run and finish the race, or to win it. I'm happy to be able to report that he finally did run and complete it very creditably.

Benefits of exercise: After about 25 minutes of continuous exercise, your body has used up most of the available glycogen stored for energy in your muscles and begins to burn fatty acids (cholesterol and triglycerides). So if you have elevated levels of either of these, try to extend your aerobic activities beyond the 30 minutes minimum that we now recommend.

Here is where exercise will save you BIG BUCKS, as well as enormously enhance your enjoyment of life.

There is considerable evidence that those who do aerobic exercise daily don't have as many respiratory infections as others. One theory is that exercise stimulates the immune system. Another is that the mild elevation in body temperature that occurs during exercise actually kills germs.

> *A patient of mine, who is a university professor, was putting in 60 plus miles per week with a goal of finishing the race in less than three hours. He developed a stress fracture in one tibia (the larger bone of the lower leg) three weeks before the race. He said he was going to run it even if his leg fell off. Having almost been to that point once myself, I certainly sympathized with him. I put him on an exercise bike with as much resistance as he could take for up to three hours a day to maintain his conditioning, tapering the week before the race, but no running at all. He did run and finished in just a little over three hours, not quite reaching his goal but being a very happy man.*

I suspect that both of these theories are correct. I know from personal experience in dealing with thousands of throat cultures over the years that bacteria do not grow as well if the incubator temperature is inadvertently set even no more than 1/2 to one degree above its usual 98.6 degrees.

Those with high blood pressure are able to control their pressures more easily with <u>less of the expensive medicines</u> if they exercise at least 30 minutes per day.

Those with diabetes will control their diabetes much better if daily exercise is a part of their treatment program. Those with a family history of diabetes may be able to <u>keep from getting diabetes</u> themselves if they start daily exercise when they are young and keep their weight down in the normal range.

Exercise in Children

These lessons are especially important for children: First, begin exercising your children early in life. Don't let them watch TV more than one hour <u>any</u> day, and it's much better to limit TV to weekends only. Many studies have shown that TV dulls the mind (with the possible exception of Sesame Street!), and the body isn't developing either when the TV is on.

Second, keep the child's weight within the normal range for its height and age so that extra fat cells don't develop and predispose the child to obesity later in life. You can do that by restricting empty calorie foods such as sweets, mashed potatoes, chips, etc. and promoting an hour each day (with you, perhaps) of exercise. Most kids don't need much encouragement to be physically active, given the opportunities.

Third, <u>require</u> that your kids play some kind of sports in early grade school. Insist that your school have a PE program for all grades where they are taught individual, as well as, team sports. Non-contact sports are best for most in the early school years, but some kids seem to thrive more in contact type activities. One of the best team sports in early grade school is coed soccer. Another activity that is as good or better is swimming on a team.

Studies have shown that all children who play sports a) like themselves more, b) have more self-confidence, c) suffer less depression and d) are less likely to develop drug abuse problems as they grow older.

In addition, girls are a) 60 percent less likely to get breast cancer, b) less likely to become pregnant before they want to, and c) are more likely to leave a man who beats them.

A great book on kids and sports which should be required reading for all parents was written by sports psychology expert Rick Wolff: Good Sports, the Concerned Parent's Guide to Competitive Youth Sports (Sagamore 1-800-327-5557). You can send questions to him at Parent's Guide, P.O. Box 5574, New York, NY 10185-5574.

Proper Running Technique

This will minimize impact and strain and increase efficiency so that your foot is under your knee and moving backwards when it strikes the ground, and so that it also is as flat as possible when it hits the ground. If your heel hits the ground first, the impact slows you down, as well as producing more shock to the body; while if you run on your toes, there is a lot more strain on your arches and plantar fascia (the tough membrane that covers the inside of the arch and attaches to the front of the heel).

Running late in the evening when it is quiet is a good way to get an idea about whether your technique is good. If one foot makes a noticeably louder noise when it strikes the ground than the other, then that one's technique needs attention. Ideally your feet should be absolutely silent when they strike the ground (a better description might be "when they *caress* the ground"). Getting someone to videotape you from front and back and both sides, including close-ups of your feet as you go by, may give you all the information you need for improved form.

Everything should be straight ahead as you run. Hands should reach straight ahead, rather than crossing in front of your body. Elbows should be at about a ninety-degree angle when not reaching out ahead. Toes should be pointed straight ahead, or perhaps very slightly pigeon-toed when really sprinting.

Your body should be upright instead of leaning back or forward (except when running hills -- more about that below). Your abdominal muscles should be tight, stabilizing your pelvis to aid your balance and hip rotation.

Running hills can put strain on your back, as well as the arches of your feet. To minimize back strain, lean slightly forward when you go down a hill, while leaning backward maybe four or five degrees when going upward.

Going uphill definitely requires that you run somewhat on your toes. You can minimize the stress on your arches and plantar fascia by being gentle as your toes hit the ground. Then, after they have just touched the ground, exert your full force to push you up. Don't just slam your toes down like a pile driver. The key is to exert your full force just after, not just before your forefoot hits the ground.

Going downhill you can more easily maintain the almost flat foot striking the ground if you lean forward a bit (as you might if you were a skier on a steep slope). You won't quite be able to achieve the goal of having the foot under the knee when it touches the ground, but still try to come as close as you can.

If you lean backward, your heel will consistently strike first with a thud and a lot of shock on your feet, legs, pelvis, and back -- well, actually your whole body.

What level of maximum heart rate should you strive for if you aim for the best possible cardiac fitness for your age?

A new formula is replacing the one that we used for over thirty years, thanks to a careful study of people as they grow older by some researchers in Colorado. This study is particularly valuable for those over fifty but is also good for those who are younger. **The new formula for maximum heart rate is 208 minus 0.7 times your age.** The thing that is important to remember about these set age-predicted heart rates is that one's physical age is rarely the same as the actual age in years. In other words some of us are in better shape than others, and that gap tends to widen as we get older. So pay more attention to how you feel than to attaining a particular heart rate based on this or any other formula.

I guarantee you that any continuous exercise will be beneficial, regardless of how high you get your heart rate on that day. As a runner for many years I will tell you that there are days when you may feel that you can run forever, while on other days you may feel that you have to stop much sooner or go much slower because your feet are made of lead. Be sure that it is your body and not your lazy bone talking, then listen to your body! But make daily exercise a way of life and I guarantee that you will then feel as though you are really living for your whole life.

CHAPTER 39 -- EYES

Foreign Bodies

If you get a foreign body in your eye, don't rub it or you may scratch the cornea. Try to flush it out with clean water (wash your hands first so that you don't get dirt and germs in it too.) Then someone with some experience can try to remove it with a clean Q-Tip moistened with water.

If these attempts are unsuccessful, then don't wait. Get it removed right away by a professional, because if it is metal and imbedded in the cornea, you will get a chemical reaction around it as rust forms. Then scar tissue that may be hard to see around or through may form. So get the foreign body out as soon as possible, within four to six hours ideally.

Prevention by wearing protective goggles when working in environments with a lot of dust or particles (such as when grinding or sanding) is very important.

Burns

Welding or working around welders often results in actinic, or ultraviolet burns to the eyes. Same for sunburns after a day on the water or beach. These can be very painful by the time you are ready to go to bed. Patching the eye and taking pain medication will help you heal with less pain, usually within 24 hours. However sometimes a call to your doctor will be necessary, hopefully early in the evening while the drugstore is still open so that you both can wind up with a good night's sleep. He may need to dilate your pupil for pain relief, put some other medicine in your eye, and perhaps patch it.

Chemical Burns

These are a real emergency, especially if alkali is involved. You must immediately flush the eye, with clean water if possible, or even with urine if no water is available. It sounds pretty gross to think about having someone urinating in your eye, but urine is sterile and somewhat acidic, so it can literally save the eye of someone with alkali in it. I know of such a case.

Flush out the eye as quickly as you can, for as long as you can, then head for the doctor. If alkali was involved, he will irrigate the eye for probably another 30 minutes or more with sterile saline, then put in medication and patch it.

Infections

These are almost always caused by someone coughing or sneezing in your face, or by rubbing your eyes with germ-laden fingers. Most are viral and these usually get well by themselves in about three days. The viral infections have red eyes with mostly clear tearing.

Bacterial infections, on the other hand, usually secrete pus. In both cases the lids may be stuck shut in the morning.

Medicated eye drops may give relief in the viral infections, but antibiotic drops or ointment are usually needed for the bacterial ones.

Always wash your hands before touching the eyes, and after putting medicine in them so that you don't spread the germs around.

Styes

These are little pimples on the edges of the eyelids. They may be centered around an infected eyelash. If so, removing the eyelash may drain and cure it.

Chalazions

These are little abscesses inside the eyelids. These may respond to hot compresses, as styes usually do, but they often hang around and wind up needing surgical drainage. Antibiotics are not very effective.

Sore Eyes

Particularly when accompanied by headaches late in the day, these can mean that you need new glasses or contacts, or a better-lit working area; or your computer monitor screen may be too bright or too dim, or not positioned correctly. Reflections and glare are distracting, and the lettering on the screen may appear a little fuzzy.

For touch typists, the screen should be directly in front of your eyes as you sit up straight. This will also help prevent sore necks. For a fuller discussion of ideal computer ergonomics, please see the chapter on **Work-Related Injuries**.

Aids to avoiding and dealing with eyestrain include frequently looking at a far away wall or outside, actually focusing sharply at that distant point for a few seconds at a time. Another little trick is to look cross-eyed two or three times an hour. (Don't worry, your eyes won't get stuck in that position -- just close your eyes if you want to quit.). These actions allow the eye muscles to totally relax in the first case for a few seconds, and to strengthen your eye focusing muscles in the second case.

I have a pair of glasses that are actually focused exactly on the distance I sit away from the monitor. I used to have considerable tiredness after a couple of hours at the keyboard. No more. I started to pay attention to what I was recommending to my patients -- "physician, heal thyself"

Protect Your Eyes

This is very important when participating in sports which carry significant risk of injury. These include collision sports, such as football, hockey, lacrosse, and rugby; contact sports, such as baseball, basketball, soccer, and wrestling; racquet sports, fencing, and any other sport involving the use of a ball, bat, racquet, or stick.

Boxing, wrestling, and martial arts are considered very high-risk sports for eye injury because eye protection is not normally worn.

Polycarbonate protective eyewear is many times stronger than most other materials, and it also protects against ultraviolet sunrays. They can be obtained in prescription glasses. They can be combined with other protection, such as a helmet, face cage or mask, and sports goggles. **People with single eye vision especially should wear eye protection at all times.**

The following companies specialize in protective eyewear:

Black Knight USA (Viking Sports)
5355 Sierra Road
San Jose, CA 95132   1-800-535-3300
Eagle Safety Eyewear
Web address: www.eaglesafety.com

Ektelon
1 Sportsystem Plaza
Bordentown, NJ 08505-9630 1-800-283-2635

Face Guard Inc.
P.O. Box 901
Salem, VA 24513   1-800-336-9683

Itech Sports Products
825 F, rue Tecumseh
Dollard-des-Ormeaux
Quebec H9R 4T8   1-800-361-5595

Liberty Optical
REC SPECS Sports Vision Equipment
380 Verona Ave.
Newark, NJ 07104   1-800-444-5010

Shutt Sports Group
1200 East Union
Litchfield, IL 62056

CHAPTER 40 -- FAINTING

If the face is red, raise the head. If the face is pale raise the tail. Most fainting is not due to a serious condition. That said, please be aware that in a number of really serious conditions fainting is the first visible symptom. Three very common benign causes of loss of consciousness due to fainting that I have seen literally hundreds of times are:

Hyperventilation Due to Intense Excitement or Intense Anxiety

The loss of brain function in this condition is due to breathing out your body's carbon dioxide faster than the body produces it, thus lowering the level in the blood to where the brain doesn't function properly.

Just losing consciousness and lying down for a few seconds will allow the body's automatic breathing regulator in the brain stem to slow the respiration until the CO_2 builds back up.

People pass out on the parade ground on a warm day, as in a military formation.

Reviewing the troops, particularly on a holiday, usually took a long time, and inevitably there would be a few who literally fell out of the formation. What happens is that the blood in the legs doesn't return very well to the heart unless the muscles of the legs are contracting and squeezing the blood upward fairly constantly, as discussed at more length in the section on pulmonary embolism. Thus, in warm weather especially, all the blood vessels in the legs dilate to their fullest, and a very large amount of blood is trapped down there in troops who are standing at Parade Rest or Attention. When enough is taken out of the circulation that the brain isn't getting its required ration, the person faints and falls to the ground. Falling to the ground cures the problem because then the blood in the legs doesn't have to flow upwards against gravity and the brain quickly wakes up. I have seen this happen to a pregnant lady while waiting in a long checkout line at the grocery store and many other similar situations.

The respiratory centers essentially have two on-off switching areas. The one that kicks in first is the carbon dioxide center. That works just fine as the primary driver of breathing rate except for when one has emphysema, or COPD, which is usually from smoking. In that condition the blood CO_2 is chronically so high that the CO_2 center loses its sensitivity. In that case breathing then has to be driven by the center that is sensitive to the blood oxygen saturation. If someone with COPD is not carefully monitored when they get bad enough to need oxygen, the very administration of oxygen may turn off the O_2 center. In that case the person just stops breathing. And death occurs, usually in the middle of the night. This is more likely to occur in someone on home oxygen if the O_2 flow is increased too much, but I have seen it happen even in pretty good hospitals before we started putting everyone who needed oxygen in the Intensive Care Unit (ICU).

The third common cause of fainting is what we refer to as a vaso-vagal reaction.

This involves a function of the vagus nerve, which, among other things, controls heart rate. What happens is that the blood essentially just drains out of the head. It may be produced by anxiety, as in waiting in line for shots or after getting the shots, again in the military. Another example is the person who insists on sitting up and watching his or her wound repaired. The sight of the blood and interior tissues of the body causes the person to faint.

So it is best to lie down when you get a shot or a wound repaired. And don't watch someone having a wound repaired or we could be sewing you up too. Smelling salts (spirits of ammonia) usually quickly takes care of vaso-vagal faintness; so does lying down, but preferably slowly.

I was the team doctor for the high school basketball team for seven years in Warsaw, Indiana. We usually had a very good team. One of the boys from the Tigers' State Championship team after I left played for the Hickory team in the movie Hoosiers. As you may have heard, love of basketball is programmed into our DNA in that state. Every year, especially during those exciting tournament games, I would be called away from the team bench on the floor to attend at least one sweet young lady who had passed out in the stands. I usually just had her breathe into an empty popcorn bag held over her nose and mouth until the carbon dioxide built back up in her blood stream to where her brain started to function properly again, and she would be fine.

The most dramatic case I had was a young mother who assured me that she had to be there and would be fine as I repaired a laceration on her child in the ER. The child and I were doing fine, but suddenly I heard a sickening thud as the mother's head hit the floor. A nearby nurse who saw her fall said that she fell backwards in slow motion like an old Mack Sennet movie. Fortunately the ER floor was padded, and she didn't suffer any head damage, but she could have. A doctor who used to practice across the street from me had a teenaged patient who passed out after a shot as she was waiting to check out with the receptionist, striking her head on the unpadded floor hard enough to sustain a mild skull fracture.

When I was a new junior in medical school, I went to work as an extern at the Central State Hospital for mental patients in Indianapolis. That place had been the epitome of the bad snake pit mental hospitals of the late 19th and first half of the 20th centuries. It was composed of seven patient buildings on a pretty wooded campus, containing about 3,000 men and women. One of the buildings contained the truly violent and criminally insane inmates. All were locked wards when I went to work.

Dr. C. L. Williams took over as superintendent about a year and a half before I arrived, and he quickly began the slow process of bringing it into the 20th century. Doing this in spite of state budget constraints was quite a challenge. But he was up to it.

He brought in a full time recreational therapist. He brought in a semi-retired general practitioner with heart trouble to run what was called the "Sick Hospital" during the day. This was a separate building. He couldn't afford a full psychiatric staff, so he brought in four junior and four senior medical students to care for the medically sick on nights and weekends and be in charge of several wards of patients for their psychiatric needs also. I was one of the second wave of those students, which were called "externs." We lived on the campus, and those of us with wives lived in a little motel area. The wives were given full-time jobs at the hospital.

Other things Dr. Williams did:

He had the buildings fumigated (when I came, just my unlocking and opening the door of a ward would send hundreds of cockroaches scurrying for cover. By the time I left two years later, the cockroaches were totally gone.)

He had every patient undergo a physical and short mental examination. We medical students did these during our off quarters in school. What a revelation! We found all manner of disease processes. Besides that we found a number of people who were apparently well. The most extreme case I found was an 80-year-old very neat and mentally alert lady who had been at Central State for 30 years. Her little room was very tastefully decorated, and it was not locked. She had evidently had a nervous breakdown when her husband suddenly died and was committed by the court. She had no other family, so there she stayed for 30 years. When I examined her, reviewed the ward records, and talked to the long-time ward attendants, I concluded that she had probably been normal for the past 29 years! With no family the best we could do for her was to let her go shopping with her attendant friends and go home with them to stay for weekends and holidays.

When I first started working there, the summer nights were filled with the yells of tormented insane patients. During my first year, the drug Thorazine began to be used as a psychotic agent. By the time I left CSH, there were <u>no</u> night noises of any kind from patients. And all the wards except for the criminally insane were open, with patients free to come and go as they were able.

You are probably wondering by now what this has to do with fainting. You'll see in a moment. This just seemed like a good excuse to tell a story with some happy endings.

> The first night I was on call at CSH, July 3, I believe, I received a phone call from the Sick Hospital to come and repair a wound above the eyebrow on a man with Parkinson's Disease who had fallen as he tried to go to the bathroom in the middle of the night.
>
> On a July night in Indiana, the man was pretty sweaty. In addition, he was taking some medication that had a very putrid odor. In addition, he had cut an artery, so was bleeding a lot, and I had trouble getting it stopped for a few minutes.
>
> Now, I had never seen anyone sewed up before; consequently I had taken a quick look in my surgery textbook for wound repair methods before I left my room. So I was a little slow doing everything for the first time. The various odors, the lack of air-conditioning in those days, and the sight of what was in reality only two or three ounces of blood, soon led to one of the attendants who were helping to keep the patient from shaking himself off the table to turn pale and tell me that he would have to leave the room. The second attendant soon followed. In another ten minutes or so, the male nurse said that he would also have to leave.
>
> By that time, I was definitely feeling a little queasy myself; so I told him, "No, you stay here. I'm going outside!" So I put a clamp on the bleeder finally, went outside, sat down on a bench and put my head between my knees. Soon the blood came back to my brain, and I went back and did a pretty good job of stitching him up. (My grandmother taught me to sew before I was five years old, so I knew most of what I needed to know. I just didn't know what a needle holder was; so I sewed by holding the curved needle with my fingers!) I've never felt faint even for a moment since, though I'll confess that I have sometimes felt sick inside.
>
> This little story, then, is a really good example of the vaso-vagal reflex that makes people faint, as it affected four people trying to help care for one patient -- who by the way, felt no pain at all.

Fainting During Exercise

A potentially more serious type of fainting is that which occurs during exercise. We in Sports Medicine should always ask, in the sports physicals that are required before a young school pupil can participate in sports for that year, whether he or she has ever fainted or felt like fainting while exercising. This type occasionally means that the heart is not functioning as it should and needs a full cardiac evaluation before the student can be released to play.

If this type of loss of consciousness ever occurs to you as an adult, you need to head for the Emergency Room immediately. Call 911. Let me reassure you, however, that if you have been running and suddenly stop without warming down for a minute or five, and feel faint, that may be just the blood staying in the muscles instead of returning to the heart.

The key is that if you are still exercising when you faint, it may be something serious, whereas if the fainting occurs after you suddenly stop, it is very likely to be benign.

People who are anemic (for example the student who has just donated blood and then has to run to avoid being late to class) may have this problem during exercise, as may those who live at sea level and exercise too vigorously at high altitude. This type simply needs a few minutes of rest, preferably lying down.

If the face is pale, raise the tail. If the face is red, raise the head.

CHAPTER 41 -- FALLS IN THE ELDERLY

These are all too common and potentially very serious in older people. The indirect mortality rate from hip fractures, for example, is enough to constitute an epidemic. The injuries that falls cause are often the beginning of the end of a normal quality of life, as well as the first of the toppling dominoes that soon begin to fall ever faster as the elderly person becomes unable to maintain the activities of daily living that are so very important to him or her.

The long stay in bed that frequently results from broken bones below the waist has a very bad effect upon the immune system, the heart and lungs, the digestive system, the brain, and of course the muscles and joints. But also a fracture *anywhere* may have a bad effect upon the individual's abilities to cope with multiple aspects of their lives. And these injuries interfere with what the elderly value most -- their independence.

Preventing falls, then, can add literally *years* to the quality and length of lives of persons of advanced age. The people themselves need to be on the lookout for ways to protect themselves just by the use of common sense (as in, no touch football after a certain age). In addition those who love and help to at least partially care for an older friend or relative should watch for potentially hazardous things that can be changed to make the environment safer.

This chapter will provide a lot of information on what sort of things may put the older person at risk for injury due to falling along with preventive strategies.

** First, if you have in recent years had a fall, be sure to tell your doctor about it because one fall almost inevitably leads to another unless some positive step is taken in prevention.

Medications

Medications (particularly those for high blood pressure) may cause drops in your blood pressure when you stand up, thus causing you to feel a little faint and perhaps lose your balance.

Prevention: Ask your doctor to always check your blood pressure in the standing as well as sitting positions to make sure it doesn't fall too much when you stand. Normally your pressure will stay about the same or even go up somewhat when you stand up, due to the carotid sinus reflex described elsewhere in this book. Those on BP medicine, however, don't have the same reflex to raise it when you stand up.

A woozy feeling is common after a meal, when you have been quietly sitting while about half of your blood has been diverted to your stomach and intestines to take part in the digestion of the food you have just eaten.

A good trick, especially after eating but also in a church pew and elsewhere, is to always sit forward in your chair and take a deep breath or two before standing up each time. The deep breath creates a slight negative pressure in your chest and literally sucks more blood up there for your heart to pump uphill to your brain. Another trick is to bend your ankle two or three times, which causes the calf muscles to squeeze blood upward.

Other types of medications that can increase the risk of a fall, more so in the elderly, are those that affect your nervous system, such as anti-psychosis drugs, anti-depressants, anti-anxiety meds (like Valium), drugs for controlling your heart rhythm, digoxin for the heart, and diuretics.

Illnesses

Illnesses, particularly of the heart and lungs, may produce these symptoms.

Arthritic Changes

Arthritic changes in the joints, along with associated **muscle weakness** may reduce one's ability to maintain a stable balance of the body when walking around or trying to move suddenly. The quadriceps muscles of the front of the thighs are the most important in that regard. Of all the muscles in the body, they are the most important in enabling a person to be independently mobile. They weaken rapidly, within a matter of days, in any condition (as a sore knee or ankle) that keeps them from being used a lot on a daily basis.

Sit on a high chair or a counter, attaching some weights to the ankle (perhaps with a belt or a handbag), and then straighten the knee from the 90 degree hanging down position in sets of ten repetitions several times each day. This will help to maintain their strength during some injury that is restricting your walking, or to increase their strength when they are already weak by gradually increasing the weight on the ankle and/or the number of repetitions each day. Riding a stationary bicycle is also excellent for these muscles, as well as helping the mobility of both the knee and the ankle. Walking in the water is very good, as is stepping up and down on a step (as while watching TV) if your condition allows it.

Gentle stretching of the hips, knees, and ankles will improve their flexibility and your ability to move around in a coordinated fashion that reduces the risk of catching your foot on some small obstacle on the ground.

Older people tend to shuffle rather than pick up their feet as they walk. This leads to tripping over relatively small obstructions on the ground or floor. Always look where you are walking. Select glasses that have only part of the lower part of your glasses as the bifocal, with the rest set for distance vision so that you can see the floor by just tilting your head slightly. Practice picking up your feet a little when you walk.

Shoes

Your shoes, as well as certain **conditions of the feet**, may affect the way you bear your weight enough to throw you off balance unexpectedly.

High-heeled shoes, platform shoes, shoes with pointed toes, and shoes with rubber on the tips of the toes may cause you to catch the foot and trip, on the grass or a rug, for example, or lose your balance enough to fall.

Pain

Pain in an area of one or both feet can make you walk awkwardly, not in a coordinated manner. Calluses and large corns, tendonitis, heel spurs, and bursitis certainly fit this category.

Long Toenails

Long toenails may catch in the carpet, especially a shag. Foot deformities from arthritis or bunions may impair your balance. If you can't see well enough or can't bend over enough to take proper care of your feet, then you must find someone to help you, perhaps even your doctor or a podiatrist. Some barber and beauty shops have pedicure capabilities that cost a lot less than a doctor's care.

Impaired Vision

Impaired vision prevents you from being able to properly watch where you are going, something of tremendous importance in the elderly, but also of considerable interest to the rest of us. Such a problem might be from cataracts, from the need for adjustment of an eyeglass prescription, or from failure to adjust quickly enough to changes in lighting, or to other reduced contrast sensitivity, so that the person may not easily locate the edge of the stairs or curbs.

People who have problems with contrast should put brightly colored tape on the edges of steps in the home and curbs outside the house.

More on Medications:

Multiple medications may interact to cause faintness, dizziness, or drowsiness. Most drugs' doses need to be cut in half in the elderly, because many don't tolerate the full normal doses used without problems in younger people. This is especially true if the kidneys are not functioning normally. Nerve and sleeping medicines in particular need to be either greatly reduced or completely avoided in the elderly.

Hazards in the Home

Elderly people tend to shuffle instead of picking up their feet as they walk, so these are especially important:

Shag carpets and rugs.

Cluttered rooms that leave little room to move around obstacles.

Poor lighting to see possible obstacles.

Telephone cords lying across walking areas.

I had a lady in the office the other day who was wearing high-heeled shoes while walking up the wide concrete walk area in front of a new office complex. She had no reason to suspect that there was any risk to this flat and apparently smooth area, so she wasn't looking down at all. Somehow she caught the toe of her shoe in a crack about 3/4 to 1 inch wide as she stepped forward, which caused her to fall heavily onto both knees. The abrasions, bruising, and swelling she sustained kept her on crutches for several days. Fortunately she was 29 years old, suffered no fractures, and healed quickly but was still sore for about two weeks. Had she been 69 or (horrors) 79, she might still be laid up! Failure to use her vision, rather than impairment, was a cause of this accident. An attorney might argue a design flaw in the sidewalk. But that's another story!

Little rugs that slide, especially in bathrooms and kitchens and other rooms with slick floors under the rugs.

Bathtubs and showers without non-skid material on the floor of the tub, as well as bathtubs and showers without bars to hold onto pose a very high risk for falls. Actually they are risky for even young people.

Carpet that sticks up higher than the floor surface in an adjacent room -- as in walking from a room with a hardwood floor into a carpeted room.

The toes of certain types of shoes tend to catch or stick in the ground or carpet.

So, if you are relatively young yourself but have elderly house guests, do the inspection recommended above for your own house, as well as for your elderly relatives and friends.

> My kids' great aunt was eating lunch at her kitchen table, which, along with the chairs, was located on a large shag rug in the home of her much-younger sister (the kids' grandmother) whom she was visiting in Sun City, Arizona. When the phone rang, she tried to hurry to answer it. But she caught the chair leg in the rug and fell, breaking her hip, and setting in motion the chain of events that led to her death a couple of weeks later.
>
> I knew about that rug. I had caught my own chair leg on it. But I never anticipated that her younger and still vigorous sister might have an old and somewhat infirm visitor.
>
> One other thing, don't be such a slave to a ringing phone that you risk injuring yourself. After all, it may be a telemarketer.

If you feel unsteady when you walk, use a cane, a walking stick, a walker, crutches, or whatever else may be available by the time you read this.

If you need and decide to use one of the above walking aids for assistance, be sure to get training in their proper use, or they may make matters worse. A cane, for example, should be held in the opposite hand from the weak side. That way your right hand, for example, with the cane in it will go forward at the same time as the left foot, thus maintaining the normal walking balance of the body.

Exercise

Exercise, to the limit of your capability, is of the utmost importance in the elderly. As we have noted elsewhere in this book, we are aiming for at least 30 minutes of moderate physical activity each day of your life. Start with whatever you can do today, and add one minute each day till you get to 30 minutes. You don't have to stop at 30 minutes, but you should plan to do at least that much as long as you live.

If some muscle begins to hurt, back off until it feels better, perhaps doing an entirely different activity for awhile. So-called cross training is good. In this you never do the same thing two days in a row, but you still do something for at least 30 minutes. One day you may walk outdoors or on a treadmill, the next do a stationary bike, the next swim or walk in a pool, and so on. Another little gimmick is to get a pedometer, which will count the number of steps you take in a day. We are aiming for at least 10,000 steps per day.

If you are concerned about possible safety while walking, consider going to a mall, many of which open their doors early for walkers before the stores actually open.

Tai chi helps with balance, aerobic activity, and the classes provide much-enjoyed social activities. Yoga activities help to increase your range of motion of most joints, thus helping your automatic balance mechanisms, Practice standing up straight, perhaps against a wall, making your back as flat as you can against the wall while flattening your tummy muscles as much as possible for about 30 seconds at a time.

I once had a very nice <u>old</u> lady, who had terrible problems with her balance, which we had no cure for. She absolutely refused to use a cane or anything else that might "make people think I'm old!!!" She wasn't "old" she was <u>very old,</u> at about 95. But she never admitted that she might actually <u>be</u> old. I regret to have to report that she didn't use a cane when no one was around; she did fall, did break her hip, and did die very soon thereafter.

When you are talking on the telephone, practice standing and balancing on just one foot for 30 seconds at a time, alternating feet, and possibly lightly using your other hand against the wall or phone stand for balance.

Ballroom dancing, which is offered in many retirement communities, is good for the body, and your mental outlook as well.

Park at the back of the parking lot. Use the stairs instead of the elevator if you can. Almost <u>any</u> exercise is better than none.

When you are sitting, lift and straighten your lower legs 10 or 20 times or more every hour. That will strengthen your quad muscles, the most important ones for balance.

If you time your activities for a day, you may be surprised at how much time you spend sitting around doing little or nothing in the way of physical activity. That may get your attention enough to make you "stir your sticks," as one of Mark Twain's characters used to say. You will be adding to the quality, and probably also the quantity, of your life.

*Another patient in our clinic this week had been in to see me for possible Alzheimer's Disease a couple of months ago. She was brought in by her son, a college professor with whom she lived in her own room. Her long list of medications included four from the list of drugs that should not be used in the elderly (see the chapter on **Drugs in the Elderly**). I recommended that she stop taking all of them. According to her son this week, within two weeks "it was like the difference between night and day." She became mentally sharp and began to walk better, although still needing a walker. Unfortunately she decided she could do without her walker night before last and fell in her bedroom, fracturing her wrist but thank goodness not her hip.*

I have not inspected her room for possible impediments, but she is definitely another illustration of two common problems that must be paid attention to as we age or care for an aged one.

CHAPTER 42 -- FAMILY SAFETY

Beach Safety

To stay safe at the beach, don't turn your back on the ocean; beware of coming tides with occasional large, unexpected random or rogue waves; and stay off driftwood logs, especially on wet sand and in surf. This type of sudden single very large wave has claimed the lives of at least 19 people along the Oregon coast in the past ten years. Eight of the fatalities involved wave-tossed logs. Washington and northern California beaches are also at risk for these phenomena. The Oregon Parks and Recreation Department has an extensive beach safety education program. For more information, contact them at 503-378-4168, extension 302, and ask for Bob Smith.

Sleep Safety

Never sleep with your baby in your bed with you. There have been many cases where the infant somehow slipped down under the covers and suffocated. That happened to a six-month-old baby that I personally delivered.

If someone sleeps in a top bunk bed, be sure you have the short rail attachment on the side so that he or she can't roll over and fall out of bed during the night.

Carbon Monoxide

This is a colorless, odorless poison gas, which is produced by the incomplete burning of fuels, such as charcoal, coal, gasoline, methane, oil, propane, tobacco, and wood. It results when there is not enough oxygen for the fuel to burn completely and turn into harmless carbon dioxide.

Natural gas also is a potential source of poison gas in our homes, but it has an odor artificially added to it so that we can smell it when we first walk into the house. The odor goes away as our noses adapt to bad odors in just two or three minutes. So pay attention. If your nose tells you something is wrong, it probably is. Leave the door open, and go to a neighbor's home to call the gas company. Do <u>not</u> go back into the house until cleared by the gas company. It could explode.

The potential sources of carbon monoxide around our homes are an auto, gas lawn mower, or snow blower running in an attached garage, charcoal grills, fireplaces, furnaces, non-electric room heaters, stoves, and water heaters. Coleman-type heaters used for camping are potentially a problem if used inside a tent or vehicle.

I have seen numerous cases of carbon monoxide poisoning, most from improperly-adjusted or leaky furnaces.

> *I have seen the death of a beautiful young woman who lived in a trailer with her dog. She was using a charcoal grill to warm the trailer in winter. Another time a man was cooking on a charcoal grill in his trailer when his dog suddenly collapsed. He rushed outside with the dog, not knowing what was happening until the vet told him that the dog had died of carbon monoxide poisoning. When he came to me an hour or so later, he still had a dangerously high carbon monoxide level in his own blood. But he was alive and recovered completely.*

> *One tragedy I encountered during my internship was a young couple who were doing what young people do in the middle of winter in a car with the heater going. The only problem was that the car was parked in a garage with the motor running. They were discovered the next morning after the car had run out of gas. I have known of many successful suicides by this route. One which was not successful is found elsewhere in this book.*

One good thing about it, if you don't die or become unconscious, you should get completely well in a few hours as oxygen gradually replaces the gas in your red blood cells.

Prevention is usually easy, at least for the furnace. Just have the gas company check your furnace every year in September before you start using it for the winter. They offer this service for a nominal fee, and it is well worth it. Actually you will often save the cost of the call in lower gas bills because the furnace will be adjusted for maximum efficiency.

Your cooking stoves and ovens should burn with an almost-invisible blue flame. If the flame is yellow, then incomplete burning is producing carbon monoxide. This may be caused by jets that aren't adjusted properly to allow enough oxygen to mix with the gas.

In a sudden case, such as a family of ten I cared for on Christmas Day one year, the kids may be vomiting along with the headache, while some of the adults may be nauseated. Some may not have a headache, but just nausea. One or two may just not feel well in general. This family thought that they all had food poisoning.

When they called me, I told them to open all the windows and doors while I was on my way. When I entered the house my nose confirmed my phone diagnosis. But within two or three minutes my nose had adapted, and I couldn't smell anything bad anymore. (This happens even with the smell of skunks, though long-dead bodies are another story.) Within a few hours the gas company had fixed the leak, the kids weren't sick to their stomachs, neighbors had brought over Christmas goodies, and a very thankful family survived to have a late opening of presents. So it was a happy ending to what was close to a terrible family disaster.

Check vents and chimneys at least twice a year for improper connections or visible stains or rust.

The following <u>appliance malfunctions</u> may indicate improper operation, with potential gas or carbon monoxide problems:

Running out of hot water too soon.

Furnace runs all the time or can't seem to heat the house.

Accumulation of soot, especially on gas appliances.

Unfamiliar or burning odor when you first walk into the house.

The next best thing is to have carbon monoxide detectors in your house. You can get them everywhere hardware is sold. Be sure they meet the present UL 2034 or International Approval Services 6-96 standards. Also be sure the batteries are good each year. Place one near each sleeping area in homes with fuel-burning appliances, a fireplace, or an attached garage. Test them every month.

These detectors are not a substitute for smoke alarms. You must have several of those around the house too. Be sure that everyone in the family knows the difference in the alarm sounds.

Symptoms of Carbon Monoxide or Natural Gas Exposure

Headache, especially if more than one person in the house has one. These typically clear up within an hour or so after leaving home in the morning and appear again late in the evening or during the night. Along with these may be an unexplained elevated blood pressure, fatigue and lack of energy; sometimes shortness of breath is the only symptom. Dizziness and even unstable walking are other possible symptoms.

Call your plumber from a neighbor's phone. The gas company, if you call them, will not charge you for the repair if it's minor. But in most states they will have to do a pressure test after their repairs are completed. If the pressure test finds that your gas lines are leaking under pressure (more likely in an older house), you may then be liable for a repair bill up to a thousand dollars or more.

A plumber, on the other hand, will be able to find the leak, fix it, and will not be required to do the pressure test. He will test all connections for leaks and fix everything he finds under normal pressure. Just as safe, in my opinion, and likely to be much cheaper than the gas company in the long run.

Driving Safety

Never drive after drinking any alcohol. Even one drink impairs your reflex reaction time by 10%. This translates as follows: Let's assume that it normally takes thirty feet to stop on a dry road when you are traveling at 20 miles per hour and you have to stop suddenly. Your reflexes are perfect, and you stop just a foot from the other guy's bumper. No harm done, right? Maybe the other driver hears the screech of your tires, but that's all. Now suppose that

> *These rules for prevention are cast in concrete:*
> *Never burn charcoal indoors or in a closed garage.*
> *Never use a gas range or oven for heating.*
> *Never leave a car running in a garage. Don't start your car and let it warm up in the morning while still sitting in the garage, even with the garage door open.*
> *Never operate unvented fuel-burning appliances in a closed room.*
> *Never use charcoal or fuel-burning stoves, lanterns, or heaters inside a tent, trailer, or motor home.*
> *If your carbon monoxide detector goes off, you must immediately open the doors, turn off fuel-burning appliances, including the furnace, and leave the house. But if you smell the natural gas smell (natural gas currently isn't detected by most carbon monoxide detectors), just open the door and leave as quickly as possible, leaving the door open behind you. Don't light a match! Don't stop to turn off anything; don't use the telephone; and especially don't turn any electrical switch. That might make a tiny spark that could cause an explosion.*

you had just one beer 30 minutes ago. It now takes you 3 more feet to stop (10% slower reaction time). This time you stop two feet into the other car's trunk! You aren't legally drunk, but you were in an accident that wouldn't have happened without that one drink. Think about it. (See the chapter on **Alcohol** for more.)

> *While we are on the subject, I have noted (actually it has been forcibly impressed upon me) that my kids don't feel comfortable riding with me when I'm driving -- me who is rated by my insurance company as one of the safest drivers on the road! I decided to analyze why and found that my attention definitely wanders when I'm trying to catch up on their far-flung lives at holiday time. When I'm driving alone or with my wife, I'm not very good company because all my antennas and senses are out checking on what is going on around us. My attention span is considerably narrowed when I'm driving with my kids.*
>
> *As I was writing this chapter I became acutely aware of this aspect of driving safety when I rode the other night with one of the safest drivers I know. He didn't speak two words in 30 minutes. Then I realized that he wasn't being antisocial but was just concentrating on what he should have been.*

> ***Never even start the car until everyone is buckled up.*** *I had a patient who died when the car was hit as it pulled out of the driveway while she just starting to buckle up. The patient hit the door and was thrown out on the street, striking her head, with enough internal damage inside her skull to kill her. No one else in the car, all of whom were buckled up, was even slightly injured.*

Never drive while talking on a cell phone, not even the hands-free ones. Anything that takes your attention away from the full focus on the road around you increases your risk of accident. Several states have reported cell phone use involved in 25-50% of auto accidents in the past two years. Does that mean that if everyone stops drinking and using cell phones there won't be any accidents? In your dreams! But the number of accidents would sure go down for a change.

Child Safety

(See also **Protecting Your Children**)

Your children will get sick and tired of you telling them how to protect themselves before they are grown. But your absolute validation will occur when you hear your grandchildren tell you something you taught their parents 20 or 25 years before.

Dogs

As I write this, I have had to very carefully repair wounds on the face from dog bites in five little kids in the past four weeks. These were little guys whose faces were about on the same level as the mouths of the dogs that bit them. Three were family pets, and two were known neighbor dogs. The little kids were doing what they do: hugging and petting the dogs, without being mean to them as older kids sometimes are if their parents haven't taught them any better. (**Teach your kids to be kind to animals!**)

I literally grew up with a German Shepherd. My sister and I subjected that poor magnificent creature to every possible indignity, riding on her, dressing her up in human clothes, sleeping with our heads on her tummy, rolling over and over with her, and who knows what else. She was our fierce protector, but the most gentle animal I can imagine to this day. A different dog we had after her death bit my best friend when he came into our yard while my sister was there. In that case, there was no question that he thought he was protecting her.

So, don't let your kids ever play with or even touch animals that aren't their own pet, not even the dog of their best friend. Especially teach them to leave sleeping dogs alone. Teach them that they can bite.

If you have a dog, never leave your child alone with it. If the dog ever snarls at or acts any way but absolutely loving toward your child, get rid of it that very minute! If a strange or a known neighbor dog comes into your yard when your child is there, take your child in the house immediately, while at the same time warning her that she must stay away from any dog that isn't hers (or his.) Do not try to get your child to hold out her hand to touch that "nice doggie."

As I write this I have a one inch long reddish-purple scar on my right forearm where a beautiful golden retriever named Butch, the pet of a neighbor of ours and my wife's best doggie friend, bit me while I was petting him through the fence a month ago. I have petted him dozens of times and often fed him dog biscuits, and I thought we were friends. But about thirty seconds after I started to pet and rub his back this time, he suddenly snarled, jerked his head up, and took a chunk of skin out of my arm. That was only the second time in my life I had been bitten. The first time was by a pit bull who had gotten out of his yard and nailed me as I was out jogging several years ago. Dogs like me normally, probably because I like them. I don't know what happened with the golden, but he'll get no more back rubs nor dog goodies from me!

The dog bite wounds I have repaired number in the <u>hundreds</u>. And I can't stress too strongly that <u>animals have teeth for a reason</u>. It is their nature to use them for attack or defense.

Dogs can be wonderful friends, and I have had several. But they bite with little or no provocation, and we must protect our kids from that even remote possibility.

Getting Lost

When I was in the first grade we learned a song that I remember to this day about what to do if we ever got lost. "Remember your name and address, and telephone number too. Walk up to that nice policeman, the very first one you meet. Then he'll be kind, and help you find, the loved ones who wait for you." Or something like that. Anyway, teach them that people who work in stores and restaurants are likely to also be glad to help them. They should just walk in and say they are lost and ask for help. Under no circumstances should they go away with anybody who isn't a police person.

Kidnapping

Teach your kids to <u>never</u> get into the car of a stranger. That includes anyone they don't know that says he or she is a friend of the kid's parents. That includes anybody who stops to give your child a ride on a rainy day.

> *I was chagrined when a little neighbor child from a block up the street in Flagstaff refused a ride from me in a thunderstorm one day several years ago. But the little kid definitely did the right thing!*

Lightning

Summer thunderstorms are fun and exciting to watch, but lightning injures more than 1,000 people a year in our country. Here are a few of the things to avoid so that you and your family will not be part of those statistics.

Almost everyone knows to avoid lone trees, swimming pools, and golf courses in electrical storms. Also don't talk on the telephone, and don't take a bath or shower. Here's why.

Lightning occurs when the clouds build up an electrical charge so high that it has to be released to somewhere on the ground. The most likely place that it will hit is the highest point in an area, which may be the tree you are standing under.

If it does hit your tree, the very least that will happen is that you will be knocked down. If you are touching the tree, the bolt may travel down the tree till it gets to where you are touching it, then go the rest of the way to the ground through your body. That is an experience that those who have lived through it don't want to repeat. The most that can happen when the bolt hits the tree is that the tree and you will explode in flames. Never stand under <u>any</u> tree to try to keep dry if you are caught out in such a storm.

Your heart may stop but respond to a hard blow to the chest and CPR from a bystander. I have had three patients who survived in that way. <u>It is safe to help such a victim</u>. They aren't still electrified, unlike those who are touching a live electrical wire, or are in water that a live wire is down in.

Also electric utility poles have the same risk as trees. So avoid them by as many feet as possible when running by them to get out of the rain.

If you want to watch the storm and have a choice, do it from inside a building, preferably one that does <u>not</u> have a lightning rod on the roof.

Electricity loves to travel through water; so if you are at a swimming pool or an old swimming hole, get out of the water. If you are at home, stay out of the shower and bathtub. The metal pipes in the house are supposed to be grounded to divert the charge into the ground, but many contractors cut this corner.

The theory of lightning rods is that the bolt will hit the rod and travel down the wire into the ground without damage to the house. Sounds good, but our neighbor across the street in Warsaw, Indiana, had such a thing happen during a magnificent storm. About an hour later one of their kids came running over to see if we could help put out the fire until the fire department got there from across the lake. Well, we did, and the house was saved. But it had a severely burned area along the grounding wire from the metal rod on the roof all the way to the ground. It had burned completely through the wood into the attic before the smell from there alerted our friends.

Another story that did not turn out so well occurred when lightning struck the electrical pole 50 yards from my grandparents' old farmhouse in Kansas and traveled to the house on the wire. The instant fire burned the house to the ground. My grandmother didn't mind the loss of her two-week-old new kitchen nearly so much as the loss of her antique hand-pumped organ.

Remember when looking for shelter. Partially covered roofed structures such as baseball dugouts, and gazebos may have wire fences attached to them. The electrical charges can run along the fence just as it did the wire to my grandparents' home.

If you live at any kind of elevation, be sure your water pipes, as well as your electric lines, are grounded with the heaviest duty wire onto a metal rod driven deeply into the ground.

Golf courses often sound an alarm when lightning is observed anywhere near the course. A golfer in the middle of the fairway is an irresistible target on his backswing or follow-through. Get into a shack. Or just lie down in a depressed area of the ground or in a ditch (away from your clubs) so that you won't be the tallest object in the area.

> *I was standing in a storm shack at a great golf course south of Sedona, Arizona, one summer afternoon in August when a sudden storm hit. My companion and I saw a bolt hit a pine tree a couple of hundred yards down the fairway and literally explode.*

Mountains are a bad place to be in a storm. You can be buried in snow in a short time, or lightning can strike all around you. My own experience is that your hair literally stands up when the area's electrical field reaches a danger point. If that ever happens to you, get on the ground as low as possible and as quickly as possible, preferably <u>not</u> in a pool of water. Guaranteed that the lightning is coming, and you want to be as small a target as possible.

Car windows should be closed in a storm. Cars tend to be <u>relatively</u> safe because their rubber tires insulate them from direct contact with the ground. However I have known of a couple of instance where cars were struck out in a flat area.

> *My friend, whose house was struck on the lightning rod in Warsaw, came to visit us in Flagstaff, Arizona, a few years later. He took some of our kids mountain climbing on the almost 13,000-foot peak just outside of town one August day. The sky was cloudless when they started, but three hours later the monsoon storm hit. Pete counted 45 bolts that struck the mountain before it stopped. They took shelter against some massive volcanic boulders and were safe. Pete was pretty shaken up, but the kids thought it was "cool!"*

Always be especially alert when you are away from home with anyone in your family. One never knows what dangers may be lying in wait for you just around the next corner.

When approached by a vehicle with its bright lights on, always look at the stripe on the right side of the road instead of looking even momentarily at the other car's lights. That way you will not be totally blinded and will maintain your orientation on the road.

A safety engineer for a large national trucking company talked to our Flagstaff Rotary Club one Tuesday several years ago. The tip that I remember best, and which saved me from at least one accident when I was in Washington, D. C., for my step-daughter-in-law's wedding, was to <u>always use you left foot to apply your brakes</u>. The single motion with your left foot is more than twice as fast as first taking your right foot off the accelerator and then moving it to the brake pedal, then pushing on it.

I was driving slowly in a very congested area with my left foot already touching the brake pedal, when suddenly without warning a brand new Mercedes pulled out in front of me from a blind alley. My left foot hit the brake and we stopped about one coat of paint from the door of that pretty car and its embarrassed driver.

You too can save your own or someone else's life or limb. Just be alert. And always drive defensively.

One more thing: Drive also as though your wife is driving the car that you are about to cut off or honk at or give the finger to. Road rage is alive and well in Arizona. One never knows who has a gun and is ready to use it on you. Don't give anyone an excuse. Be polite. It won't cost you more than two seconds at most, and it might literally save your life.

> *When I was teaching my kids to drive, I told them to stop instantly if I said (or yelled) "stop." All three did a good job. One day as my third child was driving I saw a ball bouncing out into the street from behind a parked car. I yelled "stop!" and he did -- just three feet from a little kid who ran into the street chasing his errant ball. My son wondered how I had seen the little kid because he hadn't. I told him I saw the ball and that was enough to know what might happen next.*

> *One night after I had had a driver's license for a year or so, I was riding with my father on a two-lane road in Indiana. A car approached with its bright lights shining blindingly right in our faces. My dad did nothing except slow a little. I asked him why he didn't. He told me something very important for safe driving. "If I don't turn on my bright high beam lights, then at least one of us can see."*

Safe Driving in the Winter

1. Keep the fuel tank full. Top off before leaving on a trip, especially. Then if you get stuck in a snow bank, you can keep the motor running and the heater warm for several hours, hopefully until help comes.
2. Stay in the car if stuck or broken down.
3. Carry a red flag or "help" sign you can put out if stranded.
4. Always carry chains for the tires. Know how to put them on.
5. Carry a small shovel in the trunk, along with snow boots and extra warm clothes, and perhaps also a couple of blankets.
6. Slow down.
7. Carry extra food and water.
8. Be aware that four-wheel drive doesn't help on ice.
9. Give snow plows plenty of room, and don't follow them too closely.

CHAPTER 43 -- FIRST AID

Everyone should take first aid classes. The American Red Cross uses some of the money we give them through the United Way every year to offer free classes in First Aid. Take a first aid class with your family. Buy a first aid book from them or from the Boy Scouts of America (which at least used to be a little better than the Girl Scout one). They are full books in themselves and are, with some exceptions covered in various places in this book, beyond the scope of our treatment here.

Cleaning Out a Wound

Proper wound care is so frequent and important that I want to cover it here.

Ideally you should have Betadine (povidine-iodine), or Septisol, or Hibiclens anti-germ cleansers, plus hydrogen peroxide, plus sterile saline or water for cleaning out a wound.

But just plain soap and water and elbow grease (in Indiana that term means to scrub really hard) are enough for most wounds if you don't have one of these available. Apply the soap to as clean a cloth as you have (if you don't have a clean one, wash the one you are going to use on the wound with soap and water for two or three minutes at least, then rinse it in water and then apply soap again for use in the wound). After you have washed it out well, flush it with clean water, under a running faucet, if possible. A canteen also works, but be sure you have enough water to spare for staying alive before dumping a lot on it.

When you wash out a wound, you must not only wash the outside skin but also down in the wound as thoroughly as possible. Expect this to stir up more bleeding, but don't worry about that. (Except, if the blood is really pumping, then you may have to deal with that first, by putting direct pressure on it with as clean a cloth as possible.) Normally you will be able to deal with the bleeding as soon as you get the wound cleaned out. Don't worry about pain because the wound will be "in shock" for the first few minutes after the injury, and you won't feel much, if any, pain during that shock period. Grin and bear it. A wound that is thoroughly cleansed within a few minutes after it occurs will have a <u>very</u> good chance of healing without infection, no matter what else happens to it. Spend a good four or five minutes doing a really good job.

After the wound is cleaned out, put as clean a cloth as possible directly on it and apply direct pressure to the wound. This will stop the bleeding within a few minutes in all but the most dire circumstances. The cloth to use is, ideally, two or three layers of sterile gauze pads from your first aid kit. However we aren't always in an ideal situation, even physicians who have brought along our surgical instruments. So make do with what you have, the cleanest part of a towel, the inside layers of a handkerchief, for example, not the part touching the pocket; or your shirt tail which has been inside your pants or shorts and not exposed to the dust and dirt of the trail or the construction site, or whatever. Or a girl's slip. Or several thicknesses of toilet paper.

The Boy Scouts and Girl Scouts offer First Aid merit badges.
I taught these classes while my own kids were scouts. Then for several years after they were through with scouting, the local troop my boys had been affiliated with allowed me to hike down into Havasupai Canyon with them each year in April if I would teach the first aid skill needed to pass that merit badge, as well as deal with any medical emergencies. One year I fell and skinned my knee and required that they treat me in order to pass.
Havasupai Creek is a tributary of the Colorado River which extends south from the Grand Canyon. The canyon it flows through contains, according to National Geographic about twenty years ago, two of the ten most beautiful waterfalls in the world. I'm not sure I can adequately describe how I looked forward to those hikes each year nor how grateful I was to the troop for letting me go along.

What You Should Have in Your First-Aid Kit

1. Three inch elastic bandage for sprains.

2. Liquid soap, Hibiclens, or Betadine (also known as Povidone-Iodine, you can get small one or two ounce containers of it) for cleansing and disinfecting. Hydrogen peroxide is good to use after you have cleansed with one of these.

3. Individual sterile gauze pads in sealed packets, either 3"×3" or 4"×4", about a dozen. Put one or more of these on the wound over the Telfa pad below.

4. Telfa "ouchless" pads. These are the very best for direct application to the surface of a wound because they will come right off the next day even if soaked with dried blood. After two or three days with dried blood, however, you may need to soak it with a little hydrogen peroxide to loosen it with less discomfort.

4. Tweezers, flat end works much better at removing splinters unless they are deeply imbedded. Get a good firm grip on the splinter before starting to pull, then pull straight and fairly quickly so that it won't break off down in the wound.

5. Q-tips.

6. Sharp knife. A Swiss Army knife with whatever blades you can imagine needing is great, if your budget allows it. Be sure the blade is sharp. When cutting, <u>always point the blade away from you</u>.

7. One-half or one-inch tape. Johnson and Johnson makes the best cloth tape, while 3-M has an excellent nylon one.

9. Coban, a two-inch roll. This is a self-adherent fabric. It is no-stick to you but self-sticking to cover the gauze instead of, or in addition to, tape.

10. Two long shoestrings, as from running shoes. These can be used for a lot of things, especially for tying on splints for a possible broken bone.

11. Aircast inflatable splints. These are somewhat expensive; so let your pocketbook be your guide. "Pillow splints." If sleeping pillows are available, they make the best and most comfortable splints of all. If you wrap the pillow as tightly as possible around the possibly broken bone, above and below it, and tie it with the shoestrings and/or Ace bandage, then you have the ultimate in comfort and protection of the injury. These are certainly superior to tree branches or 2×4s for splints, but the word is, "splint them where they lie," so use whatever is available to prevent motion of any possibly broken bone before the injured person is moved. Use discretion here, however. If the person is bleeding or having trouble breathing, take care of the life-threatening things before worrying very much about a broken limb.

12. Rubbing alcohol, for both cleaning and disinfecting wounds, and the adjoining skin. It won't replace thorough cleansing with soap and water, but it is a good cleansing agent and does even kill a few germs. Soap and water doesn't kill many germs but removes the germs from the wound, and that is the most important part of wound care (after controlling the bleeding).

13. Steri-strips, 1/4 to 1/8 inch. After you clean out the wound and get the bleeding stopped with pressure for awhile, then you can cleanse the skin on both sides of the wound with the rubbing alcohol to remove leftover soap, blood, and skin oils, which helps the strips stick better. Then start on one side of the wound, usually the one that may seem to sag or be a little more relaxed than the other, and attach one strip about the middle. Then after it is well stuck to that side, put your finger on the attached end to hold it down; and pull the cut edge together. Then stick the strip down across to the other side. Try to line it up carefully to prevent a big scar, because the way you pull the edges together is the way it will heal. Don't be afraid to remove a strip that doesn't look quite right, throw it away (because the stickum will be gone) and try again.

Butterfly bandaids work almost as well. Johnson and Johnson also makes them (or made them -- perhaps they don't anymore since Steri-strips came along).

Or you can make your own, but non-sterile, butterflies out of tape. Just take a piece of your tape long enough to pull across the wound, as described above. Cut about 1/3 of the way across the width of the piece of tape twice about 1 inch apart on first one side and then the other. Then fold the cut edges across on the sticky side of the tape. Put just a small drop of alcohol or Betadine on the underside of the bridge that will be next to the wound to disinfect it. Then stick it on as above.

14. Bandage scissors. Or three- or four-inch surgical scissors. Even the best ones are not very expensive, and stainless steel ones will last forever if you don't let them get rusty or try to cut wire with them.

For traveling to remote areas, and particularly to a third world country, have the above items but add a few things, some of which you will have to have a prescription for or get from your doctor. The reason for some of these is that many of these countries are so poor that they reuse syringes and needles without sterilizing them, especially in Africa.

15. Several sterile disposable syringes, 3 ml and 5 ml, with both 25-gauge, 5/8-inch and 21-gauge, 1-1/4-inch needles.

16. A 30 ml bottle of 1% Xylocaine for local anesthetic

17. 25 or 30 2.5-mg Lomotil tablets, to be taken in a dose of two every four hours for diarrhea. The generic ones work well and are cheaper.

18. Doxycycline, 100 mg tablets or capsules. These can be taken prophylactically, one daily for diarrhea prevention, or up to twice daily after you are infected.

19. Cipro, 500 mg. These are somewhat stronger, perhaps, and certainly more expensive, than doxycycline, but cover other types of infection besides diarrhea too.

20. Acidophilus or lactobacillus pills. These are good bacteria to be taken to help restore normal GI function after you are infected, or if antibiotics have destroyed too many of your good bacteria. Probiotica is a good brand, as is Lactinex.

21. Some pain pills.

CHAPTER 44 -- FOOD POISONING

On July 29, 2000, a recall was issued for 100,000 lbs of hamburger from one processor that had been sent to eleven states because part of it was found to be contaminated with E. coli. E. coli is found in massive amounts in the large intestine of almost everyone in the world. Two strains, however, which usually are found in sick animals can and do kill people who eat food contaminated with them. (If you are interested, Serotype O157:H7 is the one seen most in our country and Canada.) It is found in undercooked beef (especially hamburger) and unpasteurized milk.

My advice is to never, never, never buy hamburger that has been ground outside of your own grocery store. Some meat processors include almost every part of the cow in the hamburger they make. If contamination occurs, then the bacteria have a longer period of time to grow and multiply before you buy the package. Your own grocery, however, is very unlikely to use anything but the cheaper and tougher muscle areas of the animal for hamburger purposes.

The only way to be absolutely certain that you and your family won't get sick is to be sure that the hamburgers are cooked all the way through. This is so much more important with hamburger than with steaks because the interior of the hamburger may contain little bits of contaminated meat while the interior of the steak cannot have been exposed to any possible contamination until your knife cuts into it. The other food that very often is contaminated (assume that it's always contaminated) is poultry, particularly chicken, with salmonella.

Another source of contamination which occurs in meat sauces and gravies in particular, is named clostridium perfringens. When meat contaminated with this is left at room temperature, the germs rapidly multiply. They produce a toxin that acts on the small intestine. That toxin is destroyed by heat at 167 degrees Fahrenheit or higher. Symptoms from this are usually abdominal cramping and diarrhea, beginning usually about 12 hours after you eat the contaminated food, but with a possible spread of 6 to 24 hours. Vomiting is unusual with this one. The diarrhea usually stops on its own within 24 hours.

Leftover food plays a big part in our lives. My favorite trick is to cook some extra meat when I prepare it on the grill and then freeze it for thawing in the microwave on another day. The important thing here is to get the food into the freezer before bacteria have a chance to grow on it. That means leftovers ideally should be put into the refrigerator or freezer, uncovered until chilled, as soon as everyone is served. You can cover or seal it after the meal is over. Then when you take it out of the freezer, you must either put it directly into the microwave before it thaws or let it thaw in the refrigerator. You must try to get meat from below 40 degrees to above 167 degrees Fahrenheit as quickly as possible to prevent any bacteria from growing and producing toxins that may not be inactivated by heat, such as staphylococcus toxins.

Many people are staphylococcus (staph) carriers, carrying the bacteria in their noses and on their hands and skin without any symptoms of illness themselves. If one of these people happens to work in the kitchen of a restaurant, there will inevitably be some of those bacteria on each of the foods that they handle. If the food is cooked within a few minutes after the contamination occurs, nothing bad will happen; because staphylococcus germs are easily killed by cooking. Also, if the food is refrigerated right away after the contamination and later taken directly from the refrigerator to the stove, the germs will be too cold to produce toxins in the refrigerator and won't have time to produce toxins after removal from the refrigerator.

Where the trouble occurs with staphylococcus as with many other food contaminants, is when the food is somehow contaminated and then allowed to sit out at room temperature long enough for the bacteria to grow and reproduce and produce toxic products that cooking will not inactivate. The symptoms of staphylococcus food poisoning are usually upper abdominal pain, and severe nausea and vomiting within 2-8 hours after eating.

Milk, cream-filled pastries, custards, processed meats and fish are the foods most likely to provide the culture mediums that staph germs particularly like for rapid growth. When I was young my mother would never let us eat any cream-filled goodies during hot weather. That is probably still a good idea.

Botulism

Botulism is caused by the toxin of another member of the clostridium family, clostridium botulinum. It is a gas forming bacteria. When the end of a can swells, it means that probably there is some gas-forming bacteria growing in the can. Throw it away, because it is highly probable that it is c. botulinum. Botulism can kill if the antitoxin is not given in time. Botulinum spores are very heat resistant and may survive boiling at 212 degrees for several hours. Pressure cooking at 250 degrees for 30 minutes, however, will kill them.

The toxins produced are very heat sensitive, so that cooking food at 176 degrees Fahrenheit for 30 minutes will protect you against botulism. Toxin production by these germs goes on even in the refrigerator. So be sure to adequately heat leftovers before eating. The following foods are possible botulism sources: home-canned foods, especially vegetables, fish, fruits, and condiments, but also poultry and red meats, as well as some milk products.

Restaurant outbreaks have come from seafood and uncanned foods, such as patty melt sandwiches, chopped garlic in oil, and foil-wrapped baked potatoes. Symptoms usually begin within 18 to 36 hours after eating the contaminated food, with nausea, vomiting, cramps and diarrhea. Nerve symptoms come a little later, with muscle weakness and paralysis starting in the head area and moving downward. Paralysis of the diaphragm may result in death.

The third bad member of the clostridium family is clostridium tetani, which causes tetanus. We all know how fatal that is. We'll talk about that later.

Listeria Monocytogenes

This is a new food poisoning addition. This germ is a big problem in so-called "ready to eat" deli meats, soft cheeses, and potato salad. The latest outbreak of this type of food poisoning peaked during the fall of 2000, with the last death in November of that year. According to printed reports it was traced by the CDC to turkey deli meat produced in Waco, Texas, by the Cargill company, and Cargill had found Listeria bacteria during testing of equipment in its Waco plant several months before the outbreak, which was suspected to have caused four deaths and three miscarriages. They hadn't notified the government of these findings but tried to fix it themselves. They failed!

Pregnant women, newborn babies and adults with weakened immune systems are those most likely to be affected. Symptoms are similar to lots of other conditions: fever, muscle aches, nausea, diarrhea. In pregnant women it can cause miscarriage, premature delivery, or stillbirth.

It is found in processed foods, raw meats, deli counter cold cuts, soft cheeses, potato salad, and uncooked vegetables.

The last previous Listeria outbreak occurred in contaminated hot dogs reportedly made by Sara Lee, with 21 deaths, including six fetuses. Present estimates of the extent of this problem are 2,500 seriously ill cases per year in the United States, with 500 deaths. This makes it relatively rare compared to other germ-caused food poisoning but very dangerous, with perhaps a 20% mortality.

This germ is different from all other food-borne disease-producing bacteria, such as salmonella because, unlike the others, it continues to grow in refrigerated foods and is thus far harder to control.

The federal government is considering regulations designed to get meat processors to eliminate the presence of Listeria. The meat industry is struggling tooth and nail with industry lobbying to fend off stronger food-safety regulations. Stronger regulations may affect their bottom-line a little but are cheap compared to the recall of the 16.7 million pounds of "ready-to-eat" poultry products that Cargill had to do in December 2000 when presented with the CDC data implicating their Waco plant.

It is <u>easily</u> prevented. **All you have to do is thoroughly cook these raw foods and ready to eat foods, such as hot dogs**. If you want to eat raw veggies too, and I think you should eat some every day, then thoroughly scrub and wash them under running water before eating. Use a clean vegetable brush, one that has been washed with dish soap and hot water, or run through a dishwasher each day.

You may have heard of most of the germs mentioned above before, but I doubt if you have heard of the one that currently is the most common cause of diarrhea among bacteria in the United States. It is Campylobactor. Here it is even more common than E. coli, which is the world leader. Person-to-person contact as the source of infection is very common, as well as food contaminated by someone with it who didn't wash his hands after going to the bathroom.

Other germs that may spread from person-to-person as well as by contaminated food or water include Shigella, which typically causes bloody diarrhea; Giardia, a parasite found in almost every river and stream and lake in our country; and Salmonella, which may also come from contact with poultry, and reptiles (such as turtles and iguanas). Viruses that cause diarrhea may spread the same ways, contaminated water and food, plus dirty hands, not adequately washed after a bowel movement, which then touch food or toys that go into someone's mouth. This is an especially frequent problem in daycare centers.

People who are ill should never be allowed anywhere near food, but they need the money and don't report illnesses to their employers in the food business. **The best, and only way in my opinion, to get people who are sick out of restaurants while ill is to pay them while they are off**. Having them get a note from a doctor would be fine in order to validate the claim, but these people are often working for minimum wages and can't afford a doctor, or may not be able to get an appointment for a couple of days.

If someone reports that he has diarrhea, or a respiratory infection, or sores on the skin, his or her employer should accept that and pay them for three or four days off. Obviously some will abuse this, but not many, and it will help *enormously* in protecting our food chain. **Combined with this approach might be a statement to the employee at the time of hiring that coming to work with an infection will be a cause for being fired**.

Some states require that all food handlers obtain a food handler's card from the county health department after an examination by a physician before they can go to work anywhere that food is handled. This should be a requirement in <u>all</u> states and should include the requirement that all who get the card also have to pass a test (like when you get your drivers license) after reading a training book about proper food preparation and prevention of foodborne illnesses (similar to the driver's manual) before they get the card.

Prevention of Food Poisoning at Home

Always rinse grapes, berries, and anything you buy in the raw state in running tap water several times before cooking and/or eating. Do the same with leaves of lettuce and other salad fixings. This not only removes additional dirt and bacteria but also pesticide residues, which have become an increasingly worrisome problem in this country. See the discussion below.

Always wash your kitchen counters with soapy hot water after every meal. Or in addition you may be able to use a "Germicidal disposable wipe" which we are now using many of our medical clinics to disinfect counter tops. Or you can use 10 percent Clorox (bleach) on all surfaces it won't damage the finish of.

*Cook all processed foods thoroughly!

Irradiation of Food

This is a relatively new technique for reducing bacteria in certain foods. The technology currently used does successfully and safely reduce foodborne bacteria. This method has been attacked for a number of supposed reasons, but extensive studies have clearly shown it to be safe, and also effective under most circumstances. One thing must be kept in mind, however, and that is that food irradiation cannot be substituted for proper and safe food growing, processing from the garden to the kitchen, and preparation for the table.

Please be aware that irradiation cannot be used to mask spoiled and unsafe foods. The physical and chemical changes that occur when food spoils cannot be affected by irradiation.

Another factor which you must know in order to feel safe with these foods is that the radiation used does not hang around for more than a few seconds -- nothing like the effects of a hydrogen bomb. **So there is no risk whatsoever of radiation food contamination.**

Another indirect benefit for those of us who are concerned about food additives and chemicals used to fumigate fresh foods, is that irradiation reduces the need for those potentially toxic products.

What food irradiation does is add to food safety, increase shelf life, reduce loss from spoilage, and allow more varieties of food to be transported to and stocked in grocery stores, so that we may have more fresh foods out of season than we have now that are not just grown locally.

Traveler's Diarrhea

This is usually caused by bacteria in the local water supply. It may be caused by several different bacteria, parasites, or viruses. Our old enemy E. coli, however, is the most common culprit. The usual reason is inadequate local water purification.

In 2002 a number of cruise ships became contaminated with Norwalk virus, which caused hundreds of passenger and crew illnesses with diarrhea. Walt Disney's ship, **Magic**, as I am writing this, has been pulled from service for total prow to stern disinfection.

Most of us know "don't drink the water," but we forget and take a soft or alcoholic drink with ice in it. That happened to me the first time I shot at the Benito Juarez Games in Mexico City.

Another thing we do is to brush our teeth with a toothbrush rinsed in the local water. Or eat fresh fruits and vegetables rinsed in local water.

> *Bottled water may offer the needed protection, but I must tell you that when I was inspecting the kitchen at one hotel in a third world country, I saw them filling up the so-called bottled water containers at the tap in the sink. A waiter at a 4-star hotel in Turkey was very upset by my demand that he let me open my bottled water myself. But I didn't get sick there, and others in our group did.*

> *The second time I shot at the Benito Juarez Games, I made it halfway back to the good old U. S. of A. on an American plane, when we were served our in-flight meal, which included what appeared to be an unusually good airline salad. I hadn't had a salad for a week and dived right into it. As I swallowed the second bite, however, the light bulb suddenly went on over my head. Too late I flashed on the fact that although our plane was from America, the salad came from Mexico City. I passed out at the end of a short surgical procedure two days later. My third time down there I finally got it right, and I've traveled to some seriously third world countries since with no problems.*

On the Airplane

That noted medical periodical, *The Wall Street Journal*, in their article <u>How Safe is Airline Water?</u> on November 1, 2002 printed the results of their survey of 14 airline flights, in which they took samples of water from the galleys and lavatories of each plane for laboratory analysis by good labs. The flights were a randomized sample all the way from a flight to Atlanta, where the CDC headquarters is, to a flight to Sydney, Australia. They were looking for possible disease-producing contamination. And boy did they find it! Their idea to do this was triggered by some poorly publicized studies from Japan and The Netherlands in which E. coli and the Legionnaire's disease germ have been found. Apparently U.S. studies have had "mixed results." The WSJ samples produced "a long list of microscopic life you don't want to drink, from

Salmonella and *Staphyloccus* to tiny insect eggs." Worse, contamination was the rule, not the exception.

Federal regs require that the water tanks of airplanes are supposed to contain drinkable water. Many, perhaps most, airlines dispense bottled water initially, but on long flights, when they run out of the bottled variety, they turn to the taps.

<u>Lessons to be learned from these tests:</u> When you drink water on an airplane, drink only that which is bottled. Bring your own bottled water, maybe several bottles, for overseas flights for use when the bottled water from the airlines runs out. Use bottled water for brushing your teeth, as you would in any third world country. Bring some disposable towelettes for washing your hands before eating.

In third world countries never eat any fruits or vegetables that you have not personally peeled. Don't eat salads.

Fish Poisoning

Fish poisoning can occur from four hundred or more different species in various tropical reefs of the Pacific Ocean, the West Indies, and even our own state of Florida. Ciguatera, Scombroid, and Tetrodo-toxin are the main ones.

Clams, mussels, oysters, and scallops along the New England and Pacific coasts from June to October may eat a poisonous little creature referred to as "the red tide." The poison is not destroyed by heat and can cause muscle weakness and even paralysis in cases of large exposure.

Chemical poisoning can occur if the fresh fruits and vegetables you eat have been sprayed with arsenic, lead, or organic insecticides. So always wash all food that you are going to eat raw with running tap water before consumption.

Cadmium-lined containers may react with the food, as may acidic liquids in pottery glazed with lead.

Virtually everyone in our country has or will consume contaminated food and/or water sometime in his or her life. These suggestions may help you to keep that consumption to an absolute minimum.

CHAPTER 45 -- FOOT PROBLEMS

The three most common foot problems are **corns, calluses, and ingrown toenails.** How can you tell a corn from a callus? Corns are like an upside down pyramid composed of very hard (cornified) material that builds up initially as a protective layer of thick skin, which becomes progressively thicker and more tightly compressed under ongoing pressure until it is like a small inverted horn. Corns tend to occur where there is continuing pressure on a bony prominence. This can be directly from the shoe, as on the side of the big or little toes, between the toes, or on the sole of the foot at the end of one of the long bones of the foot (metatarsals). And they hurt.

Calluses, on the other hand, don't usually hurt. They also are a thickening of skin in response to repeated pressure from shoes, boots, or, on the hands, from use of tools, etc. over a wider area than corns. Corns usually begin as localized calluses.

*In most cases corns and calluses of the feet can be prevented by wearing shoes that fit well.

Most shoe salespeople have no idea how to properly fit a shoe to your foot. Therefore it is necessary that you learn these few simple rules yourself. When you are going to buy a new pair of shoes: 1) Always stand with your full weight on the device the salesperson uses to measure your length and width of foot. 2) Always allow 1/2 to 3/4 inch additional shoe length beyond the end of your toes when standing. The toe box should allow your toes to spread themselves a little. 3) The foot should not be squeezed by the shoe at any spot. If the shoe isn't completely comfortable when you put it on, then your foot is what will get "broken in."

Some feet, however, have structural abnormalities (e.g., bunions), which require special attention beyond our discussion here.

Ingrown toenails are addressed in their separate chapter. They often are caused by shoes that are too narrow in the toes. Gaining weight while continuing to wear the same size shoes is a common cause. We often don't realize that we gain weight everywhere, not just in the love handles.

Treatment of corns and calluses can often be successful just by wearing different shoes that fit better, along with taping a sort of donut around the pressure point. The hole in the donut is placed over the thickened, tender spot, and the rim surrounds it to protect it from further wear and tear. Eventually normal skin may come to the area, particularly if the damage has not penetrated too deeply yet.

If you want comfort a little faster, calluses can be shaved with a clean razor blade, being careful to cut away only the thick layers a little bit at a time. When you get down to where the skin begins to feel about normal in thickness, then you can smooth it the rest of the way with an emery board or file. Be sure to wash your feet before and after trimming so that you don't introduce infection inadvertently.

There are salicylic acid plasters, which you stick just on the corn itself, being careful to avoid getting it on the surrounding normal skin. After a couple of weeks the corn may separate down deep and fall out, much as a wart sometimes does.

Corns can be cut away clear to the depths of the corn without anesthetic, but it is best to use a scalpel with a #15 blade, which you can get from many drugstores. If they don't have them in stock, most will be glad to order one for you. Some magnifying glasses to help you see the bottom of the corn are also a good idea. I have removed hundreds of these, and it is always gratifying to me when the person stands up and gets a smile on her face because it doesn't hurt to bear weight anymore.

Diabetics, particularly older ones, should not try to do the surgical care of these themselves, but instead seek medical help. The poor circulation in diabetic feet can cause amputation to be needed if any little thing goes wrong. It is certainly OK, though, to do the padding and better-fitting shoe approaches to foot care.

Diabetics often develop painful neuropathy, the treatment of which is beyond the scope of this book. Suffice to say that prevention by always maintaining the best possible control of your diabetes is the correct, though not always successful, approach.

Sore Feet in Runners

These are usually caused by the shoes -- too many miles in a pair, a pair that doesn't fit well, or poor cushioning. Not stretching before and after each run and bony parts of the foot that need some special support are other causes.

Running on your toes stresses your plantar fascia (the strong thin tendon that spreads out over the sole of your feet from the heel bone to just before the toes). Running so that your heels strike the ground too hard can bruise the heel bone. And so on. See the **Exercise** chapter for proper running technique.

There are a number of good running shoes on the market, and they are evaluated in the shoe issue of *Runner's World* once a year. For serious exercise name brands such as New Balance (which I feel is better than all the others in the multiplicity of widths and lengths available, as well as the large toe box; unfortunately my last two pairs had poor quality control), Nike, Adidas, and Reebok provide a much better value than the generic, very cheap, unknown brands found in discount stores such as K-Mart, Wal-Mart, and others.

My own experience in many years of treating runners is that shoes wear out faster than we are willing to admit. So I always have my receptionist tell runners to bring their shoes in for me to look at when they make an appointment for sore feet. Sometimes the problem is caused by changing brands of shoe with a little different weight-bearing stress that the foot is not prepared for.

In most shoes, higher price means that they will last more miles. Most shoes are good for at least 300 miles before the support portions begin to wear down. Usually the sole doesn't wear down very much before the inner support begins to lose its strength.

Often the shoe itself is still mostly good, but a new insole is needed. Spenco makes a huge variety of insoles for virtually every condition. I recommend these above all others put together. They have sizes to fit every shoe, and they last forever. Athletic stores and many pharmacies carry this brand. They are made of neoprene, which does not pick up foot odors, but can be washed many times if desired. I have some of their insoles with more than 2,500 miles on them.

They also have just flat insoles shaped for the shoe. These are good to put under your regular shoe insole to cushion the impact of each step. They also can have a hole cut in them under a tender bony prominence to take the pressure off of it. They can and should be cut back, from a half inch to the full length of your toes to allow plenty of room in the toe box of the shoe.

They have heel supports, which extend to the front end of the arch and have a built-in arch support as well as excellent heel cup. These have a plug under the heel which can easily be removed in problems with heel spurs (otherwise called plantar fasciitis).

They have full-sized insoles with arch supports. All people with high arches should wear extra arch supports to prevent strain and possible stress fractures of one or more metatarsal bones (the long bones of the foot).

Anyone, not just runners, with a foot problem should go to a store that carries Spenco and look in their catalog if the store doesn't carry a full line of their foot products. The store will be happy to order anything from the catalog for you.

* **At least 50% of the time you will save yourself a trip to an orthopedic doctor or podiatrist**.

Another tip to treat or prevent sore feet is to alternate sets of running shoes every day so that your foot muscles have slightly different stresses on successive days -- sort of mini cross training.

CHAPTER 46 -- GERD (Hiatal hernia)

** **You may never have to see a doctor again for this condition if you follow these simple instructions.**

According to the medical expense summaries for the year 2000, GERD is the most costly of all gastrointestinal diseases. Therefore **you stand to save as much here as in almost the rest of this book** if you pay close attention to what follows.

What is it? It is a condition in which the circular muscle (cardiac sphincter) at the top of the stomach, where the esophagus passes through a small hole (called the hiatus) in the diaphragm, doesn't close tightly enough like a purse string (or the muscle of the rectum, called the anal sphincter), to prevent the powerful 0.1 normal hydrochloride acid in the stomach from running back uphill (Refluxing) into the lower Esophagus) and producing an inflammation or Disease of the lower esophagus: Gastro-Esophageal Reflux Disease. You can have a hiatal hernia without GERD, but not the other way around.

Some people are just born with a pucker muscle there that is weak in the first place, and allows acid to back up when there is increased pressure from below, such as in people where there is a lot of fat in the abdomen.

Others have a hole, called a *hiatus*, in the diaphragm which is too large for the sphincter muscle to get a purchase on for tightening all the way around. When that happens any increased pressure in the abdominal cavity will push some of the stomach up into the lung cavity. That is what we call a *Hiatal Hernia*. Since that portion of the stomach that is up in the chest cavity is still producing acid, the esophagus becomes chronically inflamed and almost never heals if the hernia is large.

Over a period of years more and more of the stomach and even other portions of the contents of the abdominal cavity, such as bowel may move up into the chest cavity and become trapped there, thus reducing the lung capacity. One of my best friends had about three *feet* of large intestine up in his chest cavity before he finally complained about any symptoms! That was when he had a bowel obstruction at, you guessed it, three o'clock in the morning.

Most of those will eventually require surgery. In that case laparoscopic repair through a small tube with a telescope and a light and a channel for tiny instruments in it, has come into its own for all but the biggest ones.

Most hiatal hernias, however, are small and create their symptoms by the backup of gastric acid into the esophagus that accompanies the weakened or absent pucker mechanism (the GERD). Most do not and will not require surgery.

The wall of the stomach normally has no problem with the acid because its cells actually produce that acid. Under circumstances discussed in the chapter on **Peptic Disease**, that resistance breaks down and an ulcer results. The esophagus, however, has a lining that is very susceptible to irritation by acid. Symptoms are caused by irritation of the esophagus mostly, but also by acid working its way all way to the top at the back your throat as you lie down at night. If that happens, then some of the acid may slip down into the lungs and cause wheezing or a morning cough unrelated to smoking.

For those people who have small hiatal hernias or just weak muscles, here are the things you can do to eliminate most, and perhaps all, of your symptoms of heartburn, pain in the chest, nighttime wheezing in the absence of asthma, and other less common symptoms.

1) Reduce the acid produced by your stomach in the following ways: a) eliminate all caffeine-containing drinks. Even decaf coffee has some caffeine, some as much as 14%. Also many soft drinks including tea have caffeine. b) Eliminate alcohol. c) Eliminate all tobacco. These three things cause more hyperacidity than everything else you can think of combined.

2) If you have a large belly, lose serious weight because the fat on the inside of the abdomen creates an upward pressure on the stomach and stomach contents, which worsens the underlying condition.

3) Don't eat or drink anything after supper, or for least three hours before going to bed. (Be sure to drink adequate water earlier in the day.) If the stomach is mostly empty when you go to bed, then there won't be very much acid in the stomach for you to regurgitate.

4) Elevate the head of your bed at least four inches above the level of the feet so that gravity will help keep the acid in the stomach while you are sleeping. Six inches is even better. You can use wooden blocks under the casters at the head of the bed. Or you can put a wedge under the head of your mattress. A medical supply company whose name I don't remember makes something they called a Bedge, that some of my patients really like, to put under your mattress.

5) There are two excellent over-the-counter medications that will greatly reduce the acid in your stomach. If the above suggestions don't fully relieve your symptoms, then try Zantac, 75-150 milligrams, or Pepcid, 20-40 milligrams at bedtime.

One clue to over-the-counter medications: the dose available is usually 1/2 the usual prescription dose. In the case of Zantac a 75 mg dose is available, while Pepcid has a 10 mg size you can buy without a prescription.

If these don't work and you have to see a doctor, he will probably put you on Prilosec or Prevacid, Protonix, or the newer cousin to Prilosec, Nexium.

If nothing relieves you after faithfully following this program, then special studies, including an upper GI series and gastroscopy, with possible biopsy of the inflamed areas, may be needed. Actually an upper GI is a good place to start, because it is cheaper than a lot of other studies and gives a lot of information. **A big bang for your buck.** All you have to do is not eat or drink for about twelve hours, and then drink some chocolate-flavored barium while the radiologist takes some pictures.

Further treatment depends upon the results of the tests.

CHAPTER 47 -- GOUT

Gout is a condition where crystals from uric acid, a breakdown product of recycled red blood cells and other sources as noted below, are deposited in the tissues of various joints. They are very irritating to the body's tissues and so can set up a lot of painful swelling and inflammation of whatever joint (or sometimes more than one joint at a time) is involved. Usually, but not always, the blood uric acid level is high. The higher it is, and the longer it is high, the more likely the person is to develop gouty arthritis and/or kidney stones.

There are two different mechanisms that raise the uric acid.

The first is through increased uric production by the body through alcohol consumption, unusually stressful exercise, fructose (fruit sugar) intake, high purine intake, certain blood disorders, particularly where one has an unusually high number of red blood cells (thus one who lives at high altitude with its higher red blood cell count is at greater risk for gout), obesity, and high triglycerides (a blood fat).

The second mechanism is decreased excretion of uric acid by the kidneys. Drugs that cause this include diuretics (mainly the thiazides), low-dose salicylates given to prevent heart attacks, and cyclosporine. Kidney disease of various types can't get rid of the uric acid along with many other wastes in the blood adequately. There are certain chemicals in the blood under certain circumstances that also can bring on attacks of gout.

It is very important for your doctor to find out the cause of your gout because the treatment is different for each of the mechanisms of increased production or decreased excretion note above. Sometimes the cause is pretty obvious, and special tests may not be needed under that circumstance. However, much of the time some tests that need to be done only once need to be ordered by your doctor. Whether you are overproducing or under-excreting uric acid is determined very simply by just collecting a 24-hour urine sample and getting the total output of uric acid measured. If your output is over 800 mg/dl, then you are an overproducer. Allopurinal is the drug of choice for overproducers as well as for those with sick kidneys and kidney stones. It is also used for tophi of the skin, which I have never seen and thus won't discuss here. Underexcreters do better with probenecid on a daily basis.

Factors that may bring on an attack of gout include alcohol consumption (not necessarily to excess, although excess will bring it on quicker in those who are susceptible). Dietary indiscretions, certain drugs (particularly diuretics), an unusual amount of exercise (such as hiking down into the Grand Canyon and back), infection, radiation therapy, and surgery are other things that can trigger an attack. Transplant recipients who are given cyclosporine often have this complication.

A high percentage of gout attacks affect the joint just back of the big toe. Other areas of the foot can be involved, along with joints of the fingers, wrist, and elbow.

Making the diagnosis accurately the first time is important, because gout is a long-lasting disease with many ill effects on multiple areas of our bodies.

You and your doctor may suspect that you have gout if you have a high uric acid in the blood, if the pain and inflammation reach a peak in 24-36 hours, if the joint is red and swollen, if only one joint is involved at a time, if you have multiple attacks of sudden acute arthritis, and/or you have the attack in the joint just back from one big toe. X-rays are usually normal until you have had the condition for quite awhile, then they begin to show little punched-out holes in the bone near the joint. If your doctor sticks a needle into the inflamed joint (not usually possible in the big toe area), sucks out a little fluid, and then sees uric crystals under the microscope, that more than anything else makes an accurate diagnosis.

Treatment consists of overcoming the inflammation as quickly as possible for pain relief. (Untreated cases, at least the first few times, get a lot better in nine to ten days. Most people don't wait because they are pretty sore.) Colchicine, either by mouth or by injection, is one of the few drugs that hasn't been improved upon in the years I've been in practice. We like to give it for a week or two, certainly until the pain and swelling have gone down. Along with it we often use an NSAID, which used to be indomethacin. That causes undesirable reactions, such as GI ulcerations with bleeding, kidney poisoning, and aggravation of some nerve disorders. Thus it is better now with the new COX-II inhibitor drugs such as Celebrex and Vioxx to use one of them for a week or two, because there is less chance of side effects with them, and they are probably considerably stronger than the older anti-inflammatories.

In addition your doctor may want you to take a medicine such as probenecid (Benemid) to try to get the kidneys to put out, or excrete, more uric acid. He may order a combination of colchicine and probenecid called colbenemid for the first two weeks or so, then perhaps just probenecid. After a month on probenecid you can be started on allopurinol to slow down the production of uric acid from chemicals called purines in the blood. The reason we wait for a month is because allopurinol can bring on an acute gout attack if the blood level is very high when it is started. Taking the probenecid for a month brings it down so that allopurinal can be started at a low dose and gradually increased, usually to the 300 mg. tablet, which is then taken for a very long time, perhaps for life.

Non-Drug Approaches to Treatment: a Money Saver

If you want to help yourself possibly get along on a lower dose of allopurinol or none at all, then put yourself on a low purine diet, and in particular avoid excesses of high purine foods. This approach works best in people with reduced excretion of uric acid in the urine.

High Purine Foods

- All meats, especially organ meats such as kidneys, liver, and sweetbreads, and seafood, especially anchovies. Meat stock, extracts, and gravies.
- Asparagus, beans, cauliflower, lentils, mushrooms, peas, oatmeal, and spinach.
- Yeast and yeast extracts. Beer and other alcoholic beverages.

Please remember that overeating of foods that contain only small quantities of purines can be worse than eating just a small amount of a high purine food.

I generally just tell people with the overproduction problem to avoid anchovies, kidneys, liver, and sweetbreads, and avoid beer and any other alcoholic drink made with yeast. Then if they are still having problems, go off the other things on the list too.

In addition to the low purine diet, a regular daily exercise program of at least 30 minutes of some non-stop activity is essential. (This is just one more of the dozens of ways that daily exercise helps our good health.)

The last non-drug items are stopping all alcohol, low-dose aspirin, and diuretics if your doctor will let you.

After the initial workup, you should be able to simply return for a checkup and blood test once a year, unless your case is more complicated than 90% of them, and remain free of gout.

CHAPTER 48 -- GUN SAFETY

Whether you agree with it or not, America is a heavily armed country. It is part of our heritage, for better or for worse. And by far the vast majority of the gun owners are good law-abiding people. Some want a gun simply for self-protection. I do. Some like to pretend they are frontiersmen who have to hunt to bring home food for the winter. And an elk will certainly fill one's freezer, plus the freezers of a lot of friends and neighbors. Others like to shoot at targets, sometimes in competition, without ever hurting any creature. Again I fall into that category.

Whether you agree with laws which allow hunting or not, the fact of the matter is that the wild animal herds are in better shape in many parts of the country because of the money paid for hunting licenses that is used to control the size of the herds to prevent overgrazing and starvation, and because of the efforts of sportsmen's groups such as Ducks Unlimited and Coconino Sportsmen, who help preserve the necessary habitat for the animals to thrive. Ironic, isn't it, that many animals do better because of the very people who kill and eat them. Around Flagstaff, Arizona, where I have lived for many years, the members of Coconino Sportsmen have built artificial tanks, which are actually small lakes and hold water all year round, in various areas of the forest, thus helping all the little forest creatures, not just deer and elk.

There are some misconceptions about guns which you should be aware of if you are to continue to read the frequent debates about whether private citizens should be allowed to purchase, keep, or bear firearms.

First is the term "assault weapons." The correct definition of a true assault weapon is a rifle or handgun capable of full automatic fire by just squeezing the trigger once. These are also called "machine guns" and have been closely regulated by law ever since the Al Capone days of the 1930's in Chicago.

All military rifles around the world can be made capable of full automatic fire. When those guns are sold on the civilian market for hunting or target shooting, they must be modified so that they can no longer fire more than one shot with each squeeze of the trigger, just like rifles and muskets all the way back to the middle ages. It doesn't matter if they are AK-47's or M-16's (the civilian counterpart is the Colt AR-15).

In Chicago in the '30s, my father and mother-in-law and future wife had their car blown up by a bomb attached to the starter of their car, and lived to tell about it. (But that's another story!)

Those who think no one should be allowed to own a gun will call all guns that have a military counterpart "assault weapons," even though they aren't. So the term "assault weapon" is just a propaganda buzzword.

Another set of buzzwords is "Saturday Night Special." This supposedly refers to a cheap handgun that someone can buy at a liquor store and then go rob a Circle K or shoot someone after drinking too much alcohol. (In the latter case probably the alcohol is more responsible for the mayhem than the gun.)

Let me tell you a couple of true stories about these "Saturday Night Specials."

First, my grandfather used one to defend himself, his wife, and my mother against a group of Ku Klux Klansmen who were burning a cross on his front yard and seemed to be about to do the same for their house with them in it. He stepped out onto their front porch with his cheap little handgun, according to the story my grandmother told me, and loudly stated that he would count to ten and then start shooting at anyone who was still within range. My grandmother said that they dropped their torches and started running by the time he got to "5." That little "Saturday Night Special" is one of my proudest possessions. (See page 214 for the other story.)

One more thing about gun control. I used to be frequently appointed by the Superior Court in Flagstaff to examine people in jail to help determine whether they were mentally capable of standing trial and assisting in their own defense. One such case was a man who robbed as a way of life and was about to go to jail for a long time. He told me about criminals and guns during my lengthy evaluation of him. Briefly, a criminal can always get a gun if he wants one for a "job." They have "rent-a-gun" criminal outlets in every city, where the criminal just pays for the gun for an hour or a day and then brings it back to be recycled over and over.

> *The second story involves one of my patients for whom I delivered a baby. Her husband was an abuser, and she left him soon after the baby was born because she feared for the baby's life, as well as her own. Her husband ignored the order of protection she obtained from the court, beating her whenever he could find a way to get to her. She was poor but could afford a used "Saturday Night Special," which she took home with her. Three days later her soon-to-be ex-husband broke a window beside the flimsy backdoor and opened the lock from the inside. She called 911, but he had a knife and said he was going to "carve her and the child up," according to a police friend of mine who investigated the case. To make a long story short, she shot and killed him with that "Saturday Night Special." The police arrived as quickly as they could, but couldn't have protected her in time if she hadn't protected herself. No charges were filed against her, and she became a happy, outgoing wonderful woman and mother.*

There is bumper sticker which reads, "When guns are outlawed, only outlaws will have guns!" And there is probably a lot of truth in that statement. My favorite is "Nobody ever raped a Smith and Wesson!" See the chapter on **Protecting Yourself Against Rape** for more about that.

Gun Safety

Gun safety is best taught at an early age. It is absolutely essential that small children never have any possible access to a gun, whether loaded or not. (They are all loaded.) Older children must not be allowed to have a gun in their possession unless under the immediate supervision of an adult. Whatever you have heard about the National Rifle Association (NRA) is not complete unless you are made aware of the fact that they have a Hunter Safety course for kids ten years old and older, which is outstanding. The teachers have to be certified after a training course, and I have never heard of the death of one of those kids in a gun-related accident after taking one of those classes. You don't have to want to be a hunter to take the class. I took a similar class in the Boy Scouts, and I taught it for merit badges when I was a scout leader.

I don't hunt--too softhearted. But I sure do enjoy punching holes in a target with a bullet and breaking clay pigeons with a good shotgun.

1. All guns are loaded. A friend of mine whose daughter I delivered forgot that rule and accidentally killed himself, leaving her an orphan.

2. Never point a gun at anyone unless you intend to kill him or her.

3. Before letting anyone handle any type of a gun anywhere near you, you personally must check it to be sure it is unloaded and pointed in a safe direction.

4. Always be sure that there is a backstop that is wide and high in the direction that you point a gun. If you just fire away because it looks clear, that bullet may travel a mile or

more before striking and killing someone innocently sitting in the backyard, or practicing cheerleading. I've known of both of these tragedies.

In many places now handguns are sold with trigger locks, which can and should be used whenever there may be kids around. With the lock in place, however, they are of little use for self-protection. There are also gun safes which can be kept by the bedside and opened by putting your fingers into slots which can be manipulated in a combination for quick opening in the dark. If you aren't worried about self-protection in your home, then it's a good idea to store your weapons in a locked and concealed place or an actual gun safe for their protection from theft when you are away. Also, in those cases, store the ammunition in as cool and dry an area as you can, away from the guns, so that a thief can't break in and shoot you with one of your own guns.

Many professional burglars never carry weapons so that they can easily surrender to an armed householder and won't be shot. It is <u>never</u> OK under the law to shoot someone unless in self-defense while in fear for your life. The words "I was afraid for my life" are very important when you call 911 after actually shooting someone in your house. If the person was armed, even with a small knife, you have a pretty good case for justifiable self-defense.

> A small town in Florida passed a law a very few years ago <u>requiring</u> that every home in town have a firearm in it. By some strange coincidence, the cases of burglary are now about zero for the past 5 years.

So, no matter how you personally feel about guns, there are millions of really good people in our country who feel that they want to, and maybe need to, exercise their right under the second amendment to the Constitution to keep and bear arms. Preventing bad accidents associated with that constitutional right is a part of being a good citizen. Pay attention to these suggestions and remember, **every gun is loaded!**

CHAPTER 49 -- HEAD INJURIES

Judging the seriousness of a head injury is very important in helping you to determine whether to seek medical aid or to simply observe the person yourself.

If there is no bleeding and there is no big soft lump on the skull, then the next thing that must be considered is whether there is internal damage to the brain. For many such injuries you won't need this book. It will be immediately obvious whether the person is OK or needs an ambulance for transportation to the hospital. For other cases, however, you may need the help you are getting here.

> *But concussion without loss of consciousness is far more common than most of you know. I had a case today as I write this. The patient had a lingering headache and a little nausea yesterday since a blow on the head from a falling shelf two days ago. Today the man felt well again, with no headache and normal appetite.*

Ask these questions: was there loss of consciousness? If not, then the brain is <u>probably</u> not seriously injured.

If yes, then how long was the person unconscious? Even a momentary loss means at least a mild concussion, which you can probably simply watch carefully as outlined below. Unconsciousness of five minutes or more absolutely requires transporting the person to the hospital ER right away for medical evaluation. One of 30 minutes or more is potentially very serious and needs a brain scan at the very least, along with admission to the hospital ICU.

Does the person have a headache? If so, how severe is it? Sudden headaches in the case of trauma are more likely to mean something going on in the brain than the usual headaches that people experience throughout their lives, and the severity is pretty much an excellent indicator of how severely the brain has been rattled. A mild headache that gets worse and worse needs medical evaluation. One that gets better or stays the same for a few days needs nothing except rest until it is gone.

Is the person thinking clearly?

Here is some useful information for watching someone with a head injury that may not be serious enough to require hospitalization.

First, check the person at least every two hours after the injury and keep him in bed until he is feeling and eating well. Bring the person back to the doctor's office or ER immediately if there is:

- A large, soft lump on the head.
- Unusual drowsiness (can't be aroused).
- Forceful or repeated vomiting.
- A "fit" or convulsion (jerking).
- Clumsy walking.
- Bad headache.
- One pupil larger than the other. (Be sure the same amount of light is shining in each eye).

Children

- Keep your child at rest for 24 hours.
- Clear liquids only for eight hours (Kool-aid, juice, tea, water (no milk).
- Take the child's pulse and respirations every two hours for about 12 hours.
- You may allow the child to sleep, but check its condition every one hour while awake and every two hours when asleep. See that he responds to pinch or gentle shaking and that his color, pulse, and breathing are normal. Awaken him if uncertain of his condition.

My occasional bridge partner of several years in Flagstaff came in to see me with a very severe headache one day, to the point that he couldn't play bridge that night. The physical exam was not very helpful -- no positive findings. Further questioning revealed that he had fallen and bumped his head about three months before and had had a headache, to a lesser degree than this, for several days before getting well. It hadn't disturbed his weekly duplicate bridge game. That was the clue I needed, because this is the classic story of a subdural hematoma, minimal bleeding from a small vessel initially, then serum is sucked into the clotted blood, making the clot gradually expand till symptoms appear. A scan did show such a blood clot, and our friendly neighborhood neurosurgeon quickly and easily removed the clot. My friend was back at the bridge table the very next week, winning as usual.

Call your doctor or the Emergency Room if any of the following occur:
- Severe headache that isn't helped with cool wet towel to the head.
- If the child vomits more than two or three times, or vomits clear across the room (this is called projectile vomiting).
- If there is a convulsion.

- If the child complains of weakness or is unable to move one or both arms or legs.
- If there is a peculiar gait, stumbling, dizziness, or any definitely peculiar behavior.
- If child becomes unusually sleepy or is unable to be awakened easily.
- If the child seems to be hallucinating (or "talking out of its head").

As the team doctor for the Coconino High School football team for 31 years, I have encountered players who "had their bell rung" many times. The determination about whether to let the athlete resume play or stay on the sidelines is always an extremely important one, particularly to the player, but also to the team. We who do sports medicine always err on the side of caution. But often the player can safely resume play after he has been under observation on the sidelines for several plays.

The player who is still lying on the field at the end of the play is easy. He comes out and probably won't be allowed to play again that night.

The one that is sometimes interesting is the one who is talking to his teammates about stuff unrelated to the game. On checking him, he may not even know which team we are playing. I had one of those in the big game against the Flagstaff Eagles the last game of the season one year. Our best running back was the player involved, and I took him out of the game. About 5 minutes later as I was just through taping up an ankle sprain, to my extreme embarrassment and the total joy of all the Coconino Panther fans, I saw that boy take the football on a power sweep to the left and run 35 yards for the winning touchdown! Quick recovery, eh? Fortunately all was well, and the boy did not have even a slight headache the next day.

But I learned something very important there. For the rest of my sports medicine career, whenever I took a boy out of the game for any reason, I also took away his helmet. Without a helmet, the officials won't even let a boy on the field.

CHAPTER 50 -- HEADACHES

Headaches are caused by all kinds of body conditions. An incomplete list includes measles, scarlet fever, Rocky Mountain spotted fever and other rickettsial diseases, malaria, meningitis, dehydration, high blood pressure, subdural hematoma, brain tumors, loss of sleep, brain aneurysms (little weak spots in the wall of a blood vessel that can blow out), encephalitis, hydrocephalus, metastatic cancer, concussions (both with and without loss of consciousness), tension, sinus infections, some tooth infections, alcoholic hangovers, certain wines in some sensitive people, stroke, exercise to exhaustion, an uncreative way to control unwanted impending sexual activity, and on and on. Almost any condition that can cause fever may also cause headaches.

The vast majority of recurring headaches are muscle contraction or tension headaches. These are usually located where the muscles are -- in the forehead above the eyes, in the temple areas, and the back of the head where the neck muscles are attached. Actually, those of the back of the head are really more neckache than headache since the neck muscles tighten up and are the source of the pain, but the pain may radiate into the back of the head. The portion of the head that hurts is where the neck muscles attach to it. In the most severe cases the person's shoulders are pulled up almost to the ears, and the head resembles a turtle coming out of its shell. These headaches are very painful and can be almost as incapacitating as migraines.

Fortunately they respond to treatment much better than migraines. However they may come on a daily basis for six months or more at a time.

Treatment is directed toward breaking up the muscle spasms.

Massage is a very good way to interrupt the spasms. If you have a spouse or significant other with strong but gentle fingers, then you can get some help without drugs and have quick relief.

Ice massage also is wonderful for these. Fill some paper cups with water and put them in your freezer. Then when you have this type of headache, just tear the rim off the ice cup and, holding the cup with a towel or dry wash cloth, firmly rub the tight and sore muscles with the ice for 10 to 15 minutes. Or do it till the area feels numb, then for five minutes more. With ice the area may hurt more for a few minutes and you'll want to quit. But stay with it, and the pain will improve and perhaps go away completely.

With either type of massage, rub in the direction of the muscle fibers for the full length of the muscle rather than across them.

Often there is a focus of irritation called a trigger point. That spot causes the whole muscle to fire off and go into spasms. This can happen, for example, in one of the trapezius muscles in the back of the neck; these are pretty big muscles on each side that extend out to the point of each shoulder and halfway down the upper back as well as up the neck to attach on the skull. Ice massage is especially good for trigger points. So is acupuncture by a well-trained acupuncturist (not your friendly neighborhood chiropractor).

So is biofeedback, which includes relaxation techniques and actually helps you to train your muscle to relax. This is a much under-appreciated and under-used modality which has huge benefits.

Relaxation techniques all involve muscle tensing and relaxing and deep breathing. The chapter on **Staying Fit Mentally** has a copy of a relaxation technique that I have offered for many years to stress and migraine headache sufferers, with at least a small amount of improvement in most people who do the exercises faithfully. They are particularly good for preventing muscle contraction headaches, especially those due to stress. The relaxation exercises help more for prevention, and during the pre-headache phase. Once you become good at relaxing your body with these, you will be able to at least partially relax all your muscle from the top of your head to the tips of your toes in only ten seconds. I can do it in the space of one deep breath.

For headache prevention, do these relaxation techniques for five up to ten minutes two to three times a day and just before you are about to get into any situation which you suspect may become stressful.

From the medication standpoint, small doses of tricyclic antidepressants, such as amitryptiline (Elavil) 12.5 to 25 mg once or twice a day, with few or no side effects, are a very helpful addition to the relaxation exercises described above. These medications are also used in migraine sufferers but usually in considerably larger doses. This combination will not only reduce the amount of pain and discomfort with an attack but also reduce the headache frequency. These are much more effective in the long run, even though they require a prescription, than ibuprofen-containing and other over-the-counter pain relievers. Overuse of those, along with narcotics, can trigger rebound attacks, especially in chronic stress and migraine headaches.

Narcotics, of course, must be totally avoided because you will very quickly become hooked on them and encounter the rebound headaches also as the drug wears off.

Beta blocker medications such as propanolol or atenolol, which reduce the body's production of certain chemicals in response to stress, are often given in small doses on a daily basis for prevention. Calcium channel blockers are also sometimes used, but I personally have had less success with them than with the others mentioned. Neither of these is good for treatment after the headache is already there. They are often used on an as-needed prophylactic basis when you know you are going to be undergoing something stressful.

Migraines

Keep a headache diary to see if there are things that seem to trigger an attack, such as the onset of a monthly period, a certain food, stress, fatigue, hot or cold weather or other environmental factors, medications, or foods. Or more smoking than usual. Or smoking at all. Treatment medications include caffeine, cafergot, ergotamine, double or triple strength Espresso or other very strong coffee, Feverfew, and the new -triptan family of medicines (Imitrex was the first of these and is still quite good, while Zomig is one example of a newer one). Some people want narcotics for relief, but as noted above, this is not a good thing. Addiction to these drugs is a very real concern in those with chronic and recurring pain of <u>any</u> type.

Preventing migraines or reducing their frequency can often be accomplished by relaxation exercises on a daily basis, beta blocker medications such as atenolol (which is pretty inexpensive), tricyclic antidepressants such as Elavil (amitriptyline), valproic acid, calcium channel blockers (which I haven't had as much success with as others have reported) and non-steroidal anti-inflammatory medications (NSAIDs), such as Naprosyn (Aleve is the over-the-counter name) up to 1,100 mg daily. There is some concern about the kidneys when using the NSAIDs for a long time. Methysergide and phenelzine sulfate are often used in severe cases.

Studies are underway now for preventive use of Prozac, riboflavin, and magnesium. Prozac is fairly expensive, though just became available in generic form, and requires a prescription (as do all those above except feverfew and caffeine and Naprosyn in the OTC size), but riboflavin and magnesium are cheap. Stay tuned for further info on those.

Neurontin, usually used for seizure prevention, is now being found to help in preventing certain types of migraine.

In women of childbearing age caution is necessary because several of these drugs used for prevention can cause birth defects if you get pregnant while you are taking them.

A Good Treatment Program

I would start with relaxation exercises twice a day, then add feverfew daily if still having the headaches after a month. It takes about a month before any of these reach their full effect and you can tell whether they are working or not.

Avoidance of certain foods may help. The following list is not all-inclusive but is a good place to start:

Caffeine (but it's OK to try it a few times when an attack is coming on to see whether it helps)

Cheese, particularly the sharp ones

Chocolate

Wine and other alcohol

Tobacco in any form is not a food but should be avoided.

Also anything you can do to make the muscles in spasm do some active work will cause the spasms to get better. So first tightening, then relaxing, your affected muscles is good. Bring your shoulders up your ears while you tighten the back of your neck as hard as you can for at least 10 to 15 seconds, take a deep breath, let the breath out and let your shoulders fall. Rolling your shoulders forward as though you are rowing a boat, and then rolling them backwards as though you are rowing the boat the other way is also good technique.

Migraine headaches are often preceded by an "aura," which can be any number of strange sensations, many of which are visual.

If you consistently experience an aura before the pain actually starts, then you have a pretty good shot at taking something that will either totally head it off or greatly reduce the length of the headaches. Reducing the time they last can be a big thing because I have known a lot of people who were totally out of commission for three or four days at a time with one.

Danger Signs

Certain types of headaches are signs of something bad going on inside your head. For this reason people who have new onset bad headaches should be evaluated with a brain scan of some type soon after the onset of these head problems.

The people who most need the brain scans are those who are older than 40 when recurring headaches start. The recurring ones can be due to a brain tumor, hydrocephalus, leaking aneurysm and others as noted at the beginning of the chapter.

People with migraines get used to having bad headaches, but they always follow the same pattern. If, however, a headache with a different pattern becomes severe with no apparent cause, like a fever, and doesn't respond to your usual medication, then see your doctor.

The worst headache you ever had is probably an emergency and should be evaluated in a hospital Emergency Room. Same for severe headache accompanied by projectile vomiting.

A sudden severe headache with the pain centered between the eyes, that is worse when you bend forward is probably an emergency also. Both this and the ones above can be a swelling or rupturing aneurysm, which, if caught before it actually ruptures, can be totally cured with few or no after effects. Or you can die.

Any kind of a headache accompanied by any defect in the vision of either eye needs a scan as soon as possible but may not be an immediate emergency. That set of symptoms often means a pituitary tumor.

A perhaps not-so-severe headache that develops within a few weeks after a blow on the head may be a subdural hematoma that needs surgery quickly.

Headaches are literally "a headache" for any doctor who has to try to figure out whether you have something really bad, or just a bad headache with no serious underlying condition. He will need all the help he can get to distinguish among all of the myriad of possibilities. So go to him prepared to give a very accurate history, along with your thoughts on possible causes.

CHAPTER 51 -- HEART ATTACKS

A heart attack usually occurs when one of the blood vessels of the heart becomes suddenly closed to the passage of blood. This means that part of the heart muscle is deprived of oxygen and other less important nutrients that it needs to continue to contract normally while pumping blood out to the body. For reasons we won't go into here, the left side of the heart is almost always the side where the vessels involved in a heart attack become obstructed. Thus organs that are supplied from the left side muscle (the left ventricle), which are actually every organ in the body except the lungs, suddenly are deprived of some of their blood supply.

How much loss there is depends upon whether one or more of the three primary coronary arteries are closed, whether one or more of the others is also compromised to some degree by fat in the vessel walls, and whether there have been some new vessels growing into the area in response to the diminishing blood supply if the larger vessel opening has been reduced slowly over a long period of time. We call this "collateral circulation," and the presence of such additional circulation explains why a relatively young person who has a first heart attack is much more likely to die with that attack than someone older who has developed his or her coronary artery obstruction slowly enough to allow new small arteries to grow into the area needing more blood before the main vessel finally closed.

It is very common for me to find the scars from an old myocardial infarction on an EKG in an older person with no heart symptoms, or very minor ones. These silent heart attacks did not produce enough blood deprivation to cause major symptoms. And the patient did not die.

When an area of the heart becomes oxygen starved for any reason, its electrical status becomes compromised, and it may cause the heart to do some bad things that can cause death even without any death of part of the heart muscle. The main event is ventricular fibrillation. That is why police in many cities now carry a defibrillator in their car trunks.

The symptoms noted below are a result of blood deprivation. Loss of consciousness from failure of supply to the brain occurs only in the most grave heart attack situations, such as ventricular fibrillation.

Symptoms of a Heart Attack

- Chest pain. This often feels like a gorilla sitting on your chest, but can feel like just a dull ache, or feel like gas in the chest or upper abdomen. But it doesn't feel sharp and stabbing. That kind of pain is something else. The pain or discomfort can be felt in the chest only, or going up into the neck, or can be felt going down the inside of the left and/or right upper arm. This is the textbook picture, but it can also be felt going down into the stomach area, or even one or both legs in rare cases. It can also be felt in the jaw or feel like a toothache.
- Sweating. This is very common. Beads of sweat may break out on the face and neck, even in a cool room.
- Pallor. You may turn pale, especially if you are also sweating.
- Nausea. But usually no actual vomiting.
- Shortness of breath. Or shallow breathing.
- Dizziness or feeling faint.
- Feeling of indigestion. The person may be popping antacid tablets.
- Denial. This can be fatal, because it may cause too much delay in seeking medical help.

What to do when you get these symptoms? Call 911. Tell them your symptoms so that they will send the paramedics instead of the police. Leave the phone off the hook. You don't need to give your address unless you are using a cell phone. They automatically have the address of any fixed phone you are calling from. Go to the front door, if you can, and leave it open. Take an aspirin to help slow the possible clotting of blood in the arteries of your heart. Then just lie down and wait. It shouldn't take over 6 or 7 minutes in most places.

Do _not_ drive yourself to the hospital. You may have a cardiac arrest on the way and drive into another car or people on the sidewalk and kill others, while eliminating any possible chance of saving yourself.

On the afternoon of the day I am writing this, I sent a man to the hospital via a 911 call by ambulance with an apparent heart attack. He was in his son's pediatrician's office when he began to note low anterior chest pain, which almost immediately went to his left arm. He felt dizzy. The pediatrician sent him immediately to our urgent care clinic.

That was mistake number one. What he should have done was to call 911 right then and there. The second mistake was in sending him somewhere besides a hospital emergency room. We see a lot of heart attacks in our urgent care clinics, but valuable time is saved by going directly to an ER.

While the man was driving himself to our clinic, he just had to have a cigarette. That was mistake number three. Any of these mistakes could have resulted, directly in the case of the cigarette, or indirectly through time wasted by the pediatrician's suggestions, in a preventable death.

After the cigarette he began to also have pain moving up into his neck. Then he arrived with his son at our clinic, and mistake number four never happened. We saw him immediately, gave him nitroglycerin and an aspirin, and started him on oxygen, all as we called 911. They took him straight to the hospital, leaving us to care for a very scared little boy until grandma arrived. A later phone call from his wife told us that he had arrived at the hospital in good shape and was doing well in ICU. It wasn't his time to go!

Can you <u>believe</u> someone who thinks he is having a heart attack smoking a cigarette while driving himself to emergency care?! Perhaps that is the ultimate in denial. Or a poorly concealed death wish.

CHAPTER 52 -- HEART FAILURE

This is the cause of almost all cardiac deaths that don't occur from an acute myocardial infarction (MI, heart attack). What happens is that the heart muscle weakens, from too much scarring from repeated heart attacks, from the stress of poorly-controlled high blood pressure, from myocarditis, or from too little blood available to the muscle for other reasons. When the heart muscle gets thin and weak, it can't pump the blood as strongly as it used to, and blood may then back up in the circulation.

When that happens, it often affects one side of the heart more than the other. We often refer to right-sided and left-sided heart failure in those cases.

Right-sided failure often is the direct result of lung disease, such as emphysema, which causes high pressures in the pulmonary arteries over a period of time. Eventually the heart muscle decompensates and symptoms other than those of the lung disease begin to appear.

The most striking features of right-sided failure are related to the backing up of blood waiting in line, so to speak, to pass through the right side of the heart and into the lungs where it gives up its carbon dioxide and gains a fresh load of oxygen to carry over into the left side of the heart and then out into the muscles and organs of the body.

When the blood backs up, it causes swelling and congestion in the legs first, with swelling of both feet and both ankles. This swelling is different from most of the swelling we have become accustomed to in our lives, because it consists mainly of water in and just under the skin. If you push on the swollen area with your finger, it will produce a depression or pit in the skin which doesn't go away for a short time after you let go. We call this "pitting edema." Some old people who just sit with their legs hanging down all day long get this same type of swelling by the end of the day without having heart failure. We call that "dependent edma."

Some long distance travelers who don't do the exercises I recommend in the chapter on **Pulmonary Embolism** also get this kind of swelling without having heart failure. People with a large blood clot in the main vein of one leg often get this kind of swelling after a few days. But in the case of the blood clots there is usually just one foot and ankle that swells. *Swelling of this type in just one foot or ankle should always make you suspect a possible blood clot, and you must see a doctor immediately.

The organs of the abdomen begin to swell after the blood has been backing up for awhile. The liver in particular can enlarge to two or three times its normal size. Symptoms may arise in the GI tract from the congestion of blood, with bleeding from the engorged mucous membranes in some cases, and cramps or other pains from the stretched capsules of some organs. Over a long time the stretching discomfort often goes away, but some symptoms stay. The congestion also overwhelms the kidneys so that they may need a stimulant, or diuretic, such as Lasix (furosemide) to make them get rid of the excess water that is accumulating in the system.

Left-sided failure is probably the most common, mainly because most heart attacks (MI's) involve the left side of the heart, and thus more scarring occurs there. Normally the left ventricle is the more muscular because it has to push blood all over the body, while the right ventricle just sends its blood to the adjacent lungs. However after one or two MI's have left behind little but scar tissue, the muscle wall thins dramatically and blood may begin to back up into the lungs, causing congestion in the tiny air sacs (which is why it is called "congestive" heart failure).

As the back-pressure of the blood in the tiny blood vessels of the smallest air sacs (which we call alveoli) builds up, the blood begins to leak through the vessel walls into the air spaces. At that point the person is in serious trouble, and it can get worse very rapidly, with pulmonary edema resulting. People with pulmonary edema literally begin to drown in their own secretions. Cough initially may produce white phlegm, but as the condition worsens even more it becomes blood-tinged and then grossly bloody. The patient gets very short of breath, and begins to lose brain function. At that time the sick person has no more than a few hours at most to live if treatment isn't started promptly.

*Anyone who coughs up bloody phlegm must see a doctor immediately. Don't wait till morning!

Dramatic measures are called for if the person is to be saved. Somehow the total amount of blood in the circulation must be reduced, and quickly. Treatment options include several of the following steps: giving intravenous diuretics to cause the kidneys to quickly put out a lot of urine, giving oxygen by nasal tubes so that each red blood cell that is pumped out by the failing heart has a full load of oxygen on board, and/or oxygen by IPPB (Intermittent Positive Pressure Breathing) which exerts external pressure on the small air sacs in the lungs to reverse the out flow of fluid from the blood vessels while also providing needed oxygen, IV digoxin (Lanoxin) to make the heart muscle pump stronger and more efficiently very quickly, and possibly tourniquets on all four extremities to hold back as much blood as possible from reaching the heart until some of the other measures can begin to take hold.

In addition we may withdraw a pint of blood, just as one does when donating blood to reduce the body's fluid overload.

(The practice of "bleeding" people 200 and more years ago gained popularity from the dramatic improvement when it was tried in congestive heart failure. No medical people really knew what they were doing or why they were succeeding, so they tried it for everything for a long time. George Washington, for example, probably met his maker too soon because of unwarranted and excessive "bleeding.")

Digoxin (Lanoxin) is derived from digitalis leaf, which has been used for failing hearts for hundreds of years. In its use as a cardiac stimulant it is administered in minute doses of 0.125 to 0.25mg per tablet after the initial loading doses, and its level in the blood should be monitored by periodic blood tests to be sure that the level remains within a very narrow range. Too low a level is of no value, while too high a level is poisonous. But it is a wonderful drug. I had a patient whose liver was enlarged to four time its normal size in congestive heart failure when I first met her. Under such circumstances her life expectancy was less than one year. But I put her on Lanoxin and a diuretic kidney stimulant while keeping her sodium and potassium blood levels in the normal range (diuretics cause the loss of large amounts of the minerals and potassium often has to be replaced with a tablet or two daily), then watched her closely, and she lived for a little over twenty more years!

CHAPTER 53 -- HEAT INJURIES

I live in a place where people die in the desert several times a year, from heat, exposure to the merciless rays of the sun, or just plain lack of adequate water intake. Most often it is the latter. Even those of us who are well aware that there are risks in the summer ("summer" meaning May through at least mid-October), may prepare inadequately for heat exposure. Noel Coward once wrote a song about India, "Mad dogs and Englishmen go out in the noonday sun." That statement is doubly true about the desert country of our great Southwest.

One of the times that people especially get into trouble with heat is when the days of late summer have a lot of moisture in the air, as in the monsoons in the Southwest, which occur about the time that high school and college football practice starts.

The way our temperature regulating system works involves the production of sweat, which ideally then evaporates, and the evaporation from the surface of our skin has a cooling effect on the core temperature of our bodies. If there is too much humidity in the air, as during the monsoons, then the sweat doesn't evaporate very well, and the body has more trouble cooling itself. But the body keeps on trying. So we are more vulnerable to heat injury especially when there is a lot of humidity in the air even if we are drinking a lot of fluids.

The highest risk of hyperthermia, however, occurs in those who aren't drinking enough fluids to replace those lost. When dehydration reaches a certain point, 7% in several studies, the rate of sweating decreases by 25%. This reduces the body's ability to cool itself by at least that much. This is in addition to the 50% reduction in blood flow to the skin, where the evaporative cooling occurs, when the level of 3% dehydration is reached during exercise-related heat stress.

Ideally the warm blood from inside the body flows to the surface of the skin, where the sweat evaporates to cool the body. The blood then leaves the skin capillaries as much as several degrees cooler on its trip back to the internal organs, and cools them in return before being pumped back to the skin surface again. When dehydration occurs, there isn't enough fluid in the body to allow full and unrestricted sweating, and there isn't as much blood available to flow to the skin for that part of the cooling mechanism.

The best way to tell whether athletes, both young and old, are getting enough fluids to replace their loss during exercise is to weigh each one before and after practice or training with the same clothes on and record those numbers.

For example, if a 200-pound football player weighs 6 pounds less at the end of practice than he did at the beginning, then he is 3% dehydrated and is at risk for heat injury. If that same athlete has lost 16 pounds, he is 8% dehydrated, has an elevated body temperature, and probably needs IV fluids in a hospital immediately, whether he has symptoms or not. 8% is the critical number for most people, but severe problems can develop at lower numbers also.

Signs and symptoms of heat exhaustion include flushed skin on the athlete's face and chest, chills, abdominal cramps, hairs standing up on the skin, dizziness, weakness, vomiting, and hyperirritability. As heat and dehydration increase faintness, fatigue, shortness of breath, indistinct speech, headache, and spastic muscles may also appear as signs of a worsening and more critical condition (6-8% dehydration).

There is a safety formula for marathon runners, where they are advised not to run a race if the humidity and temperature at race time exceed a certain mathematical standard. I will try to find that formula by the next edition of this book. Maybe one of my readers will be kind enough to share it with me.

I know that this was a matter for considerable concern at the Atlanta Olympics because the men's event was to be run late in the day just before the closing ceremonies, when the temperature and humidity would be at their highest for the day. Apparently the heat abated somewhat, and all was well.

I remember too well the young woman, from Portugal, I believe, who stumbled and staggered around the track, taking perhaps ten minutes to finish the last lap, in one recent Olympics. That woman was at high risk of dying from dehydration and heat injury, but no one stopped her. We admired her indomitable spirit, though my chief thought was "she may die!" But she came back four years later and won the marathon!

In the Gulf States you know you are losing fluids because the sweat just drips off of you in the heat. There is so much moisture already in the air in the deep South that sweat doesn't evaporate very much or very fast, In the Southwest, except during the monsoon months of July and August, there is so little humidity in the air that sweat evaporates before we are even aware of any moisture. Thus sometimes we forget to drink to keep up with our loss because our loss is not apparent. Once you get behind in your fluid intake, it is hard to catch up until you put yourself into a cool place.

Fluid Rules

Drink at least two quarts of water per hour when out in the sun in the summer at temperatures over 90 degrees. Increase that as the temperature climbs.

> *And at least double that figure if you are exercising as an athlete or doing hard labor, such as unloading with no assistance a truck that has been sitting outside a big store in the hot sun for 5 or 6 hours before the store people find a spot for you at their loading dock, as happened to one of my very ill patients in the summer of 2001 in Phoenix. He was very dehydrated and hadn't urinated for 14 hours when I first saw him. After some IV fluids for a couple of hours, he was transferred to a local hospital for more fluids and an overnight stay for observation.*

Salt, while helpful, is not usually a necessity, and salt tablets are not a good idea because they are too concentrated for the body to handle well. They often induce vomiting. Even though you know that sweat tastes salty, you also need to know that the more you sweat, the smaller the amount of salt that is excreted in the sweat. So, since salt tablets often make people sick at the stomach, just drink water. And it doesn't have to be cold water, just wet.

Having said that, let me assure you that Gatorade (and one or two of the Gatorade imitators) really have a good thing going with their electrolyte-balanced solutions. Given the option, drink a quart of Gatorade for every two quarts of plain water.

The absolute best way to tell whether you are drinking enough fluids is whether you are urinating every two or three hours, and especially whether your urine is almost free of color, as it should be when you are fully hydrated.

Almost every year in Arizona we hear about a high school athlete who dies from heat stroke. In almost every case it is the coach who is to blame. In the past six years through August 2001 18 high school and college football players have died of heat stroke. Three died within a week in the summer of 2001, including Korey Stringer of the Minnesota Vikings. Eighty-four have died since records started being kept in 1955, but Korey was the first from the NFL.

In the pre-season of 2003 the NFL team practicing in Jacksonville, Florida had three athletes with heat problems the first week. And they were being careful!

The ideal situation is that of the Arizona Cardinals. No matter what you and I may think about the team on the field, they have the best of all worlds for their pre-season training camp in the mountains of Flagstaff. The temperature is mild, the air is relatively dry even during the monsoons, and some high altitude training effects can be factored in too.

According to an article by Jose E. Garcia, reporting on page C6 in the *ARIZONA REPUBLIC* issue of August 7, 2001, "...His teammate, Gilbert Chavez, showed up without any fluids or food in his system on a humid day that reached 90 degrees by 5:30 a.m. Chavez vomited two hours into the practice. Hunched over and wincing in pain, Chavez, 16, a 200-pound linebacker and fullback, heard the inevitable snickers from teammates as they roasted him for his unenviable spot. After about 10 minutes, Chavez got back in time to finish a drill. "I just have to suck it in and take it," Chavez said. "Next time I'll make sure to eat and drink something before I get here."

Those of us who are team doctors, as I was for 38 years, have a responsibility to make sure that the teams we serve know what damage inadequate fluid intake can do. Every team at every practice must have water within a few yards of the players at all times and the players must be required to drink it. One boy who died of the heat had a water hose at the practice field, but it was 100 yards away from where the boys were. The boys were expected to run to the water and run back whenever they wanted a drink!

Overweight kids are much more likely to have heat problems than those of normal (or, as is frequent in high school) skinny builds. Was Gilbert Chavez overweight? The article didn't say, but my experience with high school athletes suggests that a 16-year old will probably be overweight at 200 pounds.

In the case described in the newspaper there was another tragedy that almost happened. The kid could have been on the verge of a fatal case of heat stroke. Gilbert Chavez didn't die, but he darned well could have! The coaching staff of the Marcos de Niza team of Tempe could easily have had another death on their hands.

Here is what was wrong with that episode:

First, what in the world were they doing having a two-hour practice in that heat?! Especially when another practice was scheduled for late in the afternoon. Second, vomiting is one of the symptoms of heat exhaustion. Why was the boy left to vomit by himself for ten minutes and the allowed to return to drills? (The same thing allegedly happened to Korey Stringer the day he died). Did the coaches have a death wish? Where was the trainer, for Pete's sake?!! I suspect that the team doctor must have read this article with horror. Perhaps something positive was left out of the article. But I doubt it.

IT IS ABSOLUTELY MANDATORY FOR COACHES TO BE CERTAIN THAT EVERY PLAYER, AND ESPECIALLY THE OVERWEIGHT ONES, DRINK WATER EVERY 5 OR 10 MINUTES IN HOT WEATHER. Shade should be provided during rest periods.

The *Arizona Republic* made a strong statement in its sports section in August 2003, calling the attention of athletes and coaches alike to proper preventive measures. That spread may have saved a life.

*All players must be *required* to drink at every break in the action.** That doesn't mean every 15 or 20 minutes. It means every 5 or 10 minutes. In my high school sports days, we were told just to rinse our mouths with water and then spit it out or it would slow us down or make us sick at the stomach. The thought of how many kids had to die because of that misbegotten philosophy makes me sick. Personally, I always swallowed some, and it didn't slow *me* down. Possibly because I was already the slowest guy on the team!

*Thirst is not a good indication of when to drink. By the time you are thirsty, you are already about two quarts low and probably won't be able to catch up that day.

Heat exhaustion is one of the extremes of heat stress secondary to inadequate fluid intake, but one can recover with adequate fluid replacement in a relatively short time. One with this condition is still able to sweat if he is not too dehydrated. But if dehydration is too far along for the sweat glands to no longer be able to produce sweat, the body may go suddenly into heat stroke in which the skin is hot and totally dry, the person may be talking out of his head, and the fever may quickly climb to 105 degrees or more. This person is going to die if something isn't done to cool him off immediately. Just giving cold fluids to drink isn't enough. The brain is literally cooking, and may never be normal again even if the person survives.

Get the person into the shade, or into air conditioning right now, before even calling 911 (which you must do if you can). Pour (cold) water on his clothes and fan him. Pack him in ice if available. Especially his head. Give him non-caffeine and non-alcohol-containing fluids, a few ounces at a time. Don't give salt tablets.

Symptoms of Heat Injury

Vomiting, weakness, inability to concentrate, staggering and poor coordination, paleness, or beet red face, either one, thirst, dry mouth and tongue. Headache. Rapid breathing. Rapid pulse. Maybe inability to talk properly. Loss of consciousness.

In addition to heat injury there are two other very dangerous conditions that result sometimes from the thickening of the blood as **dehydration** develops. These are heart attack and stroke.

I had a patient just a week before I wrote this who had some of the above symptoms of heat injury when I first walked into the examining room. As I was examining him, he suddenly complained of a feeling of pressure under his breastbone, along with radiation into his neck. We quickly called 911, and gave him oxygen and nitroglycerine. He was on the verge of or actually having a heart attack, and we had an ambulance there within 4 minutes. So it turned out well.

*One that did not turn so well was the great aunt of my kids. She had fallen at home jumping up to answer the telephone and tripped on the shag carpet, breaking her hip. (See the chapter on **Preventing Falls in the Elderly**.) She was doing fine post-op and her surgeon had put her on oral fluids on morning rounds, while discontinuing her IV fluids. A couple hours later, after he had signed out to another doctor for his afternoon off, she began to vomit. Her sister called me and asked what to do because she couldn't convince the nurse to call the covering doctor. I was far away in Flagstaff, Arizona, and I used all my powers of persuasion on the nurse when I finally got hold of her at the nurse's station. I asked her if she would please, in lieu of calling the doctor, to at least hang another bottle of IV fluids until her vomiting stopped. She was not impressed that I was a doctor and might know what I was talking about. Instead she firmly assured me that Aunt Toni was doing fine, and I should tell her family not to worry. To make a long sad story short, she continued to vomit, took in no fluids all that day, got dehydrated, had a massive stroke that night and died a day or two later.*

CHAPTER 54 -- HERBAL REMEDIES AND OTHER DIETARY SUPPLEMENTS

Here is where you can really go to town in your role of being your own doctor.

These are marketed as dietary supplements and were deregulated in 1994. Thus there are no patient study requirements to determine whether one of these, in fact, is beneficial, or whether it is all word of mouth. With the FDA out of the picture, safety and healing capability are not guaranteed by any monitoring organization. Manufacturers don't have to test the products they make for purity or effectiveness. There is a <u>huge</u> amount of information and misinformation out there, and most folks are feeling somewhat overwhelmed by what they hear. Also, these compounds may not require a prescription, but they aren't cheap. Estimates are that the money spent on herbal drugs and dietary supplements each year runs into the multi-billions of dollars.

So I am going to give you as much accurate and up-to-date information as I can to guide you here. Then you may decide to save your money, or you may find a preparation that is cheaper and more effective than the prescription drug you are currently taking.

Anti-Oxidants, Free Radicals, and How Not to Get Scammed

The latest trick to separate you from your money is the phrase "anti-oxidants." Every health store, nutrition department, and supermarket product now uses these buzz words. It's usually your tip-off that an expensive scam is in operation, as these products always cost much more than the traditional version. What are anti-oxidants? Vitamins E, C, and beta-carotene (a component of Vitamin A). Period. So, if you are taking that modestly priced tablet each day that contains a full assortment of vitamins and minerals, and you are eating a healthy diet low in fats and carbohydrates and high in fruits and vegetables, you are already giving your body everything it needs. Instead of paying $3.43 for a twelve-ounce bottle of "anti-oxidant power" that contains mostly red grape juice, white grape juice, and some mango or pomegranate puree, giving you a whopping 38 gram sugar high, save your health dollars. Buy apples. Buy a 67 cent can of tomato paste that has

236

high levels of anti-oxidants and practically no sugar. Mix in some olive oil, which is good for you, with the tomato paste. This makes a healthy substitute for salad dressings, mayonnaise, or Miracle Whip, which are heart attacks on a plate.

Be aware that you can overdo a good thing with anti-oxidants, as well as many other things. <u>Never</u> take more that 5,000 I.U. of Vitamin A or equivalent, nor more than 800 I.U. of Vitamin E. Excessive amounts of both of these can and will do a lot more harm than good to your body because they are slowly excreted. Overdoses of Vitamin C can be immediately excreted by the kidneys and don't build up in the body's fat storage areas to potentially toxic levels. But too much Vitamin C (which is otherwise known as ascorbic acid) will produce crystals in the urine, which could lead to kidney stones.

Understand the basics so that you can make smart decisions on where to spend your health dollars. Anti-oxidants are good in the proper amounts. They help cleanse the body of free radicals. What are free radicals? Groups of atoms with extra electrons formed when oxygen reacts with certain molecules in your body. They are highly reactive, and their chief danger comes from the damage they can do if they react with important parts of your cells. These include DNA and cell membranes, which must be strong to resist infection or invasion by cancer-causing elements (carcinogens). If free radicals damage a cell, it may function incorrectly or even die. Anti-oxidants bond with free radicals to form a harmless molecule which the body can dispose of. A trace mineral, Selenium, is also important in one of the body's own anti-oxidant enzyme systems, and this should be in your daily multi-vitamin and mineral supplement in a small quantity. Drink lots and lots of tap water -- no, you don't need to waste money on designer bottled water. This is nature's own miracle anti-oxidant.

It may sound at first as though I'm trying to steer you away from all medicinal herbs and supplements. Not so, but there are more cautions than successes for many of them, and some are quite dangerous. Learn as much as you can here, then decide for yourself whether and what you want to try.

In my experience people don't tell each other very often about what failed, perhaps because they don't want to be thought dumb for trying such a thing. And all well-controlled medical studies of new drugs have a placebo effect.

Let me tell you about the **placebo effect**, which is well known to all doctors. A placebo medication works because the person thinks it is going to work. This gives us a little hint of how powerful suggestions are to our minds. Hypnosis is a good example. Most of us have seen or heard of the very unusual, even fantastic things that people can do under hypnosis. I have successfully hypnotized quite a few people, and I will tell you here and now that it <u>works</u>. If your doctor tells you that a new drug is going to make you get well, between 20 and 40% of you will proceed to get well, no matter whether it is a sugar pill or the latest and best drug on the market for the condition. So when a new drug is being tested to see whether it is really beneficial, the placebo effect is cancelled out by doing what is called a double blind, cross-over study, in which neither the patient nor the doctor know whether the patient is being given the real drug or a "sugar pill" (or placebo) that is identical in appearance to the active drug. The patients are assigned randomly, and ideally are matched as to age, sex, and economic status, along with other aspects of their lives that may be pertinent. The bottles have only numbers plus instructions as to how to take them on the labels.

> *Feeling are facts: A competitor in any activity who feels that he is going to win has a much greater chance of doing so than someone who has a different feeling. They may have each trained and prepared physically in an identical manner. Their skills may be similar. But one person will win because of his mental preparation that led him to believe that he would win. And feeling that you are going to win causes things to happen in your mind and body that make it happen, over and over and over.*
>
> *When I was at the U.S. Olympic Training Center for mental training one Labor Day weekend, we were taught that winning begins with high self-esteem. We were taught various things to enhance that feeling in ourselves that we won't go into here because that would take another whole book.*

The doses are taken by the first group of patients for a certain amount of time, with careful monitoring of signs and symptoms, along with appropriate lab tests. At the end of the first study period, which may be even as much as a year or more, the roles are reversed, and those who got the active drug at first begin to take the placebo, while the other group begins to take the active drug. Again the patients are monitored carefully to see if their condition is improved, getting worse, developing side effects, whatever, and only the computer knows that a change has taken place.

It a well-established fact that a certain percentage of people, up to as high as 40% or more in some studies, will be better on the placebo. That is our powerful minds at work. *Feelings are facts!** We'll talk more about that elsewhere. But for now just be aware that what you feel is real for you personally, if for no one else. And what you feel has an enormous effect on how your mind and body respond to all kinds of things.

Suffice it to say that each of us is a unique individual with different capabilities in many different areas of our beings. It is absolutely wrong for <u>any</u> of us to compare ourselves unfavorably to someone else. It almost a certainty that each of us has the potential to be better than most other people in the world in <u>something</u>. It may not be in what our parents have in mind. And we may have to fail a few times before we find what we do best. (Look how many times Abe Lincoln failed before he was elected president.)

Very few people wind up doing for life what they started out to do. Sometimes we don't ever figure out what we do best, and that is sad. Sometimes we get stuck in an economic situation that is hard to get out of. If you are such a case, go to night school, trade school, or junior college. If you are a single parent, trade baby-sitting with a friend or friends so you can get the additional education. It is estimated that your lifetime earnings increase by at least $100,000 for every year of post high school education. So skip the cokes and beer and tobacco to save money for additional education. I worked my way through medical school; so I know what I'm talking about. Exercise daily for twenty to thirty minutes every day (ideally at least 30), even if it is just sprinting around doing the household chores without stopping. That will clear the brain, make you a more confident person, and also make your body function more efficiently. Plus a <u>lot</u> of other good stuff discussed in the chapter on **Exercise.**

Returning from far afield to our original subject, the growth of the herbal and dietary supplement market since deregulation has been astronomical. We will dwell below at greater length on some of the top-selling herbal remedies and supplements in the U.S. as of 2003. Some I recommend, and some I don't. Many are now being studied by well-regarded medical schools.

I recommend the following dietary supplements and herbs for use in certain limited conditions:

Glucosamine, 500 mg three times daily for osteoarthritis. There have actually been some small studies done on this. So far I am not aware of any bad side effects. And the number of patients in whom it has reduced pain and improved functioning of joints that I am aware of is now in the dozens. This is not a good scientific sample, but even our neighbor's dog has started to run again since starting to use it, whereas before she could barely hobble around.

Chondroitin is usually co-promoted with the glucosamine for arthritis. Supposedly it is from shark cartilage and helps your cartilage to return to normal. It isn't so. Some studies of chondroitin done without glucosamine have shown no benefit whatsoever. That makes sense, because the shark cartilage is digested in our stomachs and thus isn't available to our joints as cartilage. I have an ongoing survey of my patients who are taking one or both of these. So far only one has reported feeling any better with the added chondroitin. Since adding chondroitin to the glucosamine considerably increases the cost, I recommend that you skip the chondroitin.

Feverfew for migraines. Also some dietary restrictions which we will discuss in the chapter on **Migraines**.

Aloe vera for first and shallow second degree burns. But it probably isn't as effective as promoted in other skin conditions.

Valerian is pretty safe and effective for insomnia.

Here is a true horror story about herbal preparations:

In Belgium, doctors followed more than one hundred patients for over eight years after they took a weight-loss preparation containing Chinese herbs, often with an appetite suppressant, such as diethylproprion or fenfluoramine and others. An herb which produces severe kidney damage, *Aristolochia*, had been accidentally substituted for *Stephania tetranda*, which is much safer. (The two are often confused -- as are many others -- and are collectively referred to as <u>mu tong</u>.) Of these people, 41% developed kidney failure and of those, 46% developed kidney cancer and another 45% had pre-cancerous conditions in their kidneys.

It is important that you be aware that other herbal preparations usually considered to be safe because they are "natural" (we will address "natural" later too) also have significant risks, e.g. cardiac shock from Ephedra, hepatitis from germander, and seizures and kidney failure from yohimbine (used for impotence problems. Better use Viagra instead.)

Always tell your doctor if you are using or thinking of using any herbal product.

Surgical complications: Ginkgo biloba and medicinal garlic are known to cause bleeding after surgery in patients who use them, and serious bleeding after gall bladder surgery and after spinal surgery were specifically mentioned. A recent study cited in the *Journal of the American Medical Association* listed eight herbs used by a lot of people which can cause problems of one sort or another. These are echinacea, ephedra, garlic, ginkgo biloba, ginseng, kava, St. John's wort, and valerian.

Drug interaction between warfarin (Coumadin), which is taken to reduce the risk of life-threatening blood clots in several areas including the heart, and Ginkgo biloba or ginseng (and many other herbs) may make your blood unable to clot at all. Warfarin also has potentially serious interactions with many conventional drugs; so one must be very careful with it. Too little effect lets the harmful blood clots occur, while too great an effect may cause stroke or other internal bleeding.

Several herbs can increase the effects of other types of drugs or reduce the ability of your body to absorb or react to a medicine as expected. Since so few studies have been done so far, we don't know nearly as much as we need to about these effects yet.

St. John's wort taken by an AIDS patient will reduce the effectiveness of the cyclosporine he is taking to control his disease, for example. Powdered psyllium seeds slow down the absorption of lithium (for depression) and digoxin (for congestive heart failure). In the case of the heart failure patient, death can result.

Avoiding surgical complications from herbs involves two approaches. First stop all herbs at least three weeks before the operation if you have that much time. Second, and this probably should be first, tell your surgeon and your anesthesiologist what herbs you are taking, if any. But don't expect that they will know for sure what complications are possible with any given herb. We don't have much accurate information about them right now. Most is word of mouth. We learn about possible complications from articles such as these, which are written after the fact mostly.

As far as ginkgo biloba is concerned, it has been used for eye diseases of older people, impotence (I will tell you right now that Viagra is better), and altitude sickness. Plus a lot of other stuff. Garlic is often taken for high blood pressure and high cholesterol. (I like garlic -- a lot. My approach to its use is that almost any excuse for eating garlic is OK. But I have had a number of patients who take it and still need prescription blood pressure medicine.) Same for high cholesterol.

Undoubtedly there are some beneficial herbs. The risks arise from the safety of the herbal product you are taking, first from its possible interaction with other medications you are taking, and second from the quality (or lack thereof) of the herb in the pill. These are very real concerns, based unfortunately on increasing numbers of mishaps involving these very concerns.

One authority refers to "The three Ms: Mislabeling, Misrepresentation, and Misuse" as the causes of these Mishaps.

One of the biggest reasons for problems with herbs is that they are composed of more than one chemical compound, sometimes a hundred or more, and thus your body's response to one of the many may be unpredictable. (Using an example we may all be familiar with -- tobacco, which causes untold misery, has over 1,000 chemical compounds in it.) Manufactured drugs, on the other hand, rarely have more than one active ingredient. The cough and cold remedies are a notable exception to that. The more active ingredients there are, the more likely an undesirable drug reaction is to occur.

Herbal remedy manufacturers produce both standardized and non-standardized products. The non-standardized ones are usually made from whole herbs and tend to vary widely in content and potency, sometimes varying even from capsule to capsule in the same batch. We'll discuss this a little more later.

Standardized herbs are, obviously, usually safer because an effort has been made by the company to at least try to put the same amount of active ingredient in each dose, while eliminating most of the other compounds. Whether they are successful or not will also be discussed below.

The latest scam in the Misrepresentation area has all the claims that old-time snake oil used to have. Its promoters say it can cure arthritis, AIDS, Ebola, the Bubonic Plague, cancer, acne, worms, impotence, and it's good for constipation! The snake oil this year, like Hadacol 50 years ago and Bay Rum of 100 years ago, (and who remembers what 150 and 200 years ago!?), is called "Colloidal Silver." Instead of being a new breakthrough cure, it is really several centuries old and has caught on over the Internet. The Food and Drug Administration banned its sale as a remedy in 1999, but it has still been available over the Web in many forms at prices as high as $20 an ounce (4 to 5 times what an ounce of pure silver is worth. As of late June 2001 the FDA and FTC have started enforcement actions against certain Internet retailers who are engaging in "fraudulent marketing of supplements and other health products."

I don't know how successful those organizations will be at protecting you and me against these and dozens of other scams; so I will tell you that the best protection against these nefarious denizens of the underworld is for each of us to keep our money in our pockets and remember the old adage, "if it *sounds* too good to be true, then it probably *is* too good to be true."

One thing for sure about colloidal silver is that it has one absolutely documented effect: it can permanently change the color of your skin. The condition is called argyria. It builds up minute particles of silver in the skin and dyes the tissues blue-gray. This color varies from person to person and darkens in the sun. We don't know yet whether it leads to anything more serious, but with all the people who have been throwing away their money on it, we probably will have some definite indications in a very few years. Once you have turned blue-gray, it is permanent. So you too can look like Count Dracula! Perhaps Hollywood can use you for a science fiction movie, but there is probably little other use for that color skin.

Chicken soup is much better. "It can't hurt!"

Until recently there haven't been very many studies done on herbs and supplements in our country because the FDA can't require any study documentation for them. And any study is expensive, so whoever is doing such a study must have some source of financial reimbursement. Medical schools would be a logical choice for a study, but they are all so financially strapped by the reduction in educational grants and medical reimbursements for charity patients that they have little left for such testing on their own.

The companies who sell these products, unlike drug companies, don't have to provide any evidence that they actually work. And they aren't going to fund such studies out of the goodness of their hearts because someone might prove that their particular brand of snake oil didn't work.

This is beginning to change drastically, for the better I think. I have reviewed the results from more than 50 different studies (most of which were small in numbers unfortunately). So reliable information is soon going to be available to you almost as reliably as to me. (See the last paragraph below in this chapter for the Web address of massive information from the NIH). I do want to mention that I don't place a great value on any study that doesn't include at least 1,000 people.

The other light at the end of this tunnel of darkness is that The National Institutes of Health (NIH) have established a National Center for Complementary and Alternative Medicine. They are aware of the growing popularity of herbs in the family medicine chest and are funding a few studies of the effects of herbal and other unconventional remedies. The first of these was reported in April 2002 on St. John's Wort and is discussed below.

When a substitute herb is used in a formula, that is Mislabeling. Sometimes herbal products, particularly some made in China, contain several or even many active chemicals. Sometimes the compounding is of poor quality. An example is echinacea, where some makers use different plant species, or different parts of the plant, so there can be no comparison from company to company. These problems are less frequent in herbs produced in Europe, Canada, and the U. S., but they also occur here all too often. French and German herbal products tend to be more reliable because 30-40% of physicians in those countries include herbal remedies in their first line medical treatments.

The other of the three Ms is Misuse, and this is overdosing, along with improper use with other drugs.

Overdosing occurs, both deliberately by the person taking the herb and by inaccurate label information. This was recently illustrated by a chemical analysis survey of 25 different ginseng preparations purchased from a large health food store, which found concentrations of the active ingredients varying from 15 to 2,000% in capsules and liquid forms. A similar survey of ephedra compounds found more than 20% discrepancy between what the label said and what the actual content was on testing in over half of the bottles tested.

I had an older patient three days before I wrote this who was taking an herbal remedy. I asked him what he was taking it for, and he said he didn't really know, that his neighbor across the street had recommended it because she thought it would be good for him. There are definitely some herbs that are good for some conditions, but I haven't heard of one yet that should just be taken like vitamins and minerals that our bodies can't live without. In most other countries, herbs are taken for a specific purpose for a short period of time, perhaps three months. What I'm leading up to is: **don't take an herb unless you have a good reason to do so.** Herbs are products that have active effects on our bodies, for good or not, and we must treat them with respect.

The United States Pharmacopoeia (since 1820) and National Sanitation Foundation are about to start quality certification for herbal products. So within a year, hopefully, you can look on a label for the familiar USP or NSF letters, and don't buy or use an herb that doesn't display it on the bottle.

One thing you must be aware of and remember with these labels is that they certify only that the product in the package is what the label says it is. It should also mean that the substance is free of contaminants, like heavy metals and pesticides (the USP testing is the most stringent and perhaps the most trustworthy). *The certification does not mean that the product works the way the advertising says it does.* Only the Betty Crocker Good Housekeeping label requires scientific data to back up medicinal claims. But to be eligible for the Good Housekeeping seal, the product has to be advertised in the *Good Housekeeping* magazine.

ConsumerLab.com began testing herbs and other supplements in 1999 and has completed over 500 such tests so far. Companies can pay them to be sure to have their products tested (as with the other seal programs). They also have to pay to use the CL label in their advertising or the bottle's label.

As you start using an herb, be sure the label contains the following information, which *is* required by the FDA: the ingredients, the number of capsules or tablets in the bottle, and the recommended dose, along with the expiration date. By all means follow the recommended dose unless your doctor says different.

Be sure the herb is fresh because fresh ones are more potent than those that are dried before processing. The activity of the compounds break down over time, much as a fresh flower decomposes.

Some herbs have been found to be contaminated with pesticides and heavy metals, as well as with other drugs. It's scary!

So <u>choose so-called organically produced herbs</u> because they are less likely to contain such contaminants as concentrated pesticides.

Be aware, however, that most of the herbal products on the market, especially those from China, are neither freshly prepared nor organic. European herbs, particularly those from Germany and Switzerland, are produced under much stricter laws for safety than most of the rest of the world. Significantly, as you will see below, China buys huge amounts of their herbs from our country. Ours aren't perfect, but they are safer than theirs.

Here are the herbal products being used the most here in our country right now, along with much *accurate*, I hope, information about what they are good for and how to use them in your own home.

Arnica

Arnica is used on the surface of the skin for bruises, sprains, insect bites, and much more. May multiply the effects of blood-thinning drugs like warfarin (Coumadin).

Astragalus

Astragalus is used as a general tonic to hopefully improve the immune system against colds and flu. It increases the effect of warfarin and thus may cause bleeding problems when used in combination.

Black Cohosh

Black Cohosh is used for menstrual cramps, non-specific menopausal symptoms, and PMS. It may be even better for skin ulcers. It increases the effect of warfarin and thus may cause bleeding problems when used in combination.

Chamomile

Chamomile is often used in the form of tea for stomach symptoms and menstrual cramps. It increases the effect of warfarin and thus may cause bleeding problems when used in combination.

Cholestin

Cholestin is supposed to lower the cholesterol. It increases the effect of warfarin and thus may cause bleeding problems when used in combination.

Coenzyme Q-10

Coenzyme Q-10 is not an herb. It is claimed to be good for gum disease, strengthening the heart, and reducing the risk of developing Alzheimer's disease later in life. It increases the effect of warfarin and thus may cause bleeding problems when used in combination.

Cranberry (Vaccinium Macrocarpon)

My grandmother used cranberry juice for urinary tract infections. So did the Indians in the time of the Pilgrims. Recent careful scientific studies have shown that the cranberry is antibacterial against most of the serious bacteria that may infect the urinary tract. These include E. coli, which is responsible for the vast majority of UTIs, Klebsiella pneumoniae, which can afflict both lungs and urinary tract, Staph aureus, which also causes boils and lots of antibiotic-resistant infections all over the body, Pseudomonas, and Proteus organisms.

One recent relatively small study showed that recurrent bladder infections were totally prevented in 73% of men and women who drank 16 oz of pure cranberry juice daily. A couple of studies have shown that cranberry compounds protect the stomach from H. pylori, which causes ulcers. Another suggests that it may help prevent gum disease by blocking the bacteria that produce plaque in the mouth. Its antioxidant effects may have some beneficial potential in preventing cancer and heart disease, at least in animal studies. These remain to be seen, however, in humans.

I think the juice cocktail is more dilute than the pure juice. So use the pure juice if you can find it at your favorite grocery. If you can find only the juice cocktail, then I suggest you ask the store manager to order you a case at a time of the juice.

The most effective dose for UTIs isn't set in concrete as of this writing. I would use 16 oz of the pure juice if you are trying to treat acute UTIs or prevent re-infection. For the other beneficial effects, I would use at least 8 oz of the pure juice. Comparisons of the various forms of cranberries available are not yet standardized. Six capsules of the extract are probably about equal to 3 oz of the juice. I haven't been able to find a comparison of the tablet form. The usually recommended doses of the capsules are 300 to 400 mg twice a day. But school is still out on the most effective doses.

Possible ill effects are mostly mild, including heartburn and diarrhea in excessive amounts, and possible kidney stones after a long time on higher doses.

Dong Quai

Dong Quai supposedly purifies the blood, whatever that means. It increases the effect of warfarin and thus may cause bleeding problems when used in combination.

Echinacea Purpurea

Echinacea purpurea is often taken as a boost to your immune system in winter and for the common cold. It is a wildflower (the purple cone flower or American flower) which is native to North America. Immigrants to our country first learned of the medicinal uses from Native Americans, who used it more than any other for a lot of things-- abscesses and other infections, burns, joint pains, snakebite, and toothaches. It is probably most effective in the tincture (dissolved in alcohol) or fresh whole herb. It was used extensively for infections until the middle of the century, when more effective antibiotics started to be developed. Now, with the germ resistance problems being encountered to antibiotics, research is being directed again toward how it can help us today.

Some of the AIDS research has rubbed off here. There is no question that Echinacea helps our immune systems in several different ways according to the results of several hundred studies around the world dating from the 1930s in Germany. If you are interested, it stimulates beneficially the activity of several cells used by our bodies in fighting off infections, namely phagocytes, lymphocytes, and natural killer cells. It also increases the production of interleukin-1, interferon, and tumor necrosis factor, and limits the production and/or the effectiveness of spreading factor (hyalouronidase), which breaks down cell walls and thus aids the spread of infection.

Usage includes prevention and treatment of the common cold, urinary tract infections, and vaginal yeast infections -- plus a lot more. Its ability to prevent infections is less impressive than in helping to shorten recovery and reduce the severity of symptoms.

Dosage. The tincture (alcohol-based liquid) is probably the most effective. The juice is extracted from the above-the-ground portions (aerial portions) of the plant, purified, and "standardized to contain a minimum of 2.4% fructofuranosides." This is taken in!/2 tsp (2 1/2 ml) two to three times a day. I believe that this is more likely to be effective than the ones below, but time and more scientific studies will tell. A dry powdered extract (standardized to 3.5% echinasides) at 300 mg per day, and a blended tea, dose variable so far, are being used also.

Possible ill effects: may aggravate autoimmune disorders. These include collagen disorders, multiple sclerosis, rheumatoid arthritis, and those on immunosuppressive therapy (as in organ transplants).

Those with hay fever may get an allergic reaction to it, such as hives, asthma attacks, swelling shut of the throat (anaphylaxis), and swelling around the mouth (angioedema). Some of these can be quite bad. People who have allergies to certain plants and flowers in the family of chrysanthemums, daisies, marigolds, and ragweed.

It increases the effect of warfarin and thus may cause bleeding problems when used in combination.

Ephedra

Ephedra alkaloids are too dangerous to <u>ever</u> use, even once. They have been tried by probably thousands of athletes in an effort to enhance their competitive performance. It was listed as the cause of death for Baltimore Orioles pitcher Steve Bechler on February 17, 2003. The so-called "health" supplements for athletes that contain it right now, with approximate amounts of chemicals which come from the ephedra plant, are BetaLean, 20 mg, Metabolife 356, 12 mg; Ripped Force, 25 mg; Ripped Fuel, 20 mg.; and Xenadrine RFA-1, amount unknown. These are all outlawed by the Olympic Committee.

Ephedrine is the active ingredient in all of these. In the pure form it is a mild stimulant that constricts blood vessels and which is often used for this purpose in cold and sinus remedies to open up stuffy noses. It must be avoided in those who already have high blood pressure, diabetes, and heart disease but may not have much noticeable effect on other people in the small doses used.

When used in combination with other stimulants, like caffeine, which is common in many of these supplements, it is a truly potent stimulant which will both raise blood pressure, increase heart rate, and constrict blood vessels all over the body. The result may be heart attack or fatal irregularity, seizure, and stroke. In Steve Bechler's case, the constriction of his blood vessels interfered with his body's ability to lose heat through his skin, resulting in his collapsing of heat stroke. Bottles containing ephedra were found in the locker of Vikings tackle Korey Stringer after his death in 2001 of heatstroke. Several high school players have also died of ephedra-related conditions in the past two years.

Then we must consider the fact that there are often two or more other herbs and chemicals in these supplement that tend to multiply the stimulative effect when combined. Remember, each herb may have a hundred or more different chemical compounds. (As an illustration, tobacco has been found to have over 1,000 different compounds in it, even before the tobacco companies finish adding their witches brew of addicting chemicals.) So what we have in the supplements listed above are collections of very dangerous chemicals.

When people exercise with these on board, their heart rates and blood pressures go up. This may render them even more susceptible to ephedra's effects. The FDA has reviewed 140 cases of exercise deaths in which ephedra was in the bodies and found a very strong correlation with ephedra use and fatal stroke, heart attack, and seizures.

Possible ill effects include rapid heart, <u>high blood pressure, seizure, and **death**</u>. As this is written, over 100 deaths in our country alone have been possibly or probably related to the use of ephedra. Some are very high profile, like the Northwestern University and Minnesota Vikings football players who died after practices in the summer of 2001. But ephedra is in your neighborhood workout room as well as on the athletic fields of the world. So beware.

Conclusion: **Ephedra is far too dangerous to use even once.**

Evening Primrose

Evening Primrose is a source of GLA (gamma linoleic acid), which is an essential fatty acid, one of the good guys in the cholesterol/fatty acid family of polyunsaturated fats. Actually, it is in the Omega 6 branch of the family, which is the best of all for preventing hardening of the arteries.

GLA may not be adequately converted from linoleic acid in the body in several of the following conditions:

Atopic eczema, cyclic sore breasts (mastalgia), deficiencies of biotin, calcium, magnesium, vitamin B6, and zinc, high alcohol intake, high cholesterol, high saturated fatty acid intake (the saturated fatty acids are usually the solid fats at room temperature), and diabetes, particularly with diabetic neuropathy (one of a very few at least somewhat successful treatments for this condition; it may actually help prevent this condition if taken prophylactically). These conditions all may have true GLA deficiency, which might be corrected or improved.

If you have one of these conditions, then a supplement containing GLA may make you better. Borage Oil and Black Currant Seed oil are more concentrated sources of GLA. In order to get full GLA from Evening Primrose, your body must be able to convert linoleic acid to GLA, which it does normally. In the conditions above the body's conversion capability is impaired however; so the more concentrated sources are advised.

Do not use GLA to reduce inflammation, because it will actually work to *increase* inflammation through its effect on other chemicals of the body.

Studies show considerable benefit of evening primrose oil in Irritable Bowel Syndrome, but no help in PMS beyond the placebo effect. It relieves the symptoms of cyclic sore breasts in about half the people who take it but only 27% in women with non-cyclic soreness. Danazol is much better than evening primrose oil for these; but bromocriptine is about the same and a whole lot more expensive with more side effects.

No help with fibrocystic breast disease or fibroadenomas. Try totally avoiding all caffeine (even decaf) if you have fibrocystic disease. It will help a lot.

Very questionable whether it has any effects on attention deficit disorder, hyperactivity disorder, or rheumatoid arthritis.

Several studies have produced mixed reviews for its use in atopic dermatitis. The beneficial effects reported may actually be due to the linoleic acid portion of the evening primrose oil.

Doses: Cyclic mastalgia. Three to four grams a day (which translates to 300 to 400 mg per day of pure GLA.

Diabetic neuropathy: 4 to 6 grams a day of the oil (400 to 600 mg of pure GLA).

Possible ill effects: abdominal cramps, indigestion, loose stools, and nausea, especially in higher doses. It may lower the seizure threshold in epileptics, particularly in schizophrenics who take one of the phenothiazine family of anti-schiz drugs. So, **don't take it if you have epilepsy.** Also it has may increase the risk of complications of pregnancy, slowing the progress of labor. So, **don't take it if you are pregnant.**

Feverfew

Feverfew seems to be particularly good for migraine headaches, and I recommend it. It is also used in sort of a shotgun approach for allergies, psoriasis, and rheumatoid arthritis. It increases the effect of warfarin and thus may cause bleeding problems when used in that combination.

Garlic

Garlic is one of my favorite flavors. Use any excuse you can think of to get to take it. I particularly love the roasted buds. Medicinally it is claimed to be good for high cholesterol, high blood pressure, cancer, and diabetes. It was referred to in 5,000-year-old Sanskrit records. The active ingredient in garlic is an amino acid called allicin. This is what smells. So if you find a garlic preparation that has no odor, then it is almost certainly worthless.

Possible ill effects: May multiply the effects of blood-thinning drugs like warfarin (Coumadin) and cause bleeding problems when used in combination. Because it increases bleeding times through its effects on the blood platelets, it should be stopped at least three weeks before surgery if you have that much time. Stopping even one week before surgery will be helpful though. Be sure to tell your surgeon that you are taking it. Higher doses often cause upset stomachs. It goes into breast milk and may cause colic in infants.

Ginger

Ginger is reputed to be good for gas and indigestion. Grandmothers swore by it, therefore had to be good, right? It is also recommended for control of bad coughs. It increases the effect of warfarin and thus may cause bleeding problems when used in combination.

Ginkgo Biloba

Ginkgo biloba is promoted to improve memory, and it has been used for eye diseases of older people, impotence (I will tell you right now that Viagra is better), depression, ringing in the ears, asthma (don't even think of that use), and altitude sickness. Plus a lot of other stuff. The extract EGb 761 may increase brain circulation, and a couple of respected studies suggest that it may slow down the progression of Alzheimer's Disease. It has also been suggested that it is an anti-oxidant and thus slows down aging (exercise is better!)

Possible ill effects: May multiply the effects of blood-thinning drugs like warfarin (Coumadin) and has been known to increase headaches in some migraine-prone people.

Ginseng

Panax ginseng (also known as Asian ginseng) has been used as a medicine in China for over 2,000 years. It apparently has been very much like snake oil, Hadacol, and colloidal silver here in that it has been used to treat virtually every illness known to man over there. An interesting sidelight is that almost all of the ginseng grown in the U. S. is exported to China. It apparently is more reliably pure and unadulterated. While meanwhile we are buying Chinese ginseng! Flies in the face of reason, doesn't it?

After sifting through all the claims, there appear to be several common conditions for which it is truly useful.

Uses: Word of mouth says: extra energy, improving physical performance, improving concentration, helps dealing with stress helps ward off infections.

Actual testing studies say: No help with athletic activities, definite evidence of improved immunity, possibly even against tumors (but not cancer), does contain B vitamins, slows down blood clotting (it increases the effect of warfarin and thus may cause bleeding problems when used in combination), and reduces fasting blood sugars in type 2 diabetics.

The usual dose is 100 to 200 mg standardized to from 4% to 7% of the so-called ginsenoside content. That means taking from 2 to 4 grams of the root.

The Chinese use it only for short terms of up to three months at a time. No one knows what the effects may be if taken for much longer periods.

Goldenseal

Goldenseal (also known as Hydrastis Canadensis) is mainly used for sinusitis and the common cold, often in combination with echinacea. It has been harvested so aggressively that it has become an endangered species. The active ingredient is berberine.

It is apparently somewhat active against many bacteria, fungi, and protozoa (amoebae, giardia), but not against viruses. So the studies that say it is not effective against the common cold are correct. However it apparently is active in controlling, but probably not eliminating, infections from the following bacteria: Chlamydia, Diphtheria, E. Coli, Gonorrhea, Leishmania, Pseudomonas, Salmonella, Shigella, Staphylococcus, Trachoma of the eye, and Treponema pallidum (syphilis). It concentrates in mucous membrane-type tissue like the bladder, intestines, and throat, so it is especially effective in diseases such as cystitis, sore throats, and intestinal parasites.

Since most of the goldenseal sold in our country is for common cold prevention and treatment, you can save big bucks by not buying it for that purpose.

There is word in the underground that it will mask illegal drugs in the urine if you have to have a drug test. It isn't so!

Doses: For intestinal diseases: 250 to 500 mg three times a day for two to three weeks and no more.

To make a concentrated liquid for a gargle (for sore throats), simmer 1/2 to 1 gram of the dried rhizome or the root in 5 ounces of water for 10 minutes, let cool a few minutes, and strain it. The same recipe works well to use it for a mouthwash or tea.

The liquid extract dose is 0.3 ml up to 1 ml three times a day.

The tincture dose is 2 to 4 ml three times a day.

Possible ill effects: Unlike most of the other herbs here, it reduces the effectiveness of warfarin, so that your blood may clot unexpectedly and possibly disastrously.

Grape Seed Extract

Grape seed extract (also known as Vitis vinefera) is the source of PCOs (procyanidolic oligomers for the chemists among you readers), plant antioxidants reported to be more than 50 times stronger than vitamins C and E. It also apparently has considerable beneficial activity as an antioxidant scavenger of free radicals, both water and fat-soluble types. In addition the PCOs seem to reduce the effect of certain enzymes, such as collagenase, elastase, and hyalouronidase, which can break down some connective tissues in our bodies.

The conditions for which you may find this substance helpful are blood vessel disorders such as capillary fragility (which causes easy bruising), along with diabetic retinopathy and macular degeneration.

It has been reported that the average U. S. diet contains about 25 mg per day of antioxidant flavinoids. An intake above 30 mg daily may be associated with reduced cardiovascular deaths.

To use Grape Seed Extract for general health or its antioxidant effects, the dose is 50 mg per day. To use it for treatment of blood vessel or cardiac conditions the dose is 150 to 300 mg per day.

Possible ill effects: almost none. I could find no reports of bad drug reactions or side effects. But use it with care if combining with another herb or herbs.

Pine Bark Extract

Pine bark extract is another herb used for its PCO effects. Compared to pine bark extract, grape seed extracts contain 92-95% of the active ingredient, while pine bark extracts normally contain 80-85%. **Grape seed extracts are much cheaper.**

Green Tea

Green tea is taken with the hope of preventing cavities in your teeth and also cancer. It is also supposed to be good for gum disease. It increases the effect of warfarin and thus may cause bleeding problems when used in combination.

Guar Gum

Guar gum is definitely a laxative. Along with Goldenseal and Psyllium it reduces the effectiveness of warfarin, so that your blood may clot unexpectedly and possibly disastrously.

Guggul

Guggul may help lower cholesterol, a little. It increases the effect of warfarin and thus may cause bleeding problems when used in combination.

Hawthorn

Hawthorn is used for angina pectoris and hypertension. It increases the effect of warfarin and thus may cause bleeding problems when used in combination.

Horse Chestnut

Horse Chestnut is supposed to be good for diarrhea, swelling of the ankles, varicose veins, and hemorrhoids. It increases the effect of warfarin and thus may cause bleeding problems when used in combination.

Juniper

Juniper is promoted to improve your appetite and increase urine output. It increases the effect of warfarin and thus may cause bleeding problems when used in combination.

Licorice

Licorice is another one for all conditions: viral sore throats and upper respiratory infections, high cholesterol, symptoms of menopause, and ulcers. It increases the effect of warfarin and thus may cause bleeding problems when used in combination.

Kava

Kava (also known as Piper methisticum and intoxicating pepper) came from islands of the South Seas, where it has been used in various ceremonies for all of known history. The active ingredient is a group of closely related chemicals called kavalactones, which come from the root of the plant. Each plant has a somewhat different concentration of the kavalactones in its roots, perhaps because of soil and shade conditions. This concentration ranges from 3-20%; so it is very important for you to obtain standardized doses if you use it. Be aware that even the standardized tablets or capsules vary by as much as 40%; so you must be sure to look at the label and get the same amount each time.

Uses: Short term treatment of anxiety in doses from 15 to 25 mg three times a day. Full effects are not felt for two weeks or more. It may have some pain-relieving effects. It has some muscle relaxing and sedative effects, in a dose of about 200 mg just before bedtime.

Possible ill effects: Dizziness. Headache. Stomach and intestinal problems. In doses higher than those recommended above (be aware that one average bowl of kava at a kava-using ceremony will contain about 250 mg of kavalactones, and usually several bowls are taken at a party), the ill effects are more frequent. In long term users of high doses there may be liver damage, as well as a scaling dermatitis, and yellowing and thickening of the skin. One study reported acute hepatitis in a few people who had used normal doses for only three or four weeks.

European sources report that Switzerland has banned the sale of kava compounds, and several other countries began to restrict its sale in some ways in November and December 2001. The reasons were given as reports of increasing numbers of kava-related cirrhosis, hepatitis, and liver failure. In our country the FDA has put out an alert to doctors to report any ill effects found in kava users.

*Do not, under any circumstances, take kava in any form if you know you have liver disease, or drink alcohol more than one drink just occasionally. Do not take kava if you are taking any medications that may adversely affect the liver (male hormones and non-steroidal anti-inflammatory drugs are examples of such). Do not take kava if you are taking any drug that may depress the nervous system.**

Milk Thistle

Its silymarin extract reduced elevated blood sugars in a significant number of people in one small study. If the label says it is standardized, it will be more likely to be effective.

Possible ill effects: it may accentuate the effect of your diabetic medication and bring your blood sugar level dangerously low if not carefully checked and doses of diabetic drugs adjusted accordingly. It increases the effect of warfarin and thus may cause bleeding problems when used in combination.

Psyllium

Psyllium is not actually a laxative, but is used in a number of combinations for constipation. Along with Goldenseal and Guar gum it reduces the effectiveness of warfarin, so that your blood may clot unexpectedly and possibly disastrously.

Red Clover

Red Clover is another used for menopausal symptoms. It increases the effect of warfarin and thus may cause bleeding problems when used in combination.

Reishi

Reishi is used as a dietary supplement in people with cancer. Somehow it is supposed to aid the circulation. It increases the effect of warfarin and thus may cause bleeding problems when used in combination.

Saw Palmetto

Also known as Serenoa repens, saw palmetto may reduce urinary retention problems in those with enlarged prostates, thus improving night sleeping. Again our Native American friends used these berries for urinary problems, and they began to be used for benign prostatic hypertrophy (BPH) early in the last century. In Europe saw palmetto extract is used more for mild BPH than any other medication. It is about as effective as the prescription drug Proscar but much cheaper, with fewer side effects. It also is less likely to produce impotence than Proscar.

Possible ill effects: may cause stomach cramps, nausea, vomiting, diarrhea, or dizziness. There are no drug or food interactions known at the present time.

Feel free to use it when you start having to get up in the middle of the night to urinate as you get older. The usual dose is 160 mg of the standardized extract twice a day. Crude berries and non-standardized fluids probably won't produce as good a result for you. Consult your doctor for a yearly prostate exam and PSA after age 50.

Turmeric

Turmeric is an anti-arthritis herb. It increases the effect of warfarin and thus may cause bleeding problems when used in combination.

St. John's Wort

St. John's Wort is being used mostly for depression, or as a "mood enhancer."

BUT the first National Institutes of Health report compared the active ingredient of the plant, hypericum, with a placebo for eight weeks. At the end of that time only 24% of those on St. John's wort had what was called "a full response" (meaning a complete lifting of depression) as against a full response of 32% in the placebo group. One of the companies that makes SJW pointed out in a press release that SJW had the same effect as "some prescription ant-depressant drugs." The rest of the story is that the widely used drug for depression, Zoloft, in 1/2 the usual therapeutic dose, also had a little less than the placebo effect. That presumably would change with the full Zoloft dose. I personally have prescribed the higher dose of Zoloft pretty successfully for depression.

The study involved only about 340 people, so I don't consider it conclusive. But it certainly makes one pause before recommending SJW for depression. And it is a strong statement for the power of our minds. Feelings are facts.

Another concern aside from its effectiveness above is the result of another April 2002 study reported at a cancer meeting in San Francisco. It seems that taking SJW while undergoing chemotherapy with the frequently used drug Irinotecan apparently reduces the effectiveness of the anticancer drug. It also increases the effect of warfarin and thus may cause bleeding problems when used in combination.

Further new evidence indicates that SJW probably interferes with the effects of birth control pills in preventing ovulation and may be responsible for unwanted pregnancies.

There are a large number of other drug interactions just coming to light. The worst is interference with drugs being used successfully to treat AIDS, but also with drugs used in organ transplants.

Valerian

Valerian (Valeriana officinalis) has been used for insomnia since at least 100 A.D. according to ancient literature. It has been officially approved for this purpose in Germany. It may take up to 4 weeks to reach full benefit for inducing sleep and then must continue to be taken daily to maintain the full benefit.

It is about as effective for insomnia as the benzodiazopine (Valium, Librium, and Xanax) class of tranquilizers without the next-day drowsiness and habituation to outright addiction produced by those drugs. You <u>can</u> take it just occasionally when you need it, but this requires a little higher dose than when you take it each night. Take it a half hour to an hour before bedtime. Also read the chapter on **Insomnia.**

Having said that, I must hasten to tell you that I don't think you should drive a motor vehicle or operate machinery within 8 hours after a dose of valerian. And if you have been taking it, especially in higher doses, for a month or more on a daily basis, don't just suddenly stop it. You might have undesirable withdrawal symptoms. I know you aren't supposed to have to, but just to be on the safe side, taper off gradually over three to five days, a lower dose each day.

Average dose ranges are 250 to 450 mg of a water extract; 400 to 900 mg of an alcohol extract, and 2,000 to 3,000 mg (2 to 3 grams) of the dried leaves decocted to tea form.

Possible ill effects: liver damage has been reported in 4 cases where other drugs were also involved. Possible contamination also was considered to be a possibility in those cases. Similar to Goldenseal, Valerian may cause elevated blood levels of certain antibiotics (particularly erythromycin), anti-fungus meds, the statin anti-cholesterol drugs, and some others. I don't know whether it affects warfarin (Coumadin).

Don't mix it with alcohol or benzodiazopines. Don't use in pregnant women, children, or mothers who breast feed.

Herbal and Supplement Lessons to Live by

In conclusion, herbal remedies have been with us for thousands of years and probably are here to stay. Supplements are more recent but also are probably going to be around for a long time. They all work best for relatively minor conditions for short periods of time -- up to no more than three months at a time as a rule. One exception is glucosamine, which may be taken for a long time, apparently without ill effects, for arthritis.

Taking one herbal medicine at a time is best, and considerable care should be taken if you are also taking prescription medication. Mixing multiple herbs is as bad an idea as mixing herbs and prescribed drugs. You have to be very careful.

Don't take <u>any</u> herbs or supplements if you are on Coumadin (warfarin).

Avoid high doses of all herbs, especially above those recommended here.

Prefer European herbs as more reliable and consistently safe.

And always tell your doctors and pharmacists what herbs you are taking.

The list of drugs used by athletes who are trying to gain an unfair edge on their competition is long, and we won't discuss them here. Except to say that many have unwanted and often-unexpected side effects (such as sudden death with ephedra, and liver disease and cancer from anabolic agents).

Diuretics can cause serious salt and potassium disturbances, plus some other troublesome things like charley horses (muscle cramps) during competition.

Various hormones, many of which do, indeed, enhance performance and thus are banned by the Olympics, include the ones you have heard of, like growth hormone, thyroid, the andros, and testosterone, plus many others just out of the laboratory.

Stimulants include amphetamine, cocaine, ephedrine, and terbutaline (which is used often for asthma).

Creatine and protein are <u>not</u> banned by the Olympics.

For a voluminous database of material on complementary therapies, go to the Internet to the <u>International Bibliographic Information on Dietary Supplements (IBIDS)</u> at http://ods.od.nih.gov/databases/ibids.html.

CHAPTER 55 -- HYPERTENSION (HIGH BLOOD PRESSURE)

The cause is almost always hereditary to at least some degree. Other contributing causes include tobacco use of any kind, obesity, diabetes, and ongoing high stress.

The insidious thing about high blood pressure is that in most cases it causes no symptoms until you have your heart attack or stroke or your kidneys fail. So you must have your blood pressure taken whenever you see a doctor, or at least two or three times a year for your whole life. Then if your blood pressure starts to go up, you can get right on it before it is cast in concrete. If there is a family history of hypertension, then start your kids having their pressures taken early in life.

Some people with unknown high blood pressure may have dizzy spells, headaches, be red in the face, have changes in vision, or just not feel very good in general. These occur more often when the pressure is in the higher ranges, perhaps over 200.

What is "High Blood Pressure?"

The numbers that everyone agrees are high are 140/90 or higher. The upper number (the systolic pressure) is the pressure produced by the contraction of your heart pushing the blood out through the arteries with each beat. The lower number (the diastolic pressure) is the constant pressure maintained in the arteries by their elastic muscular walls between beats. As of 2003 one cannot pass a Department of Transportation (DOT) physical exam to drive trucks and buses, among other things, if the blood pressure is above 140/90. Until then the acceptable limit was 160/90. The reason the requirement was changed by the Department of Transportation is that there were a lot of heart attacks on the road in people who had passed with the higher number.

There is a movement toward lowering the numbers needed to make the diagnosis of hypertension down to 135/85. If either the upper or the lower number is too high, then you must take steps to lower them. How far they need to be lowered is subject to some debate. I aim for 130/80 or less, both sitting and standing. Since you spend many hours each day on your feet, it only makes sense to lower the standing pressure to normal also. Ask your doctor to always check your pressure in both positions.

I have often been asked, "when is my blood pressure too low?" The answer is, when you pass out. People in the best physical condition tend to have the lowest blood pressures. One marathoner that I cared for had a normal standing pressure of 84/38. Many uninformed medical professionals might consider that too low, but he was the best-conditioned of all the many athletes I have ever known. And he never passed out! What is important is whether the blood pressure stays the same when you stand up as when you are sitting down. It should do so normally, or even go up a few points because the heart has to pump slightly harder to get the blood up to the brain, which is a foot or two higher when you stand.

So if your blood pressure falls when you stand up, then it may be too low, no matter what the numbers, and further evaluation is needed.

This sort of thing can happen when you first start taking blood pressure medicine. Your body will be used to a higher pressure, and, if the medicine drops the pressure too fast, you may feel faint when you stand up suddenly. Most of the time your doctor will start with a low dose to see how you tolerate it and to let your body adjust to the lower pressure gradually. If your pressure were 200/120, for example, and he gave you a big enough dose to suddenly make it a normal 120/70 tomorrow, I guarantee that you would faint. If, however, he gives you enough to drop the BP to 180/110 in two weeks, then adds enough to bring it down to 160/90, then to 140/85, then to 120/70, you won't usually even know you are taking anything. But you will feel better.

If you do have a tendency to feel a little faint on suddenly standing up, with or without medication, just sit on the edge of the seat or bed and take a couple a couple of deep breaths before standing up. After you stand up, take another deep breath or two before moving off. That will usually be sufficient to pump more blood to the brain and prevent the faint feeling. Remember, even people with entirely normal hearts and blood pressures may feel faint when standing up suddenly after sitting still for quite awhile.

Causes of Hypertension

First and by far the most common is heredity. Obesity is a close second, followed by tobacco use, diabetes, ongoing high stress, and being a member of the black race.

Many people have what we often refer to as "white coat syndrome," where their blood pressures are high only in the doctor's office. My feeling about this is that if the pressure is high in the office of someone whom you know is there to help you, then it is undoubtedly high in many other much more stressful situations. I believe that it is important to control it in all situations. I have been a police doctor for over thirty years, and a number of those I treated for their departments also became my private patients. Two of those in particular with hypertension come to mind. I treated their blood pressures for several years. Then they each retired in the same year. Low and behold, within a few months after retirement neither of them any longer required blood pressure medication!

Because we kept their pressures in the normal range while they were still working, they developed no organ damage and should live a normal life span.

Treatments You Can Do Yourself

These include: a low salt diet (the latest recommendation is to restrict your sodium intake to no more than 1500 milligrams daily); if you are overweight, lose the excess and keep your weight in the low normal range; do an average of <u>at least</u> 30 minutes of aerobic exercise daily; limit your alcohol intake to no more than two drinks per week; avoid caffeine; avoid tobacco, including second hand smoke; eat a healthy diet which is rich in fresh fruits and vegetables and low fat dairy products, but low in processed foods, and increase your dietary potassium. Stress reduction, including Yoga, deep breathing, and other relaxation techniques on a regular basis, are also of value.

Since it does run in families, if you have any family member with high blood pressure, I strongly suggest that you use these techniques to help prevent or slow down the development of high blood pressure in yourself. These techniques also are very valuable to use along with medication if or when you actually develop hypertension yourself.

For elderly people a recent study has shown that the need for blood pressure medicine is reduced by 30% simply through weight loss and sodium restriction.

When I started practice in 1956, we had only two classes of drugs that were of any value in the treatment of hypertension, the rauwolfia drugs, such as Serpasil (reserpine) and Raudixin, and sedatives, such as phenobarbital. The other things we did were to encourage weight loss, and restrict the salt intake; and that is still, to this day, a very effective part of the non-drug portion of the anti-hypertension programs we use.

They were used to being studied already, you see, and some of the most influential medical research in the whole world has come out of the literally hundreds that have been done there at that plant. I firmly believe that the generations of General Electric employees there deserve a group Nobel Prize in Medicine for their great contributions to our present day medical knowledge.

While I was still in medical school at Indiana University, some smart doctors in Framingham, Massachusetts did a simple study on the employees of the huge General Electric plant there. They watched how the employees ate in the company cafeteria, without trying to influence the people in any way. The people actually didn't know what was being studied that time.

This study sought to learn how each person in the study (there were over 5,000 of them) used salt: salting the food without tasting it first, salting after tasting, and adding no salt at all. What they found was that those who salted before tasting had a <u>much</u> higher incidence of high blood pressure than the average population (as determined by tables kept by life insurance companies). Those who salted after tasting had about the same incidence as the general population. And those who added no salt at all had much less hypertension than the average.

The recently-completed Dietary Approaches to Stop Hypertension (DASH) shows that drastically reducing sodium intake to 1,500 mg daily decreases blood pressure independent of all other variables, including age, race, weight, and all other dietary factors. So the good people of Framingham taught us a valuable lesson over 40 years ago.

Elderly people and African Americans are the groups likely to benefit the most from low salt diets, but the studies clearly show that <u>everyone</u> can benefit to some degree.

Suggestions for Reducing Salt

Most of us are aware that reduced table salt means reduced sodium chloride (NaCl). Be aware that sodium is one of the most active elements in our world. It combines chemically with almost everything. So almost everything we use as food contains some sodium already before anyone starts to prepare it to eat. We aim to reduce sodium, while recognizing that it is impossible to totally eliminate it (also total elimination would be bad because we all need <u>some</u> sodium in our diets, just not so much.)

Here are number of suggestions for reducing our sodium intake.

1) Use "reduced sodium" or "no salt added" products. Reduced sodium means a product has at least 25 percent less salt than the "regular" version. This is especially important for canned vegetables or sauces that often contain lots of salt.

2) Use spices instead of salt. Use more herbs, spices, lemon, vinegar, or other nonsalt seasonings to flavor foods.

3) Feel free to use salt substitutes that contain no sodium. The one most often used is potassium chloride. Look on the labels of so-called light salts.

4) Remove the saltshaker from the dining table, or at least fill it with herbs or other salt-free seasonings.

5) Also remove the saltshaker from the kitchen stove or countertop. Do not add salt in cooking. If there are members of the family who don't need salt restriction, they can add their own salt after the food is prepared.

6) When you first restrict your salt intake, be aware that food will taste different. At first, you may think it does not taste as good; but at the end of a month, I promise you, food will taste just as good. Different, but good. The taste buds in your tongue will become more sensitive to smaller quantities of salt. You may even notice that some foods taste a little sweeter because the sweetness taste buds are no longer being overwhelmed by salt. If you want to try first adding no salt for two weeks, then cutting in half the salt used in cooking for another two weeks, before totally removing the salt

shaker from your house, feel free. Any reduction in sodium will immediately begin to benefit you.

Several members of my family have hypertension; so I have been on a preventative low salt diet for more than 20 years. So far I still have normal blood pressure. I guess it' s working. I was in the worst category of the Framingham study, adding salt before tasting until the food was almost white. I even added salt to my cantaloupes, watermelons, and fresh tomatoes. Food certainly tasted different. But in two weeks my tongue was telling me that food tasted just as good, only different.

7) Use fresh, unprocessed foods as much as possible. Reduce the use of processed, canned, or foods in jars, along with convenience foods, all of which contain large quantities of sodium.

Almost all condiments, such as soy sauce, teriyaki sauce, catsup, Worcestershire, relish, mustard, and many others, are high in sodium and should be avoided if at all possible. Some of these have reduced-sodium versions, which you can use in your transition. Heinz had a low salt ketchup for awhile, and I used it and thought it tasted good. But I guess not enough others did because I haven't seen it for some time.

8) ALL cured foods, such as ham, bacon, pastrami, sausages, salami, and all those other goodies from the deli are virtual salt mines. So are those delicious smoked foods. The salt is used as a preservative in these, as well as all forms of brined foods, e.g., pickles, sauerkraut, and olives.

9) When you eat out: always ask how foods are prepared. Insist that meals be prepared without added salt, MSG, or salt rich condiments. Be aware that there are certain buzzwords on each menu, such as "in its own broth, marinade, reduction, or tapenade," that usually mean really, really salty.

Other conditions where a low salt diet is medically indicated include congestive heart failure, pregnancy (to help reduce swelling and minimize the risk of toxemia of pregnancy), liver failure, and kidney failure.

Going back to the years of the Second World War, there was only one even slightly effective drug approach to controlling hypertension: phenobarbital. President Roosevelt at Yalta with Churchill and Stalin had a systolic blood pressure over 300! He was on massive doses of phenobarbital, which certainly would have enormously diminished his reasoning capabilities. When combined with even small amounts of alcohol, his reasoning ability must have been almost nil. Churchill, in his massive history of the war, could not imagine what made Roosevelt sell the people of Eastern Europe down the river to the Soviets in their agreed post war partition of zones of control. The answer, in my opinion, is that the President was severely impaired by the phenobarbital and should have resigned from office. He died of a massive cerebral hemorrhage soon after, and Harry Truman was left to pick up the pieces and authorize the use of the Atomic Bombs.

Thus the lack of an effective non-sedating anti-hypertensive drug caused the cold war that lasted until 1990. At that time my younger son personally helped tear down the

Berlin wall with three hours of blister-raising hard work, using a hammer and chisel which he rented from an enterprising East German.

I never thought it would happen in my lifetime!

There are several different classes of anti-hypertensive drugs, each class with their own side effects. Beta blockers (atenolol, metoprolol, propanolol, and several others), particularly the older ones, may make you feel a bit drowsy while they greatly reduce your production of adrenalin and other BP-raising chemicals in your body. I like to use them in people under a lot of stress, and in people who have migraine headaches. They should not be used in diabetics, especially those on insulin, nor in asthmatics, because both conditions may need a burst of adrenalin when you are getting into trouble with too low a blood sugar or too much wheezing.

ACE inhibitors (Accupril, Prinivil, Zestril, Vasotec, and others) are often my first choice because they do so many beneficial things for multiple organs. They are excellent for lowering blood pressure, are wonderful for protecting the kidneys from damage in diabetics, and for assisting the heart in heart failure. And they are the least likely medicines to cause impotence. But they have one troubling side effect which I don't know a cure for, and that is a cough that just won't go away no matter what you do. Fortunately not many people get the cough; but if you do get one, all you can do is switch medicines.

Diuretics (hydrochlorthiazide or HCT, aldactone, diazide, furosemide, and many others) cause the body's total blood volume to be reduced, thus reducing the amount that needs to be pumped out by every beat of the heart. They may increase the risk of osteoporosis, especially since they tend to be used a lot in older people. They may also increase the risk of gout. They also cause excretion of excess sodium (good) and potassium (bad). They are particularly good for African Americans and elderly people, but people on them need potassium supplements (pills or citrus juice), and their blood sodium and potassium levels must be checked frequently.

If the potassium level in the blood gets too low, you may get muscle cramps (see **Heat Injuries** chapter), or a heart irregularity. Small doses of the thiazide diuretics may be mixed with other classes of drugs to increase their effectiveness. In those the potassium must still be watched, but less frequently.

Calcium channel blockers are used for blood pressure by many physicians, but my experience has been that they have too many possible side effects for the limited beneficial effects on blood pressure.

Angiotensin II receptor antagonists offer yet another approach to BP control, with few side effects, but they tend to be more expensive than the classes noted above.

As you can see, we have a huge assortment of very effective medicines for high blood pressure. So see your doctor at least every three to four months to make sure you stay under good control, follow the personal home program outlined above, and live a normal life. Just be sure you always take your medicine. It doesn't help you if it is in the drawer rather than in your body.

Changes in Vision -- Save Money

Often the vision is affected by uncontrolled hypertension, just as it is also in uncontrolled diabetes. So do not change your eyeglasses until your blood pressure or your diabetes are entirely normal under treatment for at least a month. Your vision may improve enough that you may not need a change. Or you will avoid having to have two prescriptions, the second when everything is back to normal.

"Curing" High Blood Pressure

I can't stress too strongly that just bringing your BP down to normal for a few weeks or months with medication does not "cure" it. Rarely is it "cured," just controlled for as long as you take your medications.

It can, on some occasions, be cured with lifestyle changes. For example, if an obese person stops all tobacco, loses down to normal weight, goes on a permanent low salt diet, and exercises without stopping for at least 30 minutes every day, that person may actually cure himself or herself.

If a policeman retires from the force to a relatively non-stressful existence, and does the things above, perhaps plus some daily relaxation exercises (see the chapter **Staying Healthy Mentally** for some good relaxation exercises), he or she may be truly cured.

For the rest of us, we have to stay on BP meds all our lives. The lifestyle changes above will reduce the amount of medication we need to take, but we will still always need medicine.

Monitoring Your Own Blood Pressure

We are getting some better quality blood pressure devices for personal use, but unless you buy a Tyco or a B-D, you will need to have yours calibrated at your doctor's office, to be sure it is accurate, or to see how many points you have to add or subtract from the reading you get to correlate with your doctor's BP cuff. The way you do that is to take your cuff in and have the doctor's assistant measure your pressure in one arm with his cuff while the doctor measures the pressure in the other with yours. Then have one of them measure it in one arm while <u>you</u> measure it in the other. There shouldn't be more than a couple points difference between the two arms. You can then be sure that your measuring technique is OK and your cuff is accurate.

Your blood pressure tends to fluctuate depending on the time of day. It may be higher soon after you get up in the morning and lower after lunch in the early afternoon. So try to schedule your doctor's appointments always for about the same time of day, and do your own home checks that way also. That way you will always have about the same frame of reference.

If you happen to be using a mercury manometer, you must be aware that your pressure won't be accurate unless the bottom of the glass tube containing the mercury is at the same level as the cuff on your arm. If the manometer is at a higher level, then your pressure measurement will show up as lower than it actually is, thus giving you and your doctor a false sense of security.

I have worked in a number of clinics where there is at least one mercury gauge attached relatively high on the wall beside the examining table. It is attached high enough to be out of reach of kids. But only your standing pressure will be accurate in those cases.

Changing Altitude with Hypertension

When you go to a much higher altitude, for just a few days, or to live, your blood pressure will go up, and you will need higher doses of your medication. If you stay there, you may find that the dose can be reduced as you become acclimated to the reduced oxygen in the air. This acclimation begins in just a couple of days as your lungs secrete a substance that helps them to absorb what oxygen there is more efficiently. Then within the next few weeks your blood count rises as your body produces more and more red blood cells to help carry what oxygen there is more completely. For example, a person living in Phoenix, Arizona, altitude averaging about 1800 feet above sea level, may have a hematocrit of 37% (% of the total blood volume that is composed of red blood cells), and that would be considered normal in Phoenix. If she moved to Flagstaff, altitude 7000 feet, her hematocrit would have to be 42-45% to be considered normal. Healthy people with normal iron and vitamin levels will increase their red blood cells by about 15% in one to three months. At the end of that time, your blood pressure will have adjusted as much as it is going to, and your medicine doses should stabilize.

If you live at high altitude and move down the mountain, you will not need as much BP medicine until you have lost your high altitude adaptation, usually in about three months. You must monitor your blood pressures at least weekly in those circumstances. Most doctors are happy to have you drop in occasionally for the nurse or medical assistant to check your pressure. Fire stations also.

We used to say that the average length of life for those with untreated hypertension was about 23 years, but that those whose hypertension was treated early and adequately could live a normal life span. The first part of that statement is really true only for those who develop high blood pressure relatively early in life. Those who develop it after about age 45 or 50 won't have that favorable an outcome.

The good news is that the second part of that statement is still true.

CHAPTER 56 -- HIGH CHOLESTEROL and TRIGLYCERIDES (HYPERLIPIDEMIA)

* **Money spent here for high-priced drugs will be returned to you many times by helping to allow you to live in good health and work as long as you want to.**

High cholesterol is felt by most authorities to be a total value of greater than 190 mg/dl. This is composed of the HDL (high density lipoprotein), which is the good cholesterol and ideally should be higher than 40 and the most important risk part of the total cholesterol, the LDL (low density lipoprotein). Its ideal level is below 100 mg/dl. The new cholesterol guidelines assign LDL goals to the following risk categories:

1. Patients who are known to already have coronary heart disease. The LDL goal is less than 100 mg/dl. In this category lifestyle changes to achieve that goal should begin at 100 mg/dl. Drug treatment should absolutely begin at or above 130 mg/dl and can begin at 100 along with the lifestyle changes. This is my approach because someone already known to have coronary artery disease is living on borrowed time. We can borrow a lot more time for him (or her) if we treat an elevated LDL almost as a medical emergency right from the beginning.

2. Patients with two or more risk factors (such as family history of heart disease or stroke and high blood pressure, tobacco user plus another, or diabetes plus obesity, see the risk list). In these people the LDL goal is now less than 130 mg/dl, and lifestyle changes should begin at or even slightly below this level. There are two subgroups of types of risk factors which may modify this group even more, but follow this and you will likely do well.

3. Patients with only one or no risk factors. Here the LDL goal is less than 160 mg/dl. Lifestyle changes and possible drug therapy should be in place above 160, but the absolute level at which drugs must be used is 190.

I'm a little nervous with anything above 160, no matter how good your hereditary is or how high your HDL is. Frankly, my approach is to treat aggressively any LDL above 130.

One new study, which hasn't yet received wide acceptance, suggests that getting and keeping your total cholesterol at or below 160 will absolutely prevent the buildup of plaque in your arteries. For those who already have some hardening of the arteries (atherosclerosis), lowering your total cholesterol to 130 or below will actually shrink those old plaques and prevent new ones from occurring.

A preliminary report from another study suggests that getting the cholesterol way down may help protect against Alzheimer's Disease. Years ago it was thought that the conditions now lumped together as Alzheimer's were mainly due to hardening of the arteries in the brain. I don't believe that aspect of senility has changed. I'm quite sure that a reduced blood supply to <u>any</u> organ, especially the brain, will reduce its ability to function normally.

In order to help you achieve these goals your doctor may help you to get a pocket sized cholesterol analyzer for you to use yourself every week or two, much as diabetics check their own blood sugars.

Lifestyle changes, besides stopping all tobacco and daily exercise of at least 30 minutes of aerobic activity, will include a reduced fat, and probably a weight-loss diet. The one outlined below is a modification of the ones I use for weight loss (see the **Weight Loss** chapter), and I highly recommend it.

Desirable lifestyle changes include in particular daily exercise for at least 30 minutes without stopping, weight loss if overweight, stopping all use of tobacco and avoiding second hand smoke.

Foods Low in Fat Content

Milk Exchanges. Each exchange equals one milk exchange and provides a little less than 1/2 oz carbohydrate and slightly less than 1/3 oz of protein. The fat content and total calories depend on the type of milk product.

Table 1: Milk Exchanges

Milk	Measure	Fat Exchanges	Calories
Buttermilk	one cup	0	80
Evaporated, undiluted skim milk	1/2 cup	0	80
Nonfat, dry milk, mixed according to directions on box	1 cup	0	80
Nonfat dry milk powder	1/3 cup	0	80

Table 1: Milk Exchanges

Milk	Measure	Fat Exchanges	Calories
Skim Milk	1 cup	0	80
Yogurt, plain, made with skim milk	1 cup	0	80

Bread exchanges. Each portion equals one bread exchange and supplies about 1/2 oz of carbohydrate and 1/15 oz of protein, for about 70 calories.

Table 2: Bread Exchanges

Bread	Measure
Bread, French, raisin (no icing), rye, white, whole-wheat	1 slice
Bagel	1/2
Biscuit or roll	1 (1/2" diam.)
Bread crumbs, dried	3 tbsp.
Bun (hamburger or wiener)	1/2
Cornbread	1"×2"×2"
English muffin	1 (2" diam.)
Muffin	1 (2" diam.)
Cake, angel food or sponge, without icing	1-1/2" cube
Cereal, cooked	1/2 cup
Cereal, dry, oatmeal is reputed to be especially good	3/4 cup
Cornstarch	2 tbsp.
Crackers, graham	2 (2-1/2" sq.)
Oyster	20 (2-1/2" sq.)
Round	6

Table 2: Bread Exchanges

Bread	Measure
Rye wafer	3 (2"×3-1/2")
Saltine	6
Variety	5 small
Flour	2-1/2 tbsp.
Matzoh	1 (6" diam.)
Popcorn, popped, no butter, small-kernel	1-1/4 cups
Pretzels (3 ring)	6
Rice or grits, cooked	1/2 cup
Spaghetti or macaroni, noodles, cooked	1/2 cup
Tortilla	1 (6" diam.)

Table 3: Vegetable Exchanges

Vegetable	Measure
Beans, baked without pork	1/4 cup
Lima beans, navy beans, etc., dry, cooked	1/2 cup
Corn	1/3 cup
Corn on the cob	1/2 medium ear
Parsnips	2/3 cup
Peas, dried (split peas, etc.) or green, cooked	1/2 cup
Potatoes, sweet or yams, fresh	1/4 cup
White, baked or boiled	1 (2" diameter)
White, mashed	1/2 cup

Table 3: Vegetable Exchanges

Vegetable	Measure
Pumpkin	3/4 cup
Squash, winter (acorn or butternut)	1/2 cup
Wheat germ	1/4 cup

Almost all fruits and vegetables, except avocados and coconuts are low in fat.

Table 4: Meat Exchanges

Meat or Poultry	Measure of 1 Exchange
Beef, lamb, pork, veal, ham, very lean,	1 oz slice
Chicken or duck, no skin, <u>baked, boiled or broiled</u>	(4"×2"×1/2")
Halibut, perch, sole, and similar fish	1 oz slice
Oysters, clams, shrimp, scallops	5 small
Salmon, tuna, crab	1/4 cup
Sardines	3 medium
Other fish, and poultry without skin	1 oz slice

Fats

Each portion equals one fat exchange and contains about 1/6 oz of fat for about 45 calories. Liquid fats (at room temperature) of vegetable origin tend to be unsaturated, while animal fats are all saturated and much more likely to clog up your arteries. The unsaturated fats are safe as far as arteriosclerosis is concerned. But all fats contain about twice as many calories per unit weight than proteins and carbohydrates and thus need to be severely restricted in weight loss diets.

Polyunsaturated fatty acids are felt to be actually good for high cholesterol problems. These are found mainly in vegetable oils and fish. Particularly good for you are those which are high in Omega-3 fatty acids. The lists below, while not complete, will give you a wide range of choices in addition to the lists of foods above in cooking for the person with high cholesterol or triglycerides.

Fish
Albacore tuna
Anchovy
Atlantic cod
Atlantic herring
Chinook salmon
Coho salmon
Greenland halibut
Mackerel
Rainbow trout

Plants
Almonds
Butternuts (dried)
English walnuts
Flaxseed
Leeks
Pinto beans
Purslane
Soybeans
Wheat germ

One or two fish-oil capsules of 750 to 1000 mg of EPA can be substituted for some of the above items.

An incompletely documented possible benefit of eating these polyunsaturated fatty acid fish is that they may also decrease the risk of prostate cancer.

CHAPTER 57 -- HMOs

The HMO (<u>H</u>ealth <u>M</u>aintenance <u>O</u>rganization) idea originated with a pretty good one out in California, Kaiser Permanente. It was conceived as a way to make the cost of insuring their employees low enough for companies to provide health insurance for all of them. It was also conceived as a way to assure good quality medical care, but with no frills. It was supposed to reduce the administrative costs of the insurance company, when in fact it wound up enormously increasing them.

The usual HMO typically pays each physician in any particular contract on a fee for service basis (which they always want to discount from the doctor's regular fee schedule) for the first 50 to 100 HMO members who select him as their primary care provider (or PCP: I <u>hate</u> that term! It is demeaning to all good decent, caring physicians).

When more than the contractually agreed-on number of patients have signed up with a physician, then he or she is paid a certain amount, called the Capitation fee for each patient's name on his list at the end of each month. (Some HMOs "forget" to list a patient on the doctor's list until the patient actually has an illness, thus defrauding the doctor out of the monthly fee he or she is entitled by contract. The big lawsuit in Miami includes stuff like this.) No matter how many times the "capitated" doctor has to see a particular patient in one month, he or she will not receive any more than the single capitation fee. This can vary from perhaps $5 to as much as $30, but will never be as much as a single non-capitated office call would be.

<u>The only way the physician can come out even, or even a little ahead under this arrangement is to have a lot of people signed up with him as their PCP (primary care provider) and to see them as infrequently as possible</u> i.e., send them to an ER or Urgent Care as often as possible. One <u>good</u> aspect of this arrangement is that a physician who chooses can see a patient several times even in one week, if need be, without having to be concerned with the patient's pocketbook, since all that is paid by the patient is the co-pay of from perhaps $1 to perhaps $15.

> *You can't <u>believe</u> the layers of administrative activity that goes on in the typical HMO. We had a great little local HMO in Flagstaff, Arizona with the absolute lowest administrative expenses in the whole country. Since it could bid lower than big swollen medical insurance companies for local contracts, it was a pain in the side of the big companies for about ten years. Finally a big company submitted a bid that they knew they would lose money on for the main income producer of the local HMO. The big company wound up losing several million dollars over the two years but succeeded in forcing our little company out of business.*

The physician usually is paid extra by the HMO for certain procedures, particularly minor surgery or wound repairs. Even that sometimes gets slipped in under the capitation fee with an unsuspecting doctor (or into the global fee negotiated with an unsophisticated Urgent Care facility).

Some HMO-physician contracts include certain "pools," where the doctor is assigned a certain number of dollars each month, for referrals for one example, or hospitalizations for another, or for lab tests of all kinds for another. At the end of the year then, if any of the doctor's "pools" have unused budgeted money, then some or all that left-over money is supposed to be paid to the doctor as a bonus.

Frequently, though, the doctor, who has a chance to make some money when he's been particularly efficient for one year, is not paid by the HMO. In other words they renege on their agreement, and this creates much bad feeling by a physician toward the HMO and unfortunately also toward most of the HMO's patients.

This type of agreement rewards a smart, well-trained, efficient, experienced doctor, but can also lead one who is unscrupulous or deep in student loan debt to skimp on needed testing and referrals.

Because of these HMO-physician sometime relationships, it is a good idea to ask your prospective new physician right up front how he is compensated before you sign up with a particular HMO. Then decide whether you can live with the arrangement in place. Be reasonable in your thinking about this. If you haven't previously had any medical insurance and have several conditions that badly need attention, then you will sorely impact any such bonus agreement and may not receive as enthusiastic treatment from a physician as if there is some other reimbursement agreement in place.

It probably is obvious by now that I do not like the HMO approach to medical practice. The HMOs think of us as the "product" they are trying to sell. They pay us as little as possible, as do most employers, but we often have little recourse in negotiations with them. The reason for that is obscure but very real.

A group of dentists in Tucson, Arizona got together to try to negotiate with a large HMO four or five years ago. They really stuck together in their negotiations. So much so that the company complained to the Federal Trade Commission that the dentists were in restraint of trade. The case went to court and there was a very large verdict against the dentists.

This was just the first such case. As of this date the following physicians groups have settled cases brought against them by the all-powerful FTC:

May 2002 -- Physician Integrated Services of Denver, and Aurora Associated Primary Care Physicians

June 2003 -- Southwest Physician Associates of Dallas-Ft. Worth

July 2003 -- Washington University Physician Network, St. Louis

So, instead of several medical or dental individuals or groups banding together for contract agreements, what we have is Dr. Carl E. Shrader in Flagstaff, Arizona trying to have some clout in negotiating a decent fee schedule with a billion dollar company. It doesn't work. What happens is that the big HMO tries, usually successfully, to divide and conquer each individual physician. First they find a young doctor who is just starting out, and they promise him a lot of patients if he will just sign up and agree to their fee schedule. He's poor, if not hungry, and agrees to do just that. Then the HMO tells the rest of us "Dr. Jones is happy with our fee schedule, so if you don't sign up with us at that rate, we'll send all our clients to him." And they do!

A colleague of mine last month told me that he was finally going to quit taking any HMO patients as soon as he could resign from his present contracts. He had just had to borrow $60,000 to pay off his accrued office debts. He said that the HMOs he was contracted with were twice that much in arrears in spite of an agreement with each that he would be paid within 30 days for all clean claims. My colleague is a fine doctor and a real gentleman. Many of his patients will miss him greatly very soon.

One HMO came to Flagstaff and signed up just one doctor (out of 104 of us). Then they had a situation where there were no specialists contracted with them for needed referrals, and a young doctor who quickly became over-worked while also being underpaid. Appointments were not available for anything that was other than life-threatening in less than two or three weeks. Everyone who needed a specialist had to go elsewhere (usually to Phoenix, 150 miles away!) or pay for his or her medical care themselves. To top it off the doctor was never paid in a timely manner, so he was not only still poor, but also very tired. This situation lasted only three or four months because the uproar was so loud from their employees that the local factory canceled its contract with the HMO and went back to an indemnity plan where everyone could choose their own physicians.

Another reason I don't like HMOs is that often the only reason that a patient is now coming to me in private practice is because I am signed up with her plan. She didn't want to leave her previous doctor with whom she had an established relationship. But she had to because he wasn't listed as a provider on the new HMO that the employer had just signed up with.

The HMO concept is underline destroying underline the doctor-patient relationship that has been built up for centuries. Instead of allowing and nurturing the long-term friendship and trust that a patient and doctor used to build up over a period of years, companies now change HMOs almost every year. That way the poor patient has to go looking for a new doctor a lot, often every year.

Never doubt for a moment that <u>every</u> HMO is more concerned about its bottom line and the incentive bonuses of its administrators than about you as a patient. Basically what HMOs do is try to recruit the most cost effective physicians, and pay them as little as they can get away with to see as many patients per day as possible. This is what capitation results in.

A jury just a couple of weeks before this was written really socked it to a big national HMO for that very thing with a multi-million dollar award. They determined that your health should not be jeopardized by the fact that his bonus increases as your medical services decrease. The jury decided that is an unacceptable conflict of interest.

In the meantime you need to know that the administrative bonuses, for the medical director, and his assistants, of a big HMO, for example, will equal or exceed $100,000 per year *minimum*, plus stock options if costs are held down. Naturally the best way, in his opinion, to hold down costs is to refuse needed medical services and prescription drugs for you, the consumer. He would <u>never</u> consider cutting his outlandish performance bonuses as a way of reducing costs!

Be aware that there may be the same conflict of interest, to a lesser degree, in the contract your doctor has with your HMO. Perhaps you might delicately ask him about any bonus arrangements if you feel he might be limiting his services or consultations for you. Don't make this confrontational or you may wind up having to look for another doctor. Better instead you should complain to your company and perhaps get a new type of insurance next year.

Better still, sign up with an indemnity medical plan that lets you choose your own doctor without the doctor having to be on a particular panel or plan. Don't sign up with an HMO if you have any choice at all.

See the chapter on **Dealing with HMOs** for further discussion of this knotty problem.

On July 10, 2002 the *Wall Street Journal* reported that the big national HMO organization would be enlisting Hollywood to help improve their badly tarnished images. I feel that money could be better spent in better services, lower co-pays, and less hassle.

As this is written there is a huge class-action lawsuit being litigated in federal court in Miami, Florida, in which doctors and medical societies have accused 10 of the largest HMOs of abusive business practices to the economic detriment of 700,000 physicians. I personally have encountered some, if not all of the shady dealings complained of in the lawsuit: delaying payment for correct (clean) claims, downcoding claims so as to appear to owe less than the doctors have billed for, and using medically dubious (to say the least) medical necessity rules. So far Aetna is the only one to have settled the case, for a reported $100 million and an agreement to reform the way it does business with doctors.

The other reported defendant insurance companies are Anthem, Cigna, Coventry Health Care, Health Net, Humana, Oxford Health Plans, Pacificare Health Systems, WellPoint Health Networks, and UnitedHealth Group, which also includes Aetna.

CHAPTER 58 -- HORMONE REPLACEMENT THERAPY (HRT)

This term usually means giving female hormones to women who are no longer producing enough of their own, either because of her time of life or because her ovaries have been removed surgically. Estrogen is what is most important to replace; and if you don't have a uterus, estrogen is all you need. And it is relatively inexpensive in the conjugated form.

If you still have a uterus, then progesterone is usually combined with the estrogen to help protect against cancer of the uterus. This can be in a cyclic fashion of taking estrogen for a number of days (from one to three months), then adding the progesterone for 10 to 14 days to prime the uterine wall for menstruation upon the withdrawal of the progesterone.

There is relatively new evidence that combinations of progesterone and estrogen in the same pill, such as Prempro (see below for more controversy on Prempro), that is taken every day, also protects against uterine cancer while allowing the lady to stop menstruating. I have some reservations about this because I think that in many cases the amount of estrogen doesn't fully replace the woman's estrogen deficiency. The arguments are that a woman really doesn't need all that estrogen but just enough to prevent hot flashes. I don't agree. In addition, <u>I do not feel it is safe to give progesterone every day</u>, no matter what the dose, and I have <u>never</u> prescribed it that way. See the discussion below about the new controversy about breast cancer and Prempro. Also, I have seen evidence that suggests that continuous progesterone may raise the blood pressure or make hypertension harder to control.

I will tell you here and now that a woman who has been on full replacement doses of estrogen (which to me means at least 0.625 to 1.25 mg of Premarin or equivalent other hormone formula, e.g. 0.05 to 0.1 mg patch per day on a cyclic or continuous basis) for any extended period of time after her own hormone production has slowed and stopped, will strongly resist anyone reducing her dose because of many other feelings of body well-being beyond just the prevention of hot flashes. I had one lady in her 80s who was still taking estrogen and menstruating lightly every month. She was a vigorous lady who looked much younger. She told me, "Dr. Shrader, you can do anything you want to with me except take me off my estrogen." She was the oldest I've had on female hormone supplements, but I've had quite a number in their 70s.

When Should You Start Hormone Replacement Therapy?

This ideally should begin while you are still producing estrogen of your own, and also still having periods. Your doctor may follow you with Pap smears that include a "squamous maturation count" in which the so-called superficial squamous cells are seen in large quantities if you are getting enough estrogen. If the level of superficial cells decreases a lot from previous levels, then you may need to start hormone replacement, usually with lower doses than you will need later, after your ovaries totally quit their hormone production. The squamous maturation count is done as a part of the Pap smear, and the lab just adds a few dollars to your bill for the extra slide they have to read. **This is a very cheap test.**

The only other test really needed may be an FSH (follicle stimulating hormone) test on your blood. This is probably most accurate if taken on the 5th day of your menstrual cycle. It is somewhat more expensive, but still pretty cheap compared to some of the tests we have to order. The higher the reading, the lower is your estrogen level, and when you get to a certain level, you should start your supplemental hormones.

If you continue to menstruate, then any abnormal cells that have appeared inside your uterus that month are shed with your period and the uterine wall starts fresh again. Uterine cancer is considered to be a disease of women who are no longer menstruating, and that is why we rarely see that type of cancer in pre-menopausal women. They shed any abnormal cells each time they menstruate.

I feel strongly that women with a uterus should continue to menstruate, much as they may dislike it, because of the enormous protective effect against cancer of periodic menstruation, whether it be once a month or only once every three months. This means taking estrogen and adding progesterone in some form the last 10 to 14 days of the cycle. In a paragraph below there is a finding that taking continuous progesterone may have a bad effect on the appearance of breast cancer.

I personally believe at this time that taking progesterone just periodically (every 1 to 3 months) to bring on a period in those who still have uterus (just as the body does naturally before menopause) is probably quite safe. But for those with no uterus, there is no reason under the sun to use progesterone.

If you are on cyclic hormone replacement and you develop an abnormal spotting or bleeding pattern, you must consult your doctor right away. Often an endometrial biopsy will be required. That involves taking a sample of tissue from the inside of the uterus right in the doctor's office, then sending it to the lab for microscopic analysis. In most such cases a simple dose adjustment will be all that is needed. However more serious or complicated conditions may occasionally be found in time to quickly cure them.

Naturally you must continue to examine your own breasts once a month, as you have (I hope) throughout your life.

There are <u>many</u> benefits to women in replacing their hormones. The one that <u>everyone</u> first agreed on is that it prevents osteoporosis, the brittle bones of old age (which is described more extensively in the **Osteoporosis** chapter) and thus improves the quality of life directly, with indirect increase in length of life through reducing hip fractures and their life-threatening complications.

The second benefit, which is really more important than the first because it actually saves lives in addition to improving the quality of life, is the reduction in "hardening of the arteries" caused by the reduction in bad cholesterol and the increase in good cholesterol produced by estrogen. In 1954, a very smart doctor published some research he had been in charge of that appeared to demonstrate conclusively that taking estrogen after the menopause prevented heart attacks. This doctor was attacked in the medical press and in meetings obliquely by others who weren't able to confirm his findings. He didn't know why they had fewer heart attacks, but he said they did.

I and a few (perhaps more than a few) other physicians around the world believed in his findings, but it was more than 30 years before some properly-designed research demonstrated that he was right, and why he was right. What estrogen does is change the cholesterol pattern in women who are taking it as a supplement, so that there is less bad cholesterol (see the chapter on **High Cholesterol**) and a higher percentage of good cholesterol. This results in a lower incidence of fatty deposits in the arteries, and therefore fewer heart attacks, and thus reduced mortality.

Present studies suggest that giving estrogen <u>after</u> a lady already has heart disease is of no value in preventing further heart disease, but only starting hormone replacement <u>before</u> heart disease develops will provide the preventive benefits. The latest data as of October 2003 says that there is a *40% reduction* **in heart attacks in women started on hormone replacement therapy early in menopause**.

Risks of taking estrogen include a higher percentage chance of blood clots and pulmonary embolus along with possible increased risks for developing breast cancer.

The clot risk can be greatly reduced by simply taking a baby aspirin every day along with your estrogen. If you smoke, the risk of blood clots is enormously increased. For that reason I don't prescribe hormone replacement in smokers. They have to quit smoking first, and I always help them with that. (See the chapter on **Quitting Smoking.**)

Breast Cancer Risk

It is important for you to be aware that as of July 9, 2002 a medical study of the effects of a daily dose of a combination of estrogen and progesterone (Prempro, manufactured by Wyeth Laboratories, a highly respected drug company) showed an unacceptable increase in the risk of developing breast cancer after five years. Because of those findings the study was stopped, and it was recommended that women stop taking the progesterone portion. Prempro has recently been offered in a much lowered dosage schedule. No studies will be available on the effects of the lower dose combination for several years.

The findings were that 30 out of 10,000 women on placebo developed breast cancer in a 5-year period, while 38 women on the estrogen-progesterone combination developed breast cancer.

The Nurses' study suggests that women diagnosed with breast cancer while on HRT have less severe cancers and a lower mortality rate than breast cancers discovered in women who are not on HRT. These findings have not yet been felt to be conclusive.

I do not recommend any continuous use of progesterone. There have been possible issues with progesterone raised in the past. It, along with estrogen, is responsible for the ebb and flow of uterine monthly bleeding throughout reproductive life. The hormones in this study are purified from the urine of female horses. Whether the source is important in the breast cancer increase or not will undoubtedly be studied further.

I think the most important fact to remember here is that this progesterone was taken *daily,* which is not the way it is produced naturally in your body. It makes sense to me that exposing your body to it every day without a rest might produce undesirable effects somewhere. My own experience of more than 40 years of using cyclic hormone replacement therapy has produced only two cases of breast cancer that I can remember in women on that program. And my memory is pretty good; especially for friends I have lost.

Other benefits of HRT involve the good health of the female genital tissues (an important aspect of sexuality at advanced and not so advanced ages), and the skin, with fewer wrinkles resulting, and better elasticity. See the chapter on **Sexuality in Older Women**.

Don't look upon estrogen replacement therapy as a total fountain of youth, but I'm convinced that many of your tissues and body parts do better if they continue to receive the estrogen stimulation they received all your life from before you started to menstruate until menopause.

Regardless of other possible reasons for taking HRT, almost all of us agree that you should take estrogen supplements if you have sleep disturbances, mood disturbances, or a change in your thinking capabilities.

It might be prudent to take the progesterone for 10 to 14 days only once every three months, thus menstruating to protect against uterine cancer only 4 times a year.

Estrogen is now available as once a day pills, once a month shots, vaginal creams for female reproductive tract health, an ointment applied to the skin periodically, and patches which are changed every three days. I believe that the pills are the cheapest.

There is a suggestion that using shots, cream, ointment, or patch bypasses the liver and may reduce the risk of blood clots in the deep veins that has been attributed to estrogen therapy. If you are at risk for clots for any reason, then it would be a good idea to take a baby aspirin every day to reduce the possible risk.

Early in my practice I encountered a 50 year-old set of identical twins. Each had had her uterus and ovaries removed about ten years previously, but in different cities with aftercare by different physicians. Neither smoked. One was placed on estrogen shots once a week right after her surgery (shots were somewhat more effective than the oral medications in those days), while the other was not given anything except some sedatives for her hot flashes. When I first met them, they lived in the same little town where I practiced in northern Indiana. They were identical twins, according to them, but the one who hadn't been given any estrogen replacement looked literally ten years older than the one who had it. I started the deficient one on the hormones, but it couldn't reverse what had already happened.

Use of alternative supplements, or so-called "natural" plant estrogens, called phytoestrogens is raising safety concerns regarding cancer of the uterus. Soy and black Cohosh have data that is too conflicting to draw any conclusions about yet.

If you have a uterus, and you take <u>any</u> type of estrogen replacement, whether of plant or animal source, you <u>must</u> also periodically take a progesterone (progestin) to allow you to have periods and protect you against cancer of the uterus.

Estrogen isn't a fountain of youth, but it certainly slows the aging process in my opinion. There are, in addition, very strong medical indications that it prolongs both length and quality of life by its beneficial effects on the blood fats and body tissues, as well as its reducing the fractured hips that often lead to an earlier demise than would be expected if no fracture occurred. The recent controversies aren't new. They date back to 1954. Only the contestants are new. They think they know better because they just did a new study. That's part of being human. But they aren't necessarily right.

There is much controversy in this area, so essentially it's every woman for herself right now. I hope that this chapter will help to crystallize your thinking.

CHAPTER 59 -- HYSTERECTOMY

Hysterectomy means the removal of the uterus (womb), which is where your baby lives and grows when you are pregnant. The uterus has a protrusion with a small tube opening into the upper end of the vagina (the love or birth canal) called the cervix. The cervix is what is scraped and stained in the Pap smears for cervical cancer.

There are many good reasons for removal of the uterus, including uncontrollable bleeding from several possible causes, uncontrollable pain during your period, prolapse of the uterus where it falls down into the vagina and may even protrude from the vaginal opening, cystocele (urinary bladder collapsing into the vagina) or rectocele (rectum collapsing upward into the vagina).

If you are late in your menstrual life (usually 40 or older), your surgeon will also remove your tubes and ovaries along with the uterus. This will prevent your ever having to be concerned about possible cancer of the ovary, which is very hard to cure.

A *total* hysterectomy means that your surgeon removed the whole uterus (sometimes the cervix is left in, and that is a *partial* hysterectomy). The term total does not refer to the tubes and ovaries. If you have your uterus body and cervix removed, along with the tubes and ovaries, then we say that you had a total hysterectomy with removal of one or both tubes and ovaries.

If your ovaries are removed, then you need to be started on estrogen replacement hormone within the first month after surgery because your female tissues (vagina and vulva and urethra, the tube from the bladder) begin to wither up and get dry after just a week or two without that female hormone that is produced by your ovaries. Some (mostly male) doctors are a little slow to start estrogen. My feeling has always been that a woman shouldn't have to wait until she gets hot flashes to start her on estrogen. So ask your surgeon how soon he or she will start you on estrogen. If the answer isn't "right away" or "within the first month" or "as soon as the stitches are healed," then you might want to consider getting another surgeon or having your family doctor start you on them.

There are several surgical alternatives to hysterectomy for women who are simply bleeding too heavily and/or irregularly. One of the latest is endometrial ablation, some incomprehensible words meaning that the lining of the uterus is removed or destroyed by electrosurgery or the application of local heat from a laser or hot fluids in a thermal balloon. Discuss the risks and benefits of these options versus hysterectomy with your doctor before deciding upon a course of treatment. These alternatives are not successful if you have fibroids as the cause of your bleeding, however. Not all GYN surgeons are trained in these procedures.

The Health Technology and Advisory Committee (HTAC) of Minnesota that evaluates new and emerging health care technologies will be happy to give you these and other reports at no charge, by calling 651-282-6374, or on the web at http://www.health.state.mn.us/htac/index.htm.

If you are bleeding too much, your doctor will almost certainly try you on hormones first because the lining of the uterus is controlled as it first grows and then sheds each month, by estrogen in the first half of the cycle and then progesterone in the second half after ovulation occurs. If the egg is fertilized and implants itself in the wall of the womb, then progesterone continues to be produced by the corpus luteum of the ovary until the placenta is large enough to take over.

Your doctor may do some tests (first a PAP smear and possibly a pregnancy test) to see what your hormone status is, then try adjusting the amount of estrogen and/or progesterone for a few menstrual cycles to see if that adjustment to your hormone balance stops the unwanted bleeding. He may want to do an endometrial biopsy, where a small plastic tube with holes in it is inserted through the cervix into the uterus and suction is applied while sterile fluid is flushed into the uterus, thus dislodging some cells from the uterine wall that are captured in the suction syringe.

The other method we mostly use to get a sample of the uterine lining is to insert a small dilator lubricated with K-Y jelly into the cervix, then follow that with a small biopsy instrument which actually scrapes a little bit of the lining membrane up into its hollow tube. This scraping is repeated at all four points of the compass, so to speak, and the tissue is then placed in formalin (a tissue preservative) for transportation to the lab. A pathologist then stains the tissue and looks at it under the microscope. He can tell, of course, whether there is cancer in the tissue, but also where in the menstrual cycle you are, and whether ovulation has occurred by that time of your cycle.

These procedures sound like not much fun, and they aren't, but I have done hundreds of them and have had only one person who needed an anesthetic for either of them. They don't normally take more than two or three minutes.

If biopsy is needed, it will provide your doctor with important information for controlling your bleeding.

Your doctor may simply give you 20 mg of Premarin intravenously if the bleeding is pretty profuse, and that is often effective within an hour or less. Then he may start you on a hormone cycle.

Sometimes, when the bleeding isn't controlled by hormones, you may need what we call a D & C, where you have an anesthetic, the cervix is dilated (the D), and the interior of the uterus is scraped until there isn't much left to bleed (the C, meaning curettage, if you care). That almost always stops the bleeding for this month. But it may recur, and that's when these other procedures and hysterectomy may have to be considered. The tissue, of course, is submitted to the pathologist for analysis and reveals the same information, but with a bigger sample, as an endometrial biopsy.

Any surgery, even in the most skilled hands, has risks and possibly serious complications. And it is very expensive. So do the other things first. Get a second opinion if you have any doubts.

After the surgery, get up and move around in your room the same day, no matter how weak you may feel. Normally the nurses are ordered to get you up, but if no one does, ask to do it yourself (with aid, of course, as you will be weak, and someone will have to temporarily disconnect the catheter that will drain your bladder for a day or two).

The results of early ambulation (a big word for getting up and walking) are enormous. First and foremost it helps to prevent dangerous blood clots from forming in your legs.

Second, it helps to prevent pneumonia, which still occurs all too often when you don't breathe deeply enough to open up the little air sacs (called alveoli) in the deepest parts of the lungs. If air can't penetrate those little sacs at least several times every hour, thick secretions that contain germs accumulate and can cause serious complications. In addition to getting out of bed early and often, deliberately breathe deeply enough to open up your lungs every five minutes when you are awake.

Third, it helps prevent leg muscle atrophy from lack of use. Atrophy begins in just 2 days of non-use.

Fourth, it stimulates your endocrine system to help your normal metabolism to return quickly. Your intestinal tract returns to normal more quickly. The psychological effects of just getting out of bed for a few minutes are large also. And in general it helps you to overcome the shock of the surgery to your system more rapidly.

> *A patient that I did a difficult abdominal hysterectomy on for widespread endometriosis had a very protective husband who refused to allow the nurses to get her out of bed in the early evening. She had had her thyroid removed in Chicago by an expensive society doctor whom all the ladies loved because he kept them in bed and allowed little or no activity after <u>any</u> kind of surgery for <u>weeks.</u> Never mind that most people go home the next after thyroid surgery. He had kept my patient down for six weeks! And her husband wasn't going to have a young doctor in a small town in Indiana do anything but pamper her for months again. Never mind that she told me that it had taken more than six <u>months</u> for her to get her strength and energy back after the thyroid lump was removed.*
>
> *These folks were very good friends of mine, to the point where my kids called them aunt and uncle. So I spent the 20-minute drive to the hospital sweating out how to deal with him. She was already on my side as we had talked about it before the surgery. Fortunately for all of us, the nurse hadn't told the husband that I was coming in, mad enough to spit nails, and he had gone home at the end of visiting hours. I walked in, checked the chart, talked to her nurse and my patient friend, then we got her slowly and gently out of bed and helped her to walk around for three or four minutes before getting back in bed. Even though she had needed a blood transfusion during and after surgery, she did just as well as anyone with a much easier case.*
>
> *At her six weeks checkup before I discharged her she told me that she had recovered fully and so much quicker than when under the care of the high-priced society doctor for her much less complicated thyroid surgery of ten years previously. She also said that she had made sure that her husband was aware of that fact too. Bless his heart, he did sheepishly apologize some time later.*

Some GYN surgeons still don't want their hysterectomy patients to get up and around very soon. There is, apparently, some concern about the vaginal repairs breaking down if they get up too soon. I have personally done over two hundred of these operations, and I will match my results against anybody's in the world. The only activities that have to be restricted are lifting and straining. Running and jumping probably aren't a very good idea either. And riding a bicycle probably should wait a couple of months if you had a vaginal repair. Swimming should probably wait 6 weeks. But walking an increasing number of minutes every day on a flat surface, light upper body stretching of a theraband, or working the pedals of an upside down bicycle with your hands are all safe and good activities. This is a long way around to saying that the more you exercise within the limits of your capability after <u>any</u> kind of surgery, the quicker your whole mind and body will return to normal, and the less likely you are to have post-op complications.

One other thing, which I don't have, a solution to is that a general anesthetic leaves a residue, during which you will find it difficult to concentrate. The number of days is directly related to the number of hours you were asleep under the anesthesia. The only thing to do for prevention is to have a spinal anesthetic whenever possible (they still sedate you but you are awake very quickly afterwards). Just don't plan on doing anything creative or making any life changing decisions for the first two to four weeks after major surgery requiring general anesthetic.

If you also have your ovaries removed at the same time as your uterus, you will need hormone replacement therapy, which means just estrogen without the progesterone in women without a uterus. Your estrogen levels drop within a few days without your ovaries around to produce it and osteoporosis begins soon; so you need to be started on the replacement, within two weeks in my opinion. Also my experience has been that the vaginal tissues heal better if hormones are not allowed to drop down below normal levels.

See the chapter on **Hormone Replacement Therapy** for a complete discussion of this important subject. Some doctors start the hormones at the time of discharge from the hospital. Others, myself included, start the supplementation at the time the stitches (or staples) are removed in a week or ten days. Some wait six weeks or six months or never start them. This attitude is doing you a disservice. Tell your doctor that you want to start the hormones right away if he or she doesn't bring the subject up.

Actually you should ask your surgeon before the surgery what his or her approach is. Then consider a different surgeon if you don't like the answers.

There is a great website for anyone who is going through this surgery. All of the women at the site are going to have or have had a hysterectomy. Your doctor and this chapter will tell you the technical side of the procedure, but the ladies here will give you a lot of personal emotional support, with suggestions for coping during your six weeks of recuperation. Just post questions on the message board, and you will get lots of responses very quickly. Try the chat room. The site is **www.hystersisters.com**

CHAPTER 60 -- IMMUNIZATIONS

These offer you the most bang for your buck. Get every one you can! You will save hundreds, if not thousands of dollars, and possibly save a life.

Smallpox

Smallpox, which killed millions of north and south American Indians, as well as Indonesians and others when they came into contact with explorers from Europe, has been officially declared to be eliminated from our world, and we no longer vaccinate for it. We do, however, have a stockpile of 14,000,000 doses of the vaccine frozen at the CDC just in case a terrorist organization finds a way to grow and spread it again. More is in production as this is written. I personally think that we should continue to vaccinate our kids for smallpox, but there were occasional bad side effects that we no longer have to worry about if we don't vaccinate. Smallpox is spread person to person. See the chapter about possible **Biological Warfare Threats**.

Anthrax

Anthrax, another possible terrorist biological weapon, is immunized against in our armed forces to the tune of about 180,000 doses per year. It isn't yet available for the general public, although the cases in Florida in September and October 2001 may push us toward that capability. Certainly farmers should have that option. Anthrax is spread by inhaled airborne spores or spores that contact the skin, usually from infected animals, but not person to person.

The Florida and Washington cases were spread by deliberately-contaminated mail. Therefore Governor Jane Hull of Arizona recommended while she was in office that **no one, from now on, should open any mail from someone they don't know.**

I agree with her, because it takes only one or two anthrax spores to kill a person. That means that from now on no one should open any third class mail, solicitations, contests, and so on. Terrorist mail is likely to be <u>very</u> attractive and hard to not open. If there is no return address, don't open it. If a hand-written address looks as though English is not the addressor's primary language, don't open it and consider calling the FBI. Complicating this approach to safety is the fact that your new credit cards often come in envelopes that look like third class mail. So we are vulnerable.

Influenza

Influenza is spread person to person and is responsible for many deaths every year, especially in elderly people and those whose immune systems are deficient. Having a flu shot every year in the fall will greatly reduce your risk of getting the flu and its many complications, especially in older people, which means people over 50, and people with high risk conditions. These high risk conditions include adults as well as children with chronic lung or heart disorders, including kids with asthma. Also all diabetics, people with kidney disease or impaired immune systems, children and teenagers (six months to 18 years) on long-term aspirin therapy, and pregnant women who will be in their fourth to last month of pregnancy during the flu season.

Flu vaccine is also recommended for health care professionals, employees of nursing homes and chronic-care facilities, household contacts of and family members of high-risk people, and for anyone else who wants to reduce his or her chances of catching the flu.

Flu is not a potential terrorist weapon, but is the "gift" of the people of Hong-Kong to the world every year. Immunizations can start as soon as the new vaccine is distributed every September or early October and can continue even after the first cases show up in a community. Protection begins within a week and reaches its peak in two weeks.

The CDC estimates that having a flu shot results in a cost **savings of $47 per person immunized each year.**

SARS

SARS, the new respiratory distress disease from Asia, scares me. It is spreading exponentially, as Influenza does, and we don't have a vaccine against it. We also don't have a test for it that can be administered in the office or clinic. Lab tests currently take up to ten days to be reported. By that time the person is dead or recovering, and has exposed dozens, if not hundreds, of other people.

It seems to me that there is a finite population that our world can support without new biological epidemics occurring, and we have exceeded that number. That, perhaps, makes the chapter on **Contraception** even more important.

Pneumonia

The **Pneumococcal conjugate vaccine** provides protection currently against the seven most common disease-producing strains of pneumococcus that we see in children. The adult form protects against 23 strains, and more will probably be added as the years go by. One dose is enough to theoretically last a lifetime in adults, but it is wise to get a booster if a vaccine with more strains comes out.

When I was an intern, I saw a patient, who came into the Emergency Room, was sitting up and talking to me there, though obviously quite ill, and who died on the way from the ER to the Intensive Care Unit. Cultures that we took from his blood and spinal fluid in the ER grew out pneumococcus two days later. He had not only meningitis but also double pneumonia. He never had a chance! Even if the penicillin had had time to work, he couldn't have survived. And that was when penicillin killed pneumococcus like a hot knife through butter.

The Pneumococcus in the pre-antibiotic (particularly penicillin) days was the worst killer of all the germs, causing both deadly pneumonia and meningitis. Today we are realizing every doctor's worst nightmare -- the emergence of penicillin-resistant pneumococcus. Today, however, we have a vaccine. Pneumoccal pneumonia has been called, in old medical books, "the old person's friend" because it particularly kills those who are old and infirm, those in nursing homes, those secretly praying for God to take them home. But it also kills those older folks who are still active and vigorous and loving life. So if you are over 50, take the vaccine.

In addition to pneumonia it also causes one type of strep throat and is a common cause of middle ear infections in all ages, especially pre-schoolers. There has been a shortage of the vaccine type for kids so only kids less than one year of age have received it in many areas so far. Get it for all of your kids as soon as it is available from your doctor in your area. See below.

Frankly, I recommend this vaccine for those of all ages, because it's a *bad* bug and is getting worse since it began to develop resistance to penicillin in many communities. Also, those with lung disease of any type, at any age, should take it, along with essentially the same people who need to get the flu vaccine every year.

Polio

The Rotary Clubs of the world conducted a campaign in the 1990s called Polio Plus, in which Rotary donated polio vaccine to third world countries to immunize everybody, much as we did here in the U. S. in the 1960s. The Rotary campaign was a resounding success, with polio reduced almost to the level of smallpox in most places. Unfortunately the live virus being used for protection mutated into a virulent form in a few people, and they actually got polio. So we now start out with killed virus for at least the first two shots in babies (we had to go back to shots instead of sugar cubes or drops). The killed virus provides only short-term protection, and booster shots are needed periodically. After two killed-virus shots it is then safe to give two doses of live virus drops, which then provide long-term protection for kids and lifetime protection for adults. The current recommendations, though, are for only the killed virus shots, and whether to use the oral live attenuated virus later, after you have been rendered immune by the shots, is between you and your doctor.

Tetanus is another of the most famous immunizations. I have personally seen three cases, when I was a medical student, of this terrible and totally preventable disease. They all died of respiratory paralysis complications. All muscles in the body go into spasm, and thus the breathing muscles don't work.

One estimate of its terrible toll in the Civil War was that it killed over 500,000 men who might have otherwise been saved. Amputation proved to be the best protection.

Now we start with the first shots at about two, four and six months of age, then 18 months and five years, and give boosters every ten years after the child enters school. If there is a contaminated or high-risk wound, we will give a booster if there has been a three-to-five-year time lapse since the last one.

We usually combine boosters with a dose of diphtheria vaccine in adults and children over eight years at no extra charge. In spite of these vaccine programs, there have been still occasional cases of diphtheria reported periodically in winter, at least in southern Arizona. These have responded to increased efforts to immunize against it in kids and to combine it with tetanus at no additional charge whenever a tetanus booster is needed.

Diphtheria is a really bad infection in which a membrane can grow across the back of the throat and plug up the breathing tubes. It does respond to antibiotics if discovered in time.

Whooping cough (also known to doctors as pertussis) is the fourth of the severe baby illnesses which can be prevented by the baby shots. I was involved in an epidemic of this in South Bend, Indiana soon after my internship. At that time there were a lot of little kids who hadn't gotten their shots, even though they were free to indigent children, as they are today. At that time we started giving newborns the first shots at age one month, instead of waiting till two months as was (and still is) usual. These little tykes were fighting for every breath, and it was touch and go for awhile to pull some of them through. None died in that epidemic, but some were close.

Due to some undesirable reactions to the vaccine which we used for perhaps forty years or more, a new acellular (there are no killed cells in it, thus reducing enormously the risk of an allergic reaction to foreign protein) vaccine was developed in the 1990's, and that is what we use on kids today.

Adults, in whom the disease is usually no more than a cold, are a prime source of contagion. So don't let anyone with even a runny nose around your infant; I don't care how much they want to visit and hold the child. Most adults are fine with that, but great Aunt Harriet may not be. So be prepared, and be firm.

Rotavirus, which causes an awful lot of infant diarrhea, especially in day care centers, had a great vaccine that worked really well. Unfortunately within a few months after its release, a small number of little kids showed up with intussuseption, a condition in which the bowel tries to turn itself inside out. Most kids had no problem (and no diarrhea), but those that did often had to have surgery to correct the condition. To this day no one knows how a vaccine could possibly have such an effect on the intestines. I don't even have a guess. But there were too many for it to be mere coincidence. So it is off the market.

The CDC has released figures for the effectiveness of various immunizations for the years before they were available for a particular disease and the year 2000. These numbers bear awesome proof of the enormous frontline defense of our well-being that these vaccines play.

They are reproduced in large part below, the 20th Century average cases of each vaccine-preventable disease per year as compared to the total cases for the first year of the 21st Century. The mortality rates are not listed, but they were often huge. I personally have been aware of deaths from measles encephalitis (one), tetanus (three), polio (dozens), diphtheria (two), H. flu meningitis (six, plus hundreds -- actually probably thousands -- of ear, nose, throat, and lung infections caused by this germ). I have seen perhaps four or five cases of severe heart damage from the Infant Rubella syndrome. I have not personally seen a death from whooping cough, thank goodness, but I have had colleagues with such deaths among their little patients.

Table 5: Decreases in Deaths from Diseases

	20th Century avg. annual cases	Year 2000	Percent decrease
Smallpox	48,164	0	100
Diphtheria	175,685	4	99.99
Measles	503,282	81	99.98
Mumps	152,209	323	99.80
Whooping Cough (Pertussis)	147,271	6,755	95.4
Paralytic polio	16,316	0	100
German Measles (Rubella)	47,745	152	99.70
Infant Rubella Syndrome	823	7	99.10
Tetanus	1,314	26	98.00
H. flu, type B & others	20,000	167	99.10

Certain vaccines have been supposedly implicated in certain diseases, and some people use those word-of-mouth cases as an excuse to avoid immunizing their children.

Don't let this describe you! Don't let anyone talk you out of immunizing your kids. The benefits outweigh the possible risks by thousands of percentage points.

The next table lists alleged problems which, on very careful analysis, have turned out not to be related in any way to vaccinations, but instead are really caused by something else:

Alleged problem	Vaccine supposedly involved	
Chronic encephalopathy	DTwP	No correlation
Chronic arthritis	Rubella	No correlation
Multiple Sclerosis	Hepatitis B	No correlation
Diabetes	HIB, Hepatitis B	No correlation
Crohn's Disease	MMR	No correlation
Mercury toxicity	Many	No correlation
Autism	MMR	No correlation

There have been true, though very rare, safety problems with a few vaccines. Those that we currently are aware of are listed in the next table:

Problem	Vaccine	Frequency
Guillain-Barre Syndrome	Influenza	
Paralysis (VAPP)	Oral Polio (but not the inactivated form)	1 in 500,000?
Intussuseption	Rotavirus	
Anaphyphylaxis (severe allergic reaction)	MMR (gelatin allergy), Influenza (egg allergy)	
Thrombocytopenia (lack of blood platelets)	MMR	

Even though, as you can see from the top table, the risk of giving a particular vaccine is far less than the risk of not giving it, the vaccine makers, in consultation with the CDC have been taking steps to reduce even further the possible risks to your own child.

One such step has been to remove or greatly reduce the use of thiomersal as a very effective preservative in vaccines. This was in response to the concerns raised by some physicians about possible mercury toxicity. These concerns have apparently been proven groundless, but the vaccine companies have responded to those concerns anyway by reducing to trace amounts, or totally removing, all thiomersal from the vaccines that contained it.

Before you have your child undergo vaccination, please read and consider this information, as well as the Vaccine Information Statements which must, by Federal law, be provided to you before you consent to all the immunizations.

Let me again point out that the risks of illness from these diseases are so much higher than the risks of a vaccine-related reaction as to be almost out of sight. Still, you have the right to refuse. If you do refuse to have the vaccinations, your child will have some protection from so-called herd immunity. In other words, if everyone else is immunized, then your child may not be exposed. That, of course, breaks down when enough others feel the same way (witness the 81 cases of measles in one outbreak among unvaccinated kids in 2000). Also, remember that we have several millions of illegal aliens residing all over our country who may bring these diseases with them.

From the standpoint of your pocketbook, having your children and yourself immunized against every disease for which we have a vaccine **will save you more money than virtually everything else in the health field except stopping smoking.**

Here is the list of currently recommended childhood immunization schedules for the United States.

Age at: Vaccine	First dose	Second dose	Third dose	Boosters
Hepatitis B	Birth to 2 mos.	1 month to 4 mos.	6 - 18 mos.	11-12 years if series wasn't finished
Diphtheria, Tetanus, Pertussis, (DTaP)	2 mos.	4 mos.	6 mos	15-18 months, pre-school ages 4-6, Diph-Tet @ 11-18 yrs. Then Tet every 10 yrs, more often if a dirty wound
H. influenzae, type b	2 mos.	4 mos.	6 mos	12-15 months

Inactivated Polio	2 mos.	4 mos.	6-18 mos.	?
Pneumococcal Conjugate	2 mos.	4 mos.	6 mos	12-18 months
Measles, Mumps, Rubella (MMR)	12-15 months			11-12 years if 1st dose given too young
Varicella (Chickenpox)	12-18 months			11-12 years if 1st dose given too young
Hepatitis A (in selected high exposure areas)	24 mos to 18 years			?

The pneumococcal conjugate vaccine has been in short supply and has almost all been used for the little guys so far. As soon as <u>all</u> preschoolers have received it, our incidence of middle ear infections will drop to probably no more than 10% of current levels. That's because it is by far the main cause of these infections now.

So, if <u>any</u> of your children, but especially your preschoolers, haven't had it, ask your doctor to give it to them. And if any of your kids, no matter what age, have had infected ears, <u>get the vaccine!</u>

CHAPTER 61 -- IMPOTENCE AND OTHER MALE SEXUAL DYSFUNCTIONS

Impotence involves the inability to get an erection (hard on), inability to maintain erection, or inadequate erection. It does not necessarily mean inability to ejaculate. It is also referred to as Erectile Dysfunction.

A Saudi Arabian male college student came to me with a problem that had him seriously considering suicide. He was 19 years old, a time when premature ejaculation is common, but not the total inability to get any erection. That, however, was his problem. The joker in the deck was that he had brought a harem of eight or 10 girls with him to school; and now he was unable to perform after having already been sexually active for several years. Since he was a sheik's son, the girls tried very hard to please him. I don't know how he found time to study! The cure for his problem was simpler than most: give the girls (and himself) a week off. He was a very grateful patient.

Inability to get an erection on command is a common occurrence, and by itself should not be a source of worry. It _is_ an unpleasant shock to a man who has never had a problem before. Thus the following possible causes should be considered. The list is not intended to include all possible causes. There are a dozen more at least. But these are the most common ones I see.

Alcohol can reduce potency at <u>any</u> age.

As men get older, many things can affect your sexual potency. Stress, depression, tobacco use, diabetes, reduced circulation from other causes to the organ often called anything except penis (pecker, prick, dick, organ, tool, Dewitz, or Johnson), a wife who lets herself go to pot, medications of various types, particularly antihypertensive and mood altering drugs, lack of physical conditioning, marital discord, having an extramarital affair, especially if you feel guilty about it, general ill health, low testosterone levels in your blood, which often occurs in men from about age 50 on, or some endocrine disorders, such as hypothyroidism.

Various medications, particularly those for high blood pressure, may affect your ability to get an erection. If you are hypertensive and have a problem, ask your doctor if you can try an ACE Inhibitor. These rarely affect your potency.

As a matter of fact, if you have a problem and the answer does not jump out at you from these pages, ask your doctor if your health or your medications might be interfering with your sex life. Then work with him as a partnership to improve the situation.

Treatments vary from the obvious to the obscure.

Viagra has gotten the most press coverage the past few years, mainly because it really works. Basically what it does is to increase the blood supply to the penis so that erection can occur, and continue to occur in many cases for an hour or more. The dose needed varies from 25 to 50 to 100 mg, taken 15 to 30 minutes before you want to make love. The stuff is expensive, but the good news is that the 100 mg tablet costs the same as the 25 mg one. So if you can get by with the 25 or 50 mg dose, ask your doctor to give you a prescription for the 100 mg pills, then use a razor blade to cut them in halves or quarters. Side effects are few. If you're using nitroglycerin or other nitrates for coronary insufficiency, then don't take Viagra. It can cause death in those cases. For most other medical conditions it is safe and mostly successful, often very successful.

Also in many cases involving simple lack of use for a long time, as in someone who has lost a spouse perhaps, the Viagra just gives you a jump start and your own normal functions often return to the point where you no longer need the Viagra.

Just released is the new one -- Levitra. I haven't prescribed it because no one has asked for it, and I don't need it myself; so I know only what I have read in the new drug monthly, which isn't enough to write about here. I'm sure I will cover it fully in next year's edition.

Always have the druggist give you a list of possible side effects when you have the prescription filled for this and all other medications. Some side effects such as a temporary blue tint to peripheral vision, you may find to be no problem. Others may be undesirable. Always ask your doctor whether you can safely use Viagra -- don't just borrow one from a friend if you're older, especially if you have any chronic medical conditions.

There is an injection into the base of the penis.

There is a ring around the base to hold back the blood outflow and thus mechanically maintain an erection.

There is a new small soft pellet which is put up into the penis. This is the MUSE, a tiny pellet smaller than the size of the lead on a pencil that is inserted with a small plunger up into the tube of the penis and gently massaged for a few minutes to aid absorption. It dissolves immediately and causes dilation of the blood vessels in the penis very quickly, within five to ten minutes, thus producing an erection sufficient for lovemaking, which can last for the next 15 or up to 30 minutes in some cases. It is claimed to be successful in 66% of men with vascular disease, diabetes, surgery or trauma, including even radical prostate cancer surgery. I think it would also be successful in smokers. It is not supposed to have any drug interactions.

You must not use MUSE with a pregnant woman unless you use a condom barrier because the medication can harm the baby by uterine stimulation. You should be checked by a physician to be sure of the correct dose and to be sure your blood pressure does not drop significantly.

Other male sexual dysfunctions include rapid or **premature ejaculation**, which I define as being unable to hold back ejaculation as long as you want to. It is most common to seek medical aid for it when you repeatedly are unable to hold back your coming until your bedmate can also reach an orgasm. Some women take longer to reach orgasm than others, for a variety of reasons, some due to their anatomy, some to inadequate foreplay, some due to ineptitude on the part of their male partners. This tends to be very frustrating for both partners and can lead to serious misunderstandings if left untreated for a very long time. Most of the sorts of men who make good partners in general are desperate to help their ladies to enjoy the sex act as much as they do. Most men, though often with some limits, will willingly accept suggestions from their partners as to what turns them on, and how to make it better.

The causes of this problem in most cases are usually easily improved or corrected. Some cases require more help than others. Infrequent love-making is a common one. Unfortunately, for those whose partners live with them, infrequency of intercourse leads to the bad cycle of premature ejaculation by the man and a frustrated female partner, who then would just as soon avoid love-making as much as possible, which then means that premature ejaculation is more likely when she can't avoid her husband's overtures any more, and thus she is again frustrated, often to the point of anger and/or tears. So the vicious cycle repeats over and over, sometimes to the point of separation or divorce.

Treatment requires having an understanding partner who is ready and willing non-judgementally to help. The female portion of this couple must repeatedly allow and encourage erection to occur any way she wants to make it happen, then firmly squeeze the penis hard with her hand until the erection goes down. She must do this on a daily or even several times a day basis, without going ahead with vaginal insertion or allowing ejaculation to occur, for at least a full week, up to perhaps even three or four weeks in tough cases. This teaches the man some measure of control over when he comes.

When you begin vaginal insertion, then try a few thrusts and totally withdraw until you feel no premonition of orgasm, then insert your penis again and repeat this several times. If ejaculation is premature, then start over for a few days and then try again. Soon you will both notice improvement. If not, then other things can be tried.

Another suggestion is to masturbate several hours or a day before attempting lovemaking. This definitely will reduce the hypersensitivity of your penis and enable you to hold back much longer while you stroke and caress your significant other in the places that turn her on until she gets nice and wet. Then you can progress to vaginal insertion, but slowly and gently until she is ready for more vigorous thrusting. She will let you know. It is nice to wait until she comes, then you can just let nature take its course.

Another suggestion, especially if you are successfully holding back long enough now, is to make love much more frequently. It is tough when both of your days have been stressful and you are tired. You may agree that on a regular basis you will just "fool around" for a few minutes before you fall asleep without any expectation of vaginal sex unless you <u>both</u> want it.

It is especially common for someone who has been widowed or divorced and sexually inactive for several years to have problems with premature ejaculation the first few times with a new love. Also difficulty in obtaining an erection is common in older men. The old adage "use it or lose it" certainly applies to our mechanisms for making love. Masturbation is as good as conubial lovemaking in preserving your normal sexual capabilities if you are widowed or otherwise single.

There are shops (one I have used with success for a couple of patients is located on Bourbon Street in New Orleans) which sell elastic rings to put around the penis to restrict blood outflow. The rings that have little knobby protrusions may irritate a snug vagina but titillate one relaxed by having children. Vibrators are novel and effective methods of masturbation. To be continued.

For some men circumcision is therapeutic. The head of the penis is exposed to air and the touch of clothing and thus loses some of its extreme sensitivity.

Excessive alcohol intake just prior to lovemaking is probably the most common cause of premature ejaculation in those without a steady girlfriend.

Back to Erection Problems (Erectile Dysfunction)

Question: What's a nooner? It's making love at noon.

When I was in the US Air Force, I was Medical Officer of the Day (MOD) periodically, which meant that I ran the hospital for that 24-hour period. One Sunday morning about 3:00 AM a very drunk second lieutenant came into the dispensary of our hospital and demanded that he be given a circumcision right then and there. When the staff sergeant at first refused to wake me up the young lieutenant pulled rank on him and made some threats that led me to be called. I was a captain, in addition to being the commander of the hospital for the next several hours, and I tended to get testy when I was awakened at 3:00 AM for any reason not involving catching a baby (I delivered over 500 of them in my two years of active duty). I also took a dim view of a junior officer giving my non-commissioned officers a hard time.

So I offered him a reasonable choice: let me do the circumcision right there without any anesthetic, or go home and sleep it off. The lieutenant was pulling down his pants, and I was reaching for my scalpel when the Air Police that my sergeant had called arrived. They gently but firmly removed and escorted him back to the BOQ (Bachelor Officers Quarters), and by morning I had thought twice about putting him on report to his colonel. I'm not sure whether he came back to the surgery department later and got his circumcision, but probably all he really needed was to limit his alcohol to one or two drinks before trying to make love.

For men past age fifty, there may be some reasons, as noted above, for less blood flow to the penis. Anything that diverts blood to somewhere else in the body leaves less available for sexual gratification. One daily occurrence is eating. When we eat, especially a big meal such as our evening meals often are, 50% of the blood in our bodies is routed to the GI tract (stomach and intestines) until the process of digestion is completed. That's why we aren't supposed to go swimming for at least one hour after eating -- we won't have enough blood available to our muscles for the heavy exertion of swimming. So we may cramp up and drown.

Same thing for intercourse. As we get older there may not be enough blood for a good strong erection after a meal even if the urge is there. So, don't try to make love for at least three hours after a meal if you are having weak erections.

Another very satisfactory solution many, and not just older people, use out of necessity is to make love on awakening in the morning, before the cares and worries of the day intrude, and when there is maximum blood available to the sex organs (your partner's too).

Question: What's a morner?
Answer: a Nooner, only sooner.

After 50, men begin to not ejaculate every time they make

love, or to ejaculate in smaller quantities. This is because as the testicles get older, they produce sperm a little slower. And the prostate produces semen (the fluid that carries the sperm from the seminal vesicles to the outside) more slowly. So after intercourse it takes longer to fill the storage tanks, so to speak, for the next time. Some medications cause the same thing in younger men. Even if you don't ejaculate, you still have almost all of the same pleasure, and your partner has just as much fun. Just don't worry about it.

For Better Lovemaking

Good physical fitness greatly improves sexual function, but not if you do so much that you get too tired before making love. A morner is good then.

Sit-ups and anything else that strengthens your abdominal muscles (abs) will improve your staying and thrusting power, both for men and women. According to "authorities" there are not many really great lovers who don't have strong abdominal muscles.

Question: What's a coolie? Answer: It's making love in the snow.

CHAPTER 62 -- INFECTIONS

Needing Antibiotics

Group A Streptococcal infections. For these, plain old penicillin by mouth, the cheapest of all the antibiotics, is still the best treatment, if you are not allergic to it. Sometimes the nasty stuff draining down the back of the throat into the stomach causes vomiting, and in those cases, a shot of penicillin is needed. The shot definitely gets the antibiotic into the bloodstream much faster than the oral route. Then you can follow up with the oral medication for ten days. It is very important to take all of the medication prescribed, and it should be for a full ten days still in the case of Strep. Usually we want to treat an infection for at least 3 days after the patient seems well, to be sure we get all of the bacteria killed. If we don't kill all the bacteria, then the next time around with the same bug, it is likely to have developed resistance to the last antibiotic used.

So it's OK to wait awhile to see if you can throw off an infection by yourself, but once you do start an antibiotic for a proven bacterial infection, be sure to take all your doctor prescribes, and go back or phone in for more if there is any doubt about whether the person or child is well.

Sometimes an initial antibiotic isn't very strong against a particular germ but does kill quite a few of them at first. Sometimes, therefore, you feel better for two or three days, then take a turn for the worse. That may mean that the germ has now become resistant to that antibiotic, and you need to switch.

Not Needing Antibiotics

* **Here is where you can save yourself a <u>bundle</u> of money!**

Your kid's runny nose: A cold usually is already starting to get better when the runny nose starts. The causes of the runny nose are several. First, it is part of the body's defense mechanism to help wash the virus out off of the membranes of the nose and sinuses, and that is usually clear and thin. After a couple or three days your body fights the infection with white blood cells which surround and kill the virus, then die themselves and are blown out with the mucus, making it white or a little yellow. So far, so good.

Now you know that everyone has bacteria in their noses all the time that don't make them sick. Those bacteria are swept away by the virus and then the mucus at first. As the virus dies off, the good bacteria grow back and make the mucus more yellow and possibly a little green. So far, still so good. So far this is normal. If your child seems to be improving, even though slowly, don't rush to the doctor for an antibiotic. Wait and see. If, however, the mucus gets to be a dark green, persists for 10 or more days, or has a foul odor, and your child begins to run a higher fever, or has an upset stomach, or seems to be getting worse after initially handling it pretty well, then that child probably needs to be evaluated by the doctor, possibly with a culture.

Cough is present 60-80% of the time in viral upper respiratory infections. It usually is mostly dry, sometimes a little moist from secretions draining down the back of the throat. The cough of a viral URI should sound as though it comes from the throat. If it sounds as though it is coming from deep in the lungs, this could be a more serious condition, and you need to see a doctor. And there will never be shortness of breath in an uncomplicated viral "upper respiratory infection" (URI).

Shortness of breath and deep chest cough -- these two symptoms mean that you must see a doctor.

Also, if your child (or yourself, for that matter) is going along well, getting better each day for five days or more, then suddenly takes a turn for the worse, that often means a secondary bacterial infection has taken advantage while the resistance is low. Those occur a lot in influenza cases, especially in smokers and the elderly. See your doctor then.

Immunizations

These offer you the most bang for your buck. Get every one you can! See the preceding chapter on **Immunizations** for further discussion, including relative risks and immunization schedules.

See also the chapter about possible **Biological Warfare Threats**.

Influenza is spread person to person and is responsible for many deaths every year, especially in elderly people and those whose immune systems are deficient. Having a flu shot every year in the fall will greatly reduce your risk of getting the flu and its many complications, especially in older people, which means people over 50, and people with high risk conditions. These high-risk conditions include adults as well as children with chronic lung or heart disorders, including kids with asthma. Also all diabetics, people with kidney disease or impaired immune systems, children and teenagers (six months to 18 years) on long-term aspirin therapy, and pregnant women who will be in their fourth to last month of pregnancy during the flu season.

Flu vaccine is also recommended for health care professionals, employees of nursing homes and chronic-care facilities, household contacts of and family members of high-risk people, and for anyone else who wants to reduce his or her chances of catching the flu.

Flu is not a potential terrorist weapon, but is the "gift" of the people of Hong-Kong to the world every year. Immunizations can start as soon as the new vaccine is distributed every September or early October and can continue even after the first cases show up in a community. Protection begins within a week and reaches its peak in two weeks.

The CDC estimates that having a flu shot results in a cost **savings of $47 per person immunized each year.**

The Pneumococcus in the pre-antibiotic (particularly penicillin) days was the worst killer of all the germs, causing both deadly pneumonia and meningitis. When I was an intern, I saw a patient, who came into the Emergency Room, was sitting up and talking to me there, though obviously quite ill, and who died on the way from the ER to the Intensive Care Unit. Cultures that we took from his blood and spinal fluid in the ER grew pneumococcus two days later. He had not only meningitis but also double pneumonia. He never had a chance! Even if the penicillin had had time to work, he couldn't have survived. And that was when penicillin killed pneumococcus like a hot knife through butter.

Today we are realizing every doctor's worst nightmare -- the emergence of penicillin-resistant pneumococcus. Now, however, we have a vaccine. The Pneumococcal conjugate vaccine provides protection currently against the seven most common disease-producing strains of pneumococcus that we see in children. The adult form protects against 23 strains, and more will probably be added as the years go by. One dose is enough to theoretically last a lifetime in adults, but it is wise to get a booster if a vaccine with more strains comes out.

Pneumococcal pneumonia has been called, in old medical books, "the old person's friend" because it particularly kills those who are old and infirm, those in nursing homes, those secretly praying for God to take them home. But it also kills those older folks who are still active and vigorous and loving life. So if you are over fifty, take the vaccine.

In addition to pneumonia it also causes one type of strep throat and is a common cause of middle ear infections in all ages, especially pre-schoolers. There has been a shortage of the vaccine type for kids so only kids less than one year of age have received it in many areas so far. Get it for all of your kids as soon as it is available from your doctor in your area. See below.

Frankly, I recommend this vaccine for those of all ages, because it's a *bad* bug and is getting worse since it began to develop resistance to penicillin in many communities. Also, those with lung disease of any type, at any age, should take it, along with essentially the same people who need to get the flu vaccine every year.

Polio   The Rotary Clubs of the world conducted a campaign in the 1990s called Polio Plus, in which Rotary donated polio vaccine to third world countries to immunize everybody, much as we did here in the U. S. in the 1960s. The Rotary campaign was a resounding success, with polio reduced almost to the level of smallpox in most places.

Unfortunately the live virus being used for protection mutated into a virulent form in a few people, and they actually got polio. So we now start out with killed virus for at least the first two shots in babies (we had to go back to shots instead of sugar cubes or drops). The killed virus provides only short-term protection, and booster shots are needed periodically. After two killed-virus shots it is then safe to give two doses of live virus drops, which then provide long-term protection for kids and lifetime protection for adults. The current recommendations, though, are for only the killed virus shots, and whether to use the oral live attenuated virus later, after you have been rendered immune by the shots, is between you and your doctor.

Tetanus is another of the most famous immunizations. I have personally seen three cases, when I was a medical student, of this terrible and totally preventable disease. They all died of respiratory paralysis complications. All muscles in the body go into spasm, and thus the breathing muscles don't work.

One estimate of its terrible toll was that it killed over 500,000 men in the Civil War who might have otherwise been saved. Amputation proved to be the best protection.

Now we start with the first shots at about two, four and six months of age, then 18 months and 5 years, and give boosters every ten years after the child enters school. If there is a contaminated or high-risk wound, we will give a booster if there has been a 3-5 year time lapse since the last one.

We usually combine boosters with a dose of diphtheria vaccine in adults and children over 8 years at no extra charge. In spite of these vaccine programs, there have been still occasional cases of diphtheria reported periodically in winter, at least in southern Arizona. These have responded to increased efforts to immunize against it in kids and to combine it with tetanus at no additional charge whenever a tetanus booster is needed.

Diphtheria is a really bad infection in which a membrane can grow across the back of the throat and plug up the breathing tubes. It does respond to antibiotics if discovered in time.

Whooping cough (also known to doctors as pertussis) is the fourth of the severe baby illnesses which can be prevented by the baby shots. I was involved in an epidemic of this in South Bend, Indiana, soon after my internship. At that time there were a lot of little kids who hadn't gotten their shots, even though they were free to indigent children, as they are today. At that time we started giving newborns the first shots at age one month, instead of waiting till two months as was (and still is) usual. These little tykes were fighting for every breath, and it was touch and go for awhile to pull some of them through. None died in that epidemic, but some were close.

Due to some undesirable reactions to the vaccine which we used for perhaps 40 years or more, a new acellular (there are no killed cells in it, thus reducing enormously the risk of an allergic reaction to foreign protein) vaccine was developed in the 1990s, and that is what we use on kids today.

Adults, in whom the disease is usually no more than a cold, are a prime source of contagion. So don't let anyone with even a runny nose around your infant; I don't care how much they want to visit and hold the child. Most adults are fine with that, but Great-Aunt Harriet may not be. So be prepared, and be firm. Worst-case scenario: make them wear a surgical mask.

The CDC has released figures for the effectiveness of various immunizations for the years before they were available for a particular disease and the year 2000. See the chapter on **Immunizations** for full evaluation numbers, along with relative risks for all vaccines.

CHAPTER 63 -- INGROWN TOENAILS

This common problem is caused in most cases by having the toe box of your shoes too narrow for the toes, thus causing pressure on the toes, which pushes the skin into the edge of the nail. Gaining weight without increasing the size (usually the width, but sometimes both width *and* length) of your shoes will squeeze your toes. We wear larger clothes but forget the feet are also larger. As the skin is pushed into the nail, we frequently cut the corner of the nail back a little to take the pressure away. That works for a little while, but almost inevitably we leave a little sharp corner uncut one time. That corner soon digs into the skin cruelly and the skin is broken, with "proud flesh" being produced. Proud flesh is the body's unsuccessful effort to close the hole in the skin and wall off the source of the irritation. The area swells and becomes often so painful that you can hardly walk.

Treatment can be accomplished at home if you start early enough.

First, get wider shoes (see the chapter on **Foot Problems**). When you try on a pair of shoes, they should feel comfortable when you stand up and walk around. There should not be any sensation of pressure on the toes or any part of the feet. The old saying (usually by the shoe salesman) is that you will break in the shoes in some period of time. What actually happens is that your feet get broken in, or broken down. Your toes get squeezed, and you get an ingrown toenail, among other things.

Please note that socks that are too small can squeeze the feet and toes even when the shoes are adequate in size. The tendency of sock manufacturers to make socks in the "fits sizes 10 to 13" mode just means that they will be comfortable for size 10 and maybe 11, but I guarantee you that they will be too tight for the larger feet. It's hard to get socks in colors in sizes above 13, so you may have to find some outfits that go with white socks if you have larger feet.

Tight socks also sometimes cause a change in the way you bear weight, so that hot spots may develop because the foot can't expand when your weight comes down on it.

Second, pack some cotton between your nail and the tender skin. Use just a small piece, and roll it under the skin by using a nail file or something similar, pushing the cotton against the nail as you roll it under the skin so as to prevent pain from the procedure. Then just change the cotton twice a day, and wash it out with soapsuds at each change. It often takes several months of packing the nail before it is completely back to normal.

Third, let the nail grow out to the end of the toe and cut it straight across instead of down along the nail from then on the rest of your life.

That should do it if it hasn't gone too far. But if you already have a big hook of nail (often just like a fish hook) sticking into the skin, that has to be removed. Most of the time you will need a local anesthetic (a shot) in order to probe deeply enough. That usually means a trip to the doctor. Once the doctor has removed the part of the nail that is sticking into the skin, then you must do the above three things afterwards in order to prevent it from coming back.

CHAPTER 64 -- ITCHING

Itching is usually caused by stimulation of tiny nerves in the surface of the skin. Anything that stimulates them can produce this. One thing that most people don't know is that if they scratch themselves anywhere on their bodies, it may cause an itch somewhere else. The reason for that is that the skin is all one organ, just like the heart and liver for example. Even though different nerves supply different areas, the skin is somehow inter-related in some other ways that are not fully understood.

So a rash due to fungus on a foot may produce a sympathetic rash up on the chest or an arm that has no fungus in it. This is called an *id* reaction. Clearing up the fungus by treating the foot also clears up the arm rash, which you haven't had to treat at all.

Likewise when one spot is irritated and itches, that may set up itching spots in one or more other areas of the body, a situation that is much more likely to occur if you scratch or rub the original spot.

What kinds of things make us itch? Fortunately almost all are benign and do not represent any kind of serious medical problem. For the benefit of the one or two hypochondriacs who may be reading this, I am not going to mention any of the occasional bad things. Besides, they are usually pretty obvious.

Poison Ivy (Also Poison Oak and Poison Sumac) This is a rash caused by the oil from (usually) the leaves of these plants. The oil contains an acid, which produces a red rash with little blisters, within 24 to 48 hours, everywhere they touched your skin. Untreated they last about 14 days. Treated, they last about 14 days, but maybe you aren't quite so miserable for that two-week period.

So be aware that these plants contain the acid in their stems and branches as well as in their leaves. And in their smoke when they are burned.

How do you keep from getting poison ivy (and the others)? First, get someone to show you what they look like. Pictures in a book are a start, but I have yet to see a picture of any of these that really looked like the real thing. Poison ivy has clusters of three pointed leaves which may have a reddish tinge to the green. An old saying is "Leaves of three, leave them be." They also often look as though they have little warts on some of them. I can't describe the others well enough to be of any value. But I know them when I see them.

> *My Dad had never had a case of poison ivy before in his life. Then one fall day after all leaves were off the trees and vines and bushes in Franklin, Indiana, he tore out all the poison ivy plants along the fence around our garden. He used gloves for all of this. Then he burned them and had a nice little bonfire. Since it was a blustery November day the smoke swirled around considerably as he raked all the various twigs and branches into the flames. All were consumed. Two days later Dad awoke in the morning with a very swollen and red face and ears and neck, which were also covered with blisters. Our old doctor told him it was the worst case of poison ivy he had ever seen. Now I have practiced for almost as many years as he, while treating literally hundreds of cases of poison ivy; and my Dad's case is the worst one I've ever seen also!*

Once you know what they look like, then you can stay away from them. One problem here in Arizona is that these don't grow in the desert, nor at high altitude in places like Flagstaff. Where they do grow is down in canyons, such as Oak Creek Canyon, and that is where all the cases I have seen in Arizona have come from. Since people who visit the canyons don't have these plants at home, as we did in Indiana, they don't know what they look like, and, indeed, may have never heard of them. So they camp in them, walk in shorts through them, break off their leaves to use instead of toilet paper, or just pet their dogs who have been romping among them and thus have a nice layer of the acid on their coats.

If you have not stayed away from them successfully, and someone with you recognizes that you all may have been exposed, take heart. All is not yet lost. If it is your first exposure to them, then your immune system may not be sensitized and thus may not produce a rash if the exposure is relatively small. I've been touched by poison ivy and oak for sure, and possibly also by sumac without ever getting a rash. But I've always taken the next precaution.

That is to always wash off thoroughly with just regular soap and water every part of your body that may have touched the plants as soon as you can after exposure. If you aren't very allergic to them, then you may have as much as a 6-8 hour window for preventive washing. If you have had a rash before, then you may have only a 2-3 hour window. Soap is an alkali and will neutralize most of any acid that you haven't mechanically washed off. Also wash your dog, before washing yourself probably. Also throw all your clothes in the washing machine before washing yourself, so that when you are clean, you won't accidentally touch something that will re-expose you.

Treating the itching rash: If Ziradryl lotion is still available in areas where there are a lot of these plants, then get some and put it on the rash several times a day. That isn't available in Arizona, probably because there isn't enough demand for it for druggists to stock it. What *is* available everywhere is Caladryl lotion, made by the same company and almost as good. Same deal -- put it on several times a day. Juice of the Aloe vera plant that you have growing in your house or yard, and cortisone-type creams, such as triamcinolone (Kenalog), may help some more but not as much as we would like. Colloidal oatmeal (Aveeno) baths or soaks are very soothing. Injections of triamcinolone may help a little, and many doctors use it. It does depress the adrenal glands for a few months after use, however, so is probably better used only for a truly miserable situation (or a bad allergy season).

> *A cautionary tale: One patient of mine knew all this stuff. He didn't take a bath after considerable exposure by his dog, but he did thoroughly wash his hands and his dog. Two days later he was in my office with a very swollen private area of his body, which also had a bunch of little blisters on it. What had happened was that when he finally was able to wash his hands, which had been thoroughly exposed by way of his pet, he forgot that he had stopped to go to the bathroom in the woods. That area didn't get washed until he took a shower the next morning, and by that time it was too late!*

Once you have removed all the acid-containing plant oil by washing yourself thoroughly from head to toe, the stuff can't do you any more harm, and it will not spread to areas that were not exposed. People have often told me that the rash "just keeps spreading", but what is happening is that all exposed areas don't develop the rash at the same speed. And in some cases there may be a sympathetic *id* reaction elsewhere, although in my experience that would be pretty rare. Once the rash develops, wash yourself thoroughly one more time just to be sure you got it all, because the 14 day limit doesn't start until all of the oil is off your skin. I don't think covering the rash helps, except when using the oatmeal soaks.

Mosquito bites. For prevention use a DEET-containing bug repellant when in mosquito country, which is most places in the world, depending on the time of year and how dry the weather has been. The best relief for the bite is the oily Campho-Phenique, which is available in all drugstores. Don't scratch them, or they may get infected.

Chiggers. These are tiny, almost microscopic little red bugs that get on your skin and bore down in. You can easily see them with a magnifying glass. They tend to accumulate anywhere there is a constriction in your clothing, such as your beltline. They are in the grass everywhere in the Midwest, and probably everywhere else east of the

Mississippi River. We don't have them in the Southwest. Unfortunately we <u>do</u> have rattlesnakes and scorpions. That's another chapter!

You can remove chiggers from your skin by just sterilizing a sewing needle in a flame, then swabbing the bite with alcohol, and picking it out gently with the tip of the needle (perhaps with the aid of a magnifying glass). Then, of course, swab with alcohol again. Or you can use Campho-Phenique, which will cut them off from oxygen, and they will die. They will also die if they burrow too deep. A little dab of flexible collodion or clear nail polish on each bite will both kill the chigger and help the itch.

When you are just desperate to scratch something, try rubbing an ice cube on the area instead. That will always provide at least temporary relief and won't prolong the vicious itch-scratch-itch-scratch cycle. Most of the time, if you can find a way to quit scratching, you will soon stop itching.

As far as itching is concerned, your fingernails are deadly weapons.

There is an all too common skin condition called dermatitis factitia, in which the skin becomes thickened and red, along with lines of scabs caused by scratching on exposed areas of the skin. The diagnosis is easy: the only places there is a rash are only where they are within reach of the fingernails, and the distance between scratch lines is the same as the distance between fingernails. Sometimes the skin is just thickened from constant rubbing without actual scratching. Little children with eczema are another example. They often scratch until they bleed.

Treatment of this type of condition requires that you stop scratching. Here are some tricks that often help. 1) Stop using all stimulants, such as caffeine, tobacco in all forms, and spicy foods (particularly hot peppers). 2) Alcohol is not a stimulant, but it too can aggravate itching. 3) Cut your own or your child's fingernails very short and file them down to the quick <u>every day.</u> 4) Wear mittens to bed so you can't scratch in your sleep. 5) Apply one of the creams from the cortisone family just before bedtime, and cover the skin immediately with Saran Wrap all night. 6) Avoid soap, except possibly Aveeno, to the affected areas. 7) Soak in a tub, or use <u>very</u> wet hand towels soaked with Aveeno colloid solution for 15-30 minutes three times a day if possible. 8) Rub the itching area with ice until the itch stops whenever possible. 9) Aloe vera juice or gel may be soothing. 10) Caladryl lotion applied several times a day may help. 11) An antihistamine, such as Tacharyl, or over-the-counter Chlortrimeton may also help to reduce the skin's sensitivity. 12) A mild sedative at bedtime, such as 50 mg of Benadryl or 3 mg of melatonin, may help you to sleep better. And if you sleep more soundly, you aren't as likely to scratch.

Good luck with these home remedies for itching. They will usually save you the cost of at least one doctor's visit.

CHAPTER 65 -- LIVER DISEASE

The liver has way over one thousand different functions in our bodies. It is a delicate chemical factory, where all sorts of compounds are manufactured from the raw materials you provide in your diet. The chemical reactions going on there provide most of the body's heat by thermochemical reactions.

When it gets sick, your whole body suffers.

The two most common chronic liver diseases are <u>Cirrhosis</u> and <u>Hepatitis C</u>. Both often end in liver transplant or death. It saddens me that both of these are almost totally preventable. Cirrhosis can be prevented by avoiding excess alcohol consumption, and hepatitis C can mostly be prevented by avoiding IV drug use with its needle sharing.

Treatment of hepatitis C with Interferon is helpful sometimes, but this is true in way less than 50% in every study I've seen. There are a couple of possibly promising experimental drugs on the horizon.

About the only thing you can do in most of the cases of these two diseases is to keep it from getting worse. If you can do this, you will have the chance of quite a few years before you get into serious trouble.

Here are the things you must do.

First and foremost you must totally stay away from all alcohol.

Second, have yourself immunized against both hepatitis A and B. This will at least avoid further injury to the liver from infections.

Third, if you are overweight, get down to your normal weight and keep it down. Fat deposits in the liver will cause more damage.

Fourth, begin and maintain a regular daily exercise program. (See the **Exercise** chapter.)

Fifth, take a daily multivitamin supplement, emphasizing especially the B complex family. But never take more than 5,000 units of vitamin A per day. Vitamin A can be poisonous to the liver in high doses.

Sixth, avoid taking any non-steroidal anti-inflammatory drugs (NSAIDs), for example, Advil, Ibuprofen, and Naproxen. Even the newer COX II inhibitors are risky.

Seventh, avoid all herbal supplements. All but one of them has been shown to be toxic to the liver in certain doses.

Be sure your affairs are in order, particularly with an up-to-date last will and testament, along with a medical power of attorney and living will.

Enjoy your life to the fullest every single day.

Hepatitis A

Hepatitis A is a very common, usually mild, viral disease of the liver, which many of us get in childhood without even knowing it. We now have a vaccine for it, and infants receive it as part of their baby shots. It is passed from person to person through fecal contamination -- mainly not washing the hands adequately after having a bowel movement or changing a dirty diaper. Care involves just treating the symptoms for a couple of weeks. The stools remain infectious for quite awhile in many cases. So take special care to use good hygiene.

Hepatitis B

Hepatitis B is also caused by a virus acquired through contact with any body fluids. Use of shared needles by drug users, as with hepatitis C, is a common source. Accidental needle sticks in health care workers are a potential hazard.

This carries a much greater risk of severe illness and long-term problems than hep A, but not so much as hep C and cirrhosis.

Fortunately there is an excellent vaccine to prevent it. All infants now are supposed to receive their first dose before they leave the hospital after birth. All health care workers are offered the vaccine before they start any job where they might be exposed to body fluids.

Treatment is symptomatic, with the same program as hep C.

See also the chapter on **Blood Borne Diseases**.

Yellow Fever

Yellow fever is another very serious viral disease of the liver which disappeared from our country when we got serious about mosquito control in the South and even Washington, D.C. An immunization is available and should be done before going to a country where the disease is still found. Consult www.cdc.gov for lists of immunizations needed for each country.

CHAPTER 66 -- LOSING WEIGHT

(Including guaranteed weight loss diets)

Read the chapter on **Obesity** along with this one for best results. Some of the information is repeated, some is presented in a different way, and some is new in that chapter.

There have been literally hundreds of diets and weight loss programs published in the past, and there will be thousands in the future. Some work. Some don't. Some are dangerous.

Examples of the latter are: use of thyroid hormone -- now outlawed in most states (the doctor who prescribes it can lose his license), Dexamyl and other amphetamine-containing drugs, such as fen-Phen. Meridia and Xenical are two more recent ones, which so far appear safer.

Breaking down weight loss into its simplest parts, the only way to lose weight is to eat less than you burn up. There are a number of ways to accomplish this, and I will discuss several in the next couple of pages.

1. Exercise daily for at least 30 minutes without stopping.

2. Don't eat between meals.

Cokes and other caffeine-containing snacks have two drawbacks: first, the caffeine causes the production of more stomach acid, thus making you more hungry; second, the calories quickly add up. I'm continually amazed at how many calories overweight people consume in the form of beverages.

To give you an example of how they add up: the amount of exercise that will burn up the calories in one can of pop or beer equals the amount of energy spent in running a mile in six minutes. I don't know about you, but it has been a long time since I could run a mile in six minutes.

If you feel you have to have beverages instead of just plain water (which has <u>no</u> calories), drink caffeine-free Diet Coke or Diet Pepsi.

3. Limit your total fat intake to no more than 30 percent of your total food intake each day. I personally think that you should go farther than that. I recommend no more than one ounce of fat in any form per day. Fat has twice as many calories as the same weight of protein and carbohydrates.

4. Eat no sweets. Make all of your carbohydrates the complex type, which require more work by your digestive system before they get into your blood stream. These include whole grain bread, cereal, fruits and vegetables, particularly raw (the cellulose is broken down by cooking), pasta, and whole grains such as rice.

5. Try these behavior modification suggestions:

a. Shop from a prepared list to avoid impulse buying. Do not shop for food when you are hungry. Buy only foods that require preparation before they can be eaten.

b. Keep all foods in the kitchen and nowhere else. There should be no food in the car or office or workroom or TV room.

c. Eat at a specified time and do nothing else at that time. Don't read or watch television while you eat.

d. Eat slowly and leave some food on the plate.

e. Serve only what is to be eaten. Don't put out family-style meals with big bowls for extra helpings.

f. If you are anxious, don't eat. Take a bath, or run an errand, or go to bed with your spouse.

g. Don't skip meals. Your body will think you are starving and reduce the rate at which you burn calories to starvation mode. Just reduce the quantities for each meal. It is especially important to eat breakfast, which, theoretically, should be the biggest meal of the day.

For children: Restrict their TV watching to no more than two hours a week. Do not allow them to eat when they watch TV. Adults should not have between-meal snacks, but kids often need them. Just be sure that the snacks are good nutritious foods, no closer than two hours before mealtime. And I firmly believe that keeping salt to a minimum in childhood, as well as later, will reduce the later development of high blood pressure or postpone its appearance for many years.

The latest dangerous diet drug was Fen-phen, which may have caused some heart damage in a few people. The thing that helped the most with Fen-phen was the frequent visits to the doctor, with the weigh-ins and positive feedback every week or two. Two of the latest drugs designed to do it for you are Xenical and Meridia. So far their biggest deterrent to general use is their high prices. Both have some side effects. Ask your druggist for a list.

Xenical prevents the absorption of fat-soluble vitamins from your GI tract. These are Vitamins A, D, E, and beta carotene. Many, possibly most, obese people have lower than normal levels of Vitamin D and beta carotene. So people who take Xenical should also take a multivitamin containing those vitamins daily at least two hours before or after a dose of the drug.

Actually, I highly recommend that everyone on a diet take an <u>inexpensive</u> multivitamin and mineral supplement daily. We will talk more about that elsewhere. Walgreen's, for example, has their A-to-Z preparation, 365 of them for only $15.99. Centrum is great but costs more. Also available are Micebrin and Micebrin T, Myadec with minerals, Theragran with minerals. Don't buy vitamins, "chelated" or otherwise, from either your doctor or a door-to-door salesman. <u>They are a total waste of money.</u>

Another thing with Xenical is that it may cause increased levels of oxalate in the urine. Therefore anyone with a history of calcium oxalate kidney stones should not take Xenical or you may get another stone. Soon.

Overeaters Anonymous is a good program. So is Weight Watchers. There are a number of them, all of which do better with frequent patient supervision. This can get expensive, but it works. Some measure out portions for the week's menu, and sell the food to you. Some include weekly meetings with others who are trying to lose. Thus there is a support group, which is also a social hour.

So-called central body obesity means that most of the fat is located in the abdomen -- the beer belly. That form of obesity is the one most likely to produce adult-onset diabetes. This type of obesity is totally preventable with exercise. But you will have to cut back on your refined carbohydrates (alcohol and sodas in particular) to get rid of it.

A loss of just 10 to 15 pounds will produce a dramatic drop in the blood pressure when you have hypertension.

Weight loss is easier said than done. Pills have been used for at least fifty years, but all so far have had one or more drawbacks. When I first started practice there was a drug put out by Smith, Kline and French called Dexamyl. It combined dexedrine (an amphetamine), which made you hyper and caused you to burn up a lot of calories, with amytal (a barbiturate) which had a sedative effect. I prescribed that to only one patient before I tumbled to what I was doing to her. She felt great and lost ten pounds in the first month. Then she found that she needed a bigger dose to produce the same effect and felt really irritable when she missed a dose by a couple of hours. It didn't take much diagnostic savvy to realize that she was becoming an addict to both of these very addicting drugs, instead of each canceling out the addictive effect of the other. I had to withdraw her slowly and carefully because barbiturate addicts can get into really serious trouble to the point of death if withdrawn from the drug too rapidly. That drug was around for ten or fifteen years before the FDA put it high enough on the controlled substances list that most doctors quit prescribing it.

As we all know, the only way anyone can lose weight is by eating less than your body burns up for a prolonged period of time -- weeks, months, even years. ALL successful weight-loss stories (programs) have one thing in common -- the person burns up more calories than he or she takes in until the desired amount of weight is lost. Then a maintenance program balancing calories (food) taken in against calories burned is used for long-term normal weight.

Because of differences in the rate at which everybody burns calories (their metabolic rate), you can't compare your food intake to someone else's. You may be burning at less than half the rate of another person.

Obesity is very closely related to the amount of time spent watching TV, starting in early childhood. So, less TV and more exercise will be our motto from now on.

The weight loss programs that really work include daily exercise -- at least 30 minutes per day of continuous exercise without stopping. This type of exercise is often referred to as aerobic or cardiovascular exercise. This can be a simple as just walking at what <u>you</u> feel is a brisk pace, or jogging, using a stationary bike (riding a regular bike on the road usually isn't aerobic exercise because you coast a lot), cross-country skiing or ski machine, using a stair master, or going up and downstairs in your home, and lap swimming (which may be the best aerobic workout of all).

The reason for doing at least 30 minutes of exercise at a time without stopping is that your muscles burn glycogen, which is conveniently stored in the muscle fibers for easy access, for the first 25 minutes of a workout. After 25 minutes, when the glycogen has been used up, the muscles start burning fatty acids, e.g. cholesterol and triglycerides, as well as stored body fat. So every minute you exercise past 25 minutes burns up some unwanted fat.

To lose one pound you have to burn up 3500 calories that you don't replace with food intake. The average 150-pound person who just sits all day burns less than 1000 calories.

1. Limit your calories first by avoiding refined carbohydrates (e.g. sugars and alcohol), which our bodies don't have to do any work to digest and go directly to fat if not burned up right after eating. Refined carbohydrates cause a "sugar rush" from a rise in your blood glucose level, which in turn causes the body to secrete higher amounts of insulin than usual. The insulin causes those carbohydrates to be immediately stored as body fat. That makes the blood sugar fall below the body's usual comfort range. When that happens, you get hungry again. A regular roller coaster.

Complex carbohydrates such as raw fruits and vegetables, whole grain breads, pasta, and rice, require several digestive steps and are thus less likely to go directly to fat because the blood sugar stays within the body's comfort range during digestion. For diabetes prevention and treatment, eating complex carbohydrates reduces the need for insulin production to control sudden elevations of blood sugar.

2. Portion control. No between-meal snacks. Don't go back for seconds. If you feel you have to always fill your plate, then use a smaller plate. Always leave some food on your plate. (That certainly goes against the grain for one such as I who grew up in the Great Depression; but you can take that leftover food and freeze it, then thaw it out in the microwave for another day.)

Here are a couple of examples of what snacks can do to a diet. One ounce of alcohol in a mixed drink, or a beer, or a can of soda, or a large tortilla, or a large slice of bread contain about 160 calories.

To give you an idea how much exercise you would have to do to successfully lose weight without also restricting food intake, consider this: if you run a mile in six minutes you'll burn the calories in that drink -- 160 calories. So skip that drink; use diet sodas ("only 4 calories") or water.

3. Keep all food in the kitchen and nowhere else. NO food in the car, office, workroom, or TV room.

4. Eating out. A full meal in a restaurant contains at least 1000 calories. So instead of a dinner entree, try ordering just an appetizer, or an appetizer and a green salad. Or split a Caesar salad with someone, and have herbal tea or decaf coffee sweetened with saccharin (Sweet and Low) or aspartame (Equal). Skip dessert at all times -- don't even take one bite or you may not be able to resist taking several more bites (at 30 to 50 calories per bite). Drink two glasses of water as soon as you sit down, before you take your first bite. Skip the bread course entirely -- not a bite.

5. Reduce caffeine consumption because it causes increased acids in the stomach, which makes you more hungry.

6. Many people know that they can restrict their intake of most foods pretty easily. But certain foods are just so-o-o good that eating even one bite, of chocolate or potato chips, for examples makes you want to eat the who-o-ole package. So you do! Usually we are talking about carbohydrates here -- the carboholic (like alcoholic) syndrome. The only solution to this is to do like the successful recovering alcoholic: avoid at all times those things that make you binge.

7. After just two weeks of faithfully following a low-calorie diet (800--1200 calories) your stomach will literally shrink and not demand so much food to make it feel full.

8. Shopping. Never go food shopping when you are hungry. Make a shopping list of just what you need to use in your diet for that week. Then don't buy anything else on impulse, especially not snacks ("maybe I could just reward myself for being so good last week.") If you are going to want to reward yourself each time you reach an intermediate goal, don't use food as the prize. Eat to live. Don't live to eat! <u>Buy only food that requires preparation before it can be eaten.</u>

9. Food is <u>not</u> love. Don't confuse food with love.

Older People

Older people worry that they will "look old" if they lose weight so that their skin sags. That certainly does happen in many cases (especially in smokers and people who have spent a lot of time out in the sun unprotected by sun blocks) but much less than expected. Particularly if the weight loss is combined with mild to moderate exercises that tone up your underlying muscles on an ongoing basis.

So, to avoid (or at least reduce) the sagging skin of later years, lose the weight while your skin is still elastic, certainly before age 50, stop the use of tobacco, and protect your skin from ultraviolet rays (see the chapter on **Skin**). Then you can reduce the urge, or need, to have cosmetic plastic surgery, none of which is ever covered by health insurance.

Weight Loss After Pregnancy

One of the highest risk factors for long term obesity in women is excessive weight gain during pregnancy. The most important part of this is prevention.

Limit yourself to a weight gain of about two pounds per month early in the pregnancy, and three pounds toward the end. If you were underweight to start with, you can gain perhaps three or four pounds more; while if you were overweight in the beginning, you should gain three or four pounds less.

Obese women should gain no more than about 13 or 14 pounds in the whole nine months. I had several obese women who, with good nutrition and exercise within their capabilities, actually had a net weight loss during their pregnancies. I watched them pretty carefully because I knew we were stretching the envelope, and they all delivered normal healthy babies.

Exercise daily, right up until you go into labor if possible.

With resumption of normal activity and eating habits, most of your weight gained during pregnancy will be lost within three months, then there will be further steady loss for another three months. Some highly motivated individuals will lose faster. This chapter is devoted to some of those who are less motivated.

Mothers who breast feed their little ones and try to follow the "Recommended Daily Requirements for lactating women" of 2,500 calories per day will almost certainly find themselves unable to lose any weight at that level. Part of this is due to the fact that a lot of women who lactate don't get very much exercise. Therefore they should eat no more than 2,000 calories worth of food per day.

One small recent study of overweight breast-feeding women produced the good news that you can have all of the above. By lowering daily calories by 500, and exercising for 45 minutes four days per week, these women lost an average of one pound per week between one month and three months after delivery. Their weight loss did not affect the normal growth of their babies as compared to the babies of a control group of mothers who did not restrict their calories, and did not exercise during the same time period.

So mothers, breast feed your little ones, eat less, and exercise for 30 minutes a day. And enjoy life more!

General Rules for Diets

Measuring food. Food should be measured. You will need standard measuring cups and measuring spoons. All measurements are level. Cooked foods are to be measured after being cooked.

Food preparation. Meats should be baked, boiled, roasted or broiled. Do not eat fried foods unless fat allowed in the meal is used.

Fat allowed in your diet may be used to season vegetables. Vegetables may be cooked in bouillon or fat-free meat broth if desired.

> One of the main goals of this book is to promote good health through natural methods. Here we want all women, who can, to breast feed their infants for as long as possible, perhaps even a year. We also want those mothers to exercise, because exercise serves many important functions for us, not just as an aid to weight loss. We also want these mothers to recover from the obesity that all too often accompanies pregnancy as soon as possible.

Food selection. Select your diet from the same foods purchased for the rest of the family- milk, vegetables, bread, meats, fats, and fruits (fresh, dried, or frozen or canned without sugar).

Many special dietetic foods should not be used unless they are figured in the diet plan. Also, they are unnecessarily expensive. Always check the labels of these foods for proteins, carbohydrates, fat, and calorie content.

Foods that should be avoided: Sugar; candy; honey; jams and jellies; syrups; pie; most cakes and cookies; pastries; condensed milk; regular soft drinks; candy-coated gum; fried, scalloped, or cream-based foods; beer, wine, and other alcoholic beverages.

Eat your meals about the same time every day. Eat only the amounts given on your diet plan and do not skip meals.

CHAPTER 67 -- THE DIETS

The exchange-type diet lists below are based on the recommendations of the American Diabetes Association and the American Dietetic Association in cooperation with the National Institute of Arthritis, Metabolism, and Digestive Diseases and the National Heart and Lung Institute of the U. S. Public Health Service, Department of Health and Human Services, plus my own experience in helping thousands of people lose serious weight.

Instructions for Daily Menu Guide Use

The foods allowed in your diet should be selected from the exchange lists. We call them "exchange diets" because you can exchange anything on one list for anything else on the same list and have the same food value and the same number of calories in the quantities specified.

For example, when your menu calls for one bread exchange, all foods on the bread exchange list may be used in the amount stated. If two bread exchanges are allowed, double the amount or add a second item from the same list. Note that 1 slice of bread equals one bread exchange. So does 1/2 bagel, 1/2 cup cooked cereal, and 3/4 cup of dry cereal. Beans, peas, corn, and potatoes, along with several other common food items also are bread exchanges in the proper amounts. The greatest aspect of this type of diet is the wide variety of foods it allows, so that you don't get tired of the same old stuff all the time.

The most success will be achieved if all the foods allowed in this plan are eaten. For best results, do not skip meals, and do not save any of the portions for the next day. When you skip meals, your body thinks it is starving and goes into the starvation metabolic mode. This mode reduces drastically the rate at which you burn food. Remember that ideal body weight is achieved with energy taken in as equal to energy burned. But if the rate at which you burn energy is reduced, as in the starvation mode (or becoming a couch potato), then it becomes hard for your body to burn up as much as you take in. So eat everything allowed on this 800 calorie diet every day, and never save calories from today to be eaten tomorrow. Unlike the tax code, there is no carryover allowed in dieting for weight control.

*You do not need to spend money on special diet foods with these diets. Just plan your weekly menu in advance, much as you probably do now. Watch for weekly specials in the supermarkets. And enjoy your better look in the mirror each week.

When you feel hungry, drink a glass of water. As a matter of fact, drinking as much as three quarts of water per day will assist your weight loss enormously.

Your stomach will shrink within two weeks on these diets, and you will soon feel full on small portions.

My patients have lost literally thousands of pounds on these diets. I firmly believe that they are vastly superior to almost all of the highly-publicized weight loss programs in all of the books in the library or bookstore.

And I positively guarantee you that if you follow this diet faithfully, every day, and do some kind of continuous exercise without stopping for only 30 minutes each day, you will lose your excess weight steadily and surely. When you get down to where you want to be, then you can gradually increase your food intake to 1200 calories per day (see 1200 cal diet below), or more as you weigh yourself daily and determine that your weight is remaining stable.

Once you have lost all you want to lose, watch your weight at least two or three times a week. If you gain 5 pounds, go back on the weight reduction diet. I promise you that it is much easier to lose 5 pounds than 45 or 50 lbs again.

All diets that allow less than 1200 calories per day are deficient in one or more vital minerals and vitamins. Therefore it is absolutely necessary for you to take a single multiple vitamin and mineral tablet every day. There are several reliable ones on the market, plus a lot that may be somewhat questionable. I feel comfortable with Walgreen's A thru Z, $15.99 for 365 of them, one daily. That is probably the best value for your money. Centrum with minerals, Myadec, Theragran with minerals, Micebrin and Micebrin T are all made by reliable companies but are more expensive. All of these are just one large tablet daily. You don't have to spend a lot of money for these supplements. All come from natural sources. Realistically our bodies don't care where the required compounds come from, just that the proper chemical formulas are present.

The following 800 calorie diet will also be repeated below along with the others for your convenience. Feel free to share these with your friends if you wish.

800 calorie diet for weight loss

Carbohydrate	2-1/2 oz (75 grams)
Protein	2 oz (55 grams)
Fat	1 oz (30 grams)

800 calorie daily menu allowances

Breakfast
1 fruit exchange (list 3)
1 bread exchange (list 4)
1 meat exchange (list 5)
1 fat exchange (list 6)
1/2 milk exchange (list 1)
*Coffee or tea one cup only

Lunch
2 meat exchanges (list 5)
1 vegetable exchange (list 2)
Vegetables as desired (list 2*)
1 fruit exchange (list 3)
1/2 milk exchange (list 1)
*Decaf coffee or tea up to two cups only

Dinner
2 meat exchanges (list 5)
1 vegetable exchange (list 2)
Vegetables as desired (list 2*)
1 fruit exchange (list 3)
1/2 milk exchange (list 1)
*Decaf coffee or tea up to two cups only

*Do not drink more than three cups of any caffeine-containing beverage in any 24-hour period. The caffeine (besides other potentially ill effects that we will talk about elsewhere) causes the production of excess stomach acid, which makes you more hungry. So it is best to drink them only on a full stomach and limit the quantities. Alcohol does the same thing, but is an absolute no-no when you are trying to lose weight because of the empty calories in each drink.

The single day sample menus below are given to illustrate correct use of the exchange lists. Your weekly menus should be planned on the basis of the daily menu guide.

Sample portions for the 800 cal diet
Breakfast

Apple juice	1/3 cup
Whole wheat toast	1 slice
Egg	one
Corn oil margarine	1 tsp
Skim milk	1/2 cup

Lunch

Cheddar cheese	two 1-oz slices
Carrots	1 large
Radishes, lettuce, etc.	as desired
Orange	one small
Skim milk	1/2 cup
Low calorie dressing	1 tbsp

Dinner

Baked or broiled chicken w/o skin	2 oz
Green beans	1/2 cup
Lettuce salad with a tomato	as desired
Banana	1 small
Yogurt, plain, mixed with the banana or a different fruit on another night as a great substitute for dessert	1/2cup

For those on reduced fat diets in addition to needing to lose weight, what you want to do is eliminate fat from animal sources as much as possible. Plug these suggestions into the proper slots in the various diets.

Meat and poultry	One exchange
Beef, lamb, pork, veal, ham, very lean	1 oz slice (4" × 2" × 1/4")

Chicken or duck, no skin, <u>baked, boiled or broiled</u>	(4" × 2" × 1/4")
Halibut, perch, sole, and similar fish	1 oz slice
Oysters, clams, shrimp, scallops	5 small
Salmon, tuna, crab	1/4 cup
Sardines	3 medium

Helpful hints:

Eat fish and poultry without the skin.

The milk you drink must all be skim (just think of it as colored water) or nonfat (which has more taste).

If you eat yogurt, make sure it's low-fat.

Use corn, soy, or safflower oil margarine instead of butter.

Fats

Each portion equals one fat exchange and contains about 1/6 oz of fat for about 45 calories. Liquid fats (at room temperature) of vegetable origin tend to be unsaturated, while animal fats are all saturated and much more likely to clog up your arteries. The unsaturated fats are safe as far as arteriosclerosis is concerned. But all fats contain about twice as many calories per unit weight than proteins and carbohydrates and thus need to be severely restricted in weight loss diets.

Milk Exchanges

Each exchange equals one milk exchange and provides a little less than 1/2 oz carbohydrate and slightly less than 1/3 oz of protein. The fat content and total calories depend on the type of milk product.

Milk	Measure	Fat exchanges	Calories
Buttermilk	one cup	0	80
Evaporated undiluted skim	1/2 cup	0	80

Milk	Measure	Fat exchanges	Calories
Evaporated undiluted whole	1/2 cup	2	170
Nonfat dry milk, mixed according to directions on box	1 cup	0	80
Nonfat dry milk powder	1/3 cup	0	80
Skim or nonfat milk	1 cup	0	80
1% butterfat	1 cup	1/2	103
2% butterfat	1 cup	1	125
Whole	1 cup	2	170
Yogurt, plain, made with skim milk	1 cup	0	80

If you desire a substitute for the milk indicated in the diet plan, choose either a milk product that contains the same number of fat exchanges or allow for the difference in the total meal plan. For example, if the diet plan calls for one cup of skim milk (no fat exchange), you can substitute one cup of 2% milk and omit one fat exchange from the total meal list.

Vegetable Exchanges

Each portion (except for vegetables marked with an asterisk) contains one vegetable exchange and supplies about 25 calories, 1/6 oz carbohydrate and 1/15 oz of protein. One serving is 1/2 cup.

*Those marked with an asterisk * can be eaten as much as desired if eaten raw. Limit the amount to one cup if cooked.

Asparagus
*Lettuce
Beans, green or yellow
Mushrooms
Bean sprouts
Okra
Beets
Onions
*Broccoli
*Parsley
*Brussels sprouts
*Peppers, green or red
*Cabbage
*Radishes
Carrots
Rutabagas
Cauliflower
Sauerkraut
*Celery
*Tomatoes
*Chicory
Tomato juice
*Chinese cabbage
Summer squash
Cucumbers
Turnips
Eggplant
Vegetable juice cocktail
*Escarole
*Watercress
Greens: beet, chard, collard, dandelion, kale, mustard, spinach, turnip
Zucchini

Fruit exchanges

Fruit may be fresh, dried, frozen or canned without syrup or sugar.

Each portion equals one fruit exchange and supplies about 1/3 oz carbohydrate, for about 40 calories.

Fruit	Measure
Apples	1 small (2" diam.)
Apple juice or cider	1/3 cup
Applesauce	1/2 cup
Apricots, fresh	2 medium
Apricots, dried	4 halves
Banana	1 small
Various berries (boysenberries, blackberries, blueberries, raspberries)	1/2 cup
Cantaloupe	1/4 (6" diam.)
Cherries	10 large
Dates	2
Figs, fresh	1 large
Figs, dried	1 small
Fruit cocktail	1/2 cup
Grapefruit	1/2 small
Grapefruit juice	1/2 cup
Grapes	12
Grape juice	1/4 cup
Honeydew melon	1/8 (7" diam.)
Mandarin oranges	3/4 cup
Mango	1/2 small
Nectarine	1 small
Orange	1 small

Fruit	Measure
Orange juice	1/2 cup
Papaya	3/4 cup
Peach	1 med.
Pear	1 small
Persimmon, native	1 med.
Pineapple	1/2 cup
Pineapple juice	1/3 cup
Plums	2 med.
Prunes	2 med.
Prune juice	1/4 cup
Raisins	2 tbsp.
Strawberries	3/4 cup
Tangerine	1 large
Watermelon	1 cup

Bread exchanges

Each portion equals one bread exchange and supplies about 1/2 oz of carbohydrate and 1/15 oz of protein, for about 70 calories.

Bread	Measure
Bread, French, raisin (no icing), rye, white, whole-wheat	1 slice
Bagel	1/2
Biscuit or roll	1 (1/2" diam.)
Bread crumbs, dried	3 tbsp.
Bun (hamburger or wiener)	1/2
Cornbread	1"×2"×2"

Bread	Measure
English muffin	1 (2" diam.)
Muffin	1 (2" diam.)
Cake, angel food or sponge, without icing	1 1/2" cube
Cereal, cooked	1/2 cup
Cereal, dry	3/4 cup
Cornstarch	2 tbsp.
Graham crackers	2 (2 1/2" sq.)
Oyster crackers	20 (2 1/2" sq.)
Round	6
Rye wafer	3 (2 1/2")
Saltine	6
Variety	5 small
Flour	1-1/2 cups
Matzoh	1 (6" diam.)
Popcorn, popped, no butter, small-kernel	1-1/2 cups
Pretzels (3 ring)	6
Rice or grits, cooked	1/2 cup
Spaghetti or macaroni noodles, cooked	1/2 cup
Tortilla	1 (6" diam.)
Beans, baked without pork	1/4 cup
Lima beans, navy beans, etc., dry, cooked	1/2 cup
Corn	1/3 cup
Corn on the cob	1/2 medium ear

Bread	Measure
Parsnips	2/3 cup
Peas, dried (split peas, etc.) or green, cooked	1/2 cup
Potatoes, sweet or yams; fresh	1/4 cup
Potatoes, white; baked or boiled	1 (2" diam.)
Potatoes, white, mashed	1/2 cup
Pumpkin	3/4 cup
Squash, winter (acorn or butternut)	1/2 cup
Wheat germ	1/4 cup

Meat Exchanges

Each portion equals one meat exchange and contains about 1/4 oz of protein and 1/6 oz of fat for about 73 calories.

Meat	Measure
Cheese, cheddar, American, or Swiss	1 oz slice 3-1/2" square, 1/8" thick
Cottage cheese	1/4 cup
Egg	1
Halibut, perch, sole, and similar fish	1 oz slice
Oysters, clams, shrimp, scallops	5 small
Salmon, tuna, crab	1/4 cup
Sardines	3 medium

Meat	Measure
Beef, lamb, pork, veal, ham, liver, chicken, duck, etc.	1 oz slice (4" × 2" × 1/4")
Cold cuts	1-1/2 oz slice (4-1/2" square 1/8" thick)
Vienna sausages	2
Weiner (hot dog), limit to not over 1 exchange per day	1 (10 per lb)
Peanut butter (omit 2 fat exchanges from the day)	2 tbsp

Fat Exchanges

Each portion equals one fat exchange and contains about 1/6 oz of fat for about 45 calories. Liquid fats (at room temperature) of vegetable origin tend to be unsaturated, while animal fats are all saturated and much more likely to clog up your arteries.

Fat	Measure
Avocados	1/8 (4" diameter)
Bacon, crisp	1 slice
Butter or margarine	1 tsp
Corn oil (an unsaturated fat)	1 tsp
Safflower oil (an unsaturated fat)	1 tsp
Cream, half-and-half (saturated fat)	3 tbsp
Heavy cream, 40%	1 tbsp
Light cream, 20%	2 tbsp
Sour cream	2 tbsp
Cream cheese	1 tbsp

Fat	Measure
French or Western dressing	1 tbsp
Blue Cheese (Roquefort) dressing	2 tsp
Italian dressing	1 tbsp
Mayonnaise	1 tsp
Mayonnaise-similar (e.g., Miracle Whip)	2 tsp
Low fat mayonnaise-similar	3 tsp
Nuts	6 small
Oil or cooking fat	1 tsp
Olives	5 small

Common Snacks and Other Foods

Snack	Exchanges	Amount
Fish sticks, frozen	2 meat, 1 bread	3 sticks
Fruit-flavored Jell-O	1 bread	1/4 cup
Ginger ale	1 bread	7 oz
Ice cream	1 bread, 2 fat	1/2 cup
Low-calorie French or Italian dressing	nil if only 1 tbsp	1 tbsp
Potato or corn chips	1 bread, 2 fat	10 large or 15 small
Sherbet	2 bread	1/2 cup
Vanilla wafers	1 bread	6
Waffle, frozen	1 bread, 1 fat	1 (5 1/2" diam)

Items That Do Not Need to Be Measured

Seasonings: Cinnamon, celery salt, garlic, garlic salt, lemon, mustard, mint, nutmeg, parsley, pepper, aspartame, saccharin and other sugarless sweeteners, spices, vanilla, and vinegar.

Other foods and beverages: Coffee or tea (without cream or sugar), fat-free broth, bouillon, unflavored gelatin, sour or dill pickles, cranberries (without sugar), rhubarb (without sugar).

In the chapter on **High Cholesterol** these fat exchanges are broken down into the so-called good fats (polyunsaturated) and bad fats (saturated). Mostly the thing to remember is that all animal fats are saturated, and most vegetable fats are unsaturated to at least some degree. There are further breakdowns into Omega 3 and Omega 6 fats for those of you with one of the more rare blood fat disorders.

GUARANTEED WEIGHT LOSS DIETS

I am repeating the instructions for each diet so that you can choose the one you want, tear out the page, and paste it on your refrigerator door for instant reference. For a sample diet illustrating just how to plug in the "exchanges," just refer to the one given above for the 800 calorie diet.

All diets that allow less than 1200 calories per day are deficient in one or more vital minerals and vitamins. <u>Therefore it is absolutely necessary for you to take a single multiple vitamin and mineral tablet every day</u>. There are several reliable ones on the market, plus a lot that may be somewhat questionable. I feel comfortable with Walgreen's A thru Z, $15.99 for 365 of them, one daily. That is probably the best value for your money. Centrum with minerals, Myadec, Theragran with minerals, Micebrin and Micebrin T are all made by reliable companies but are more expensive. All of these are just one large tablet daily. You don't have to spend a lot of money for these supplements. All come from natural sources. Realistically our bodies don't care where the required compounds come from, just that the proper chemical formulas are present.

800 calorie diet for weight loss

Carbohydrate: 2-1/2 oz (75 grams)
Protein: 2 oz (55 grams)
Fat: 1 oz (30 grams)

800 calorie daily menu allowances
Breakfast
1 fruit exchange (list 3)
1 bread exchange (list 4)
1 meat exchange (list 5)
1 fat exchange (list 6)
1/2 milk exchange (list 1)
*Coffee or tea (one cup only)
Lunch
2 meat exchanges (list 5)

1 vegetable exchange (list 2)
Vegetables as desired (list 2*)
1 fruit exchange (list 3)
1/2 milk exchange (list 1)
*Coffee or tea (one cup only)
Dinner
2 meat exchanges (list 5)
1 vegetable exchange (list 2)
Vegetables as desired (list 2*)
1 fruit exchange (list 3)
1/2 milk exchange (list 1)
*Decaf coffee or tea (up to two cups only)

*Do not drink more than three cups of any caffeine-containing beverage in any 24 hour period. The caffeine (besides other potentially ill effects that we will talk about elsewhere) causes the production of excess stomach acid, which makes you more hungry. So it is best to drink them only on a full stomach and limit the quantities. Alcohol does the same thing, but is an absolute no-no when you are trying to lose weight because of the empty calories in each drink.

1000 calorie diet

Carbohydrate: 3 oz (90 grams)
Protein: 2 oz (60 grams)
Fat: 1-1/2 oz (45 grams)
The single day sample menus below are given to illustrate correct use of the exchange lists.

Your weekly menus should be planned on the basis of the daily menu guide.

All diets that allow less than 1200 calories per day are deficient in one or more vital minerals and vitamins, as noted above. Be sure to include a daily multiple vitamin and mineral supplement as discussed under the 800 calorie diet above. The additions from the 800 calorie diet above are underlined.

Breakfast
1 fruit exchange (list 3)
1 bread exchange (list 4)
1 meat exchange (list 5)
1 fat exchange (list 6)
1/2 milk exchange (list 1)
*Coffee or tea (one cup only)
Lunch
2 meat exchanges (list 5)

1 1/2 vegetable exchange (list 2)
Vegetables as desired (list 2*)
1 fruit exchange (list 3)
1/2 milk exchange (list 1)
*Coffee or tea (one cup only)
Dinner
2 meat exchanges (list 5)
1/2 bread exchange list 4)
1 vegetable exchange (list 2)
Vegetables as desired (list 2*)
1 fruit exchange (list 3)
1/2 fat exchange (list 6)
1/2 milk exchange (list 1)
*Decaf coffee or tea (up to two cups only)

*Do not drink more than two cups of any caffeine-containing beverage in any 24 hour period. The caffeine (besides other potentially ill effects that we will talk about elsewhere) causes the production of excess stomach acid, which makes you more hungry. So it is best to drink them only on a full stomach and limit the quantities. Alcohol does the same thing, but is an absolute no-no when you are trying to lose weight because of the empty calories in each drink.

Bedtime snack (These can be added to one of the other meals, preferably breakfast or lunch, if no bedtime snack is desired.)
1/2 bread exchange (list 4)
1/2 milk exchange (list 1)

1200 calorie diet

Carbohydrate: 4 oz (120 grams)
Protein: 2 oz (60 grams)
Fat: 1-1/2 oz (45 grams)
All diets that allow less than 1200 calories per day are deficient in one or more vital minerals and vitamins. Theoretically this diet should have enough of all, but I recommend taking one of the supplements every day anyway, because I believe that the nationally-recommended minimum daily requirements are insufficient for vibrant good health. We discuss this issue a little more elsewhere under Staying Well.

Breakfast (additions from the 1000 calorie diet are underlined)
2 fruit exchange (list 3)
1 bread exchange (list 4)
1 meat exchange (list 5)

1 fat exchange (list 6)
<u>1</u> milk exchange (list 1)
*Coffee or tea (one cup only)
Lunch
2 meat exchanges (list 5)
<u>2</u> bread exchanges (list4)
1 vegetable exchange (list 2)
Vegetables as desired (list 2*)
1 fruit exchange (list 3)
1/2 milk exchange (list 1)
*Coffee or tea (one cup only)
Dinner
2 meat exchanges (list 5)
<u>1 bread exchange </u>(list 4)
1 vegetable exchange (list 2)
Vegetables as desired (list 2*)
1 fruit exchange (list 3)
1/2 milk exchange (list 1)
*Decaf coffee or tea (up to two cups only)

*Do not drink more than two cups of any caffeine-containing beverage in any 24 hour period. The caffeine (besides other potentially ill effects that we will talk about elsewhere) causes the production of excess stomach acid, which makes you more hungry. So it is best to drink them only on a full stomach and limit the quantities. Alcohol does the same thing, but is an absolute no-no when you are trying to lose weight because of the empty calories in each drink.

Bedtime snack (These can be added to one of the other meals, preferably breakfast or lunch, if no bedtime snack is desired.):
1/2 bread exchange (list 4)
1/2 milk exchange (list 1)

1500 calorie diet

Carbohydrate: 5 oz (150 grams)
Protein: 2-1/3 oz (70 grams)
Fat: 2-1/3 oz (70 grams)
All diets that allow less than 1200 calories per day are deficient in one or more vital minerals and vitamins. Theoretically this diet should have enough of all, but I recommend taking one of the supplements every day anyway, because I believe that the nationally-recommended minimum daily requirements are insufficient for vibrant good health. We discuss this issue a little more elsewhere under **Staying Well.**

Breakfast
1 fruit exchange (list 3)
<u>2</u> bread exchange (list 4)
1 meat exchange (list 5)
2 fat exchange (list 6)
1 milk exchange (list 1)
*Coffee or tea (one cup only)
Lunch
2 meat exchanges (list 5)
1 vegetable exchange (list 2)
Vegetables as desired (list 2*)
1 fruit exchange (list 3)
<u>1</u> milk exchange (list 1)
<u>1 fat exchange</u> (list 6)
*Coffee or tea (one cup only)
Dinner
2 meat exchanges (list 5)
1 vegetable exchange (list 2)
<u>1 bread exchange</u> (list 4)
Vegetables as desired (list 2*)
1 fruit exchange (list 3)
<u>1 fat exchange</u> (list 6)
<u>1</u> milk exchange (list 1)
*Decaf coffee or tea (up to two cups only)

*Do not drink more than two cups of any caffeine-containing beverage in any 24 hour period. The caffeine (besides other potentially ill effects that we will talk about elsewhere) causes the production of excess stomach acid, which makes you more hungry. So it is best to drink them only on a full stomach and limit the quantities. Alcohol does the same thing, but is an absolute no-no when you are trying to lose weight because of the empty calories in each drink.

Bedtime snack (These can be added to one of the other meals, preferably breakfast or lunch, if no bedtime snack is desired.)
1/2 bread exchange (list 4)
1/2 milk exchange (list 1)
Good luck with your weight loss. Happy eating to live, not living to eat!

CHAPTER 68 -- MASTURBATION

When I was in the seventh grade, there was a convocation in our high school gym about masturbation. Someone from a church or the YMCA (an organization I dearly love -- in fact I helped start one in Warsaw, Indiana) or perhaps a former ballplayer, came and spoke to all the boys in our small school about the *evils* of masturbation.

I had read *a lot* of books by that time, but had never seen the word and had no idea what the man was talking about. The fact that I had just skipped the sixth grade and thus was the youngest boy in my new class may have had something to do with my ignorance. Certainly my secondary physical sexual characteristics were less developed than my new male classmates, and my voice hadn't begun to change.

Finally, with considerable frustration about fifteen minutes into the talk, I finally asked one of my best friends, who was a year older, what on earth the man was talking about. He said, "you know, jacking off," and he made a motion with his hands. Actually, I had heard "jacking off" but didn't know what that was either. (I was a naïve little kid!) But I kind of got the idea.

The man said it was bad for your brain and interfered with studies. It could mess up an athlete's coordination, was bad for the wind (I already *knew* that cigarettes were bad for your wind), caused cavities, and was forbidden by the Bible. Plus a lot of other stuff that I thankfully immediately forgot.

I had no idea why the Bible said it was forbidden. My grandfather was a minister and my mother a Sunday school teacher; so I had considerable acquaintance with the bible, but couldn't recall a section about masturbation. I still can't, and I have no idea to this day why in the world the school officials would subject a bunch of young boys to such a collection of myths about their sexual urges.

The man made no mention of avoiding premarital sexual intercourse, unmarried teenage pregnancy, and sexually transmitted diseases (known in those days as VD, rather than the STDs of today.) These situations can be greatly diminished by masturbation,

338

and it would have made a lot more sense to talk about them. I gave just such a series of talks to high school kids of both sexes about four years into my medical practice.

But that man's lecture had a strong effect on me for several years, until I was far enough along in medical school to know what really happens in masturbation. And every time I masturbated, I felt guilty for a long time.

Wet dreams are certainly reduced in frequency by masturbation, as are daydreams about naked girls for most guys. Boys and men have an organ that is pretty prominent, especially at sometimes awkward times. So they are often quicker to experiment with that organ than girls, whose clitoris is partially covered at the very front of their genital area.

In women some have told me that water is their best friend if they are not in a stable relationship at a particular time. For all women before becoming sexually involved with another person, it is a good idea to become acquainted with your anatomy while lying in a tub of warm water. Perhaps use a mirror to look more closely. This is not a big dark secret. It is you, for all of your life. You need to know about yourself, if for no other reason than just keeping clean.

Then gently feel around and learn where the opening to the vagina is. The hymen is the rim of tissue on the back part of the vagina. It usually is pretty tight at first if you haven't been using a tampon during your period. Insert your finger into the opening and see how far in it goes, probably a lot farther than you expected. You can push back against the hymen firmly, and by doing that repeatedly for several weeks, you can stretch it enough that it may not be uncomfortable when you first make love.

Feel where the urine comes out just in front of the vaginal opening. Just inside the opening is often found one of the sexual "hot spots" for women's sexual pleasure during foreplay and intercourse. The other "hot spot" is right at the front of your genital area, a little pea-like spot that sticks out a little from under the overlying hood of the lips. When you are sexually excited, it swells just as the penis in a man does (only not quite so much, of course). Stimulating either or both of these "hot spots" while lubricated with warm water will rouse all but the most dormant sexual feelings. If you don't have a tub, or it isn't convenient, use warm K-Y jelly.

Guys can use K-Y jelly also, and probably should if they have been circumcised. Olive oil, mineral oil, or baby oil work just as well.

Both sexes can rent X-rated pornographic videos and masturbate to your heart's content throughout the movie. There are all kinds of X-rated stuff that you don't want your kids getting into on the Internet. You can fantasize about all manner of private thoughts while masturbating.

There are sex shops in most big cities that sell all manner of sexually stimulating equipment, for personal or mutual use. Vibrators are always a hot item.

In the case of severe injury or illness to your partner, masturbation while gently holding or caressing each other will still allow loving activities and expressions of sexuality. Sexuality does not require intercourse to be loving interplay between lovers.

Masturbation does not lead to mental illness or blindness, and there is considerable doubt about whether it really does impair athletic performance the next day, as most coaches might tell you.

One recent small study suggests that ejaculation more than five times a week by men in their twenties resulted in one-third less cancer of the prostate in those men later in life. I'm not at all sure that ejaculation in your twenties will have any possible effect upon you 30 or 40 years later. But I do believe that continuing to ejaculate later in life may well help to keep the tissues of the prostate healthier. Perhaps it may flush out pre-cancer cells, just as continuing to have periods on hormone replacement therapy after menopause in women causes cancer cells to be shed so that cancer of the uterus cannot occur.

In addition, I believe that continuing to ejaculate may help slow down the development of benign prostatic hypertrophy (BPH).

I have heard it said that one meets a better class of person when masturbating than one can meet in a bar. Certainly safer. Don't go trolling at a bar just because you are horny. Don't be afraid to get acquainted with yourself.

CHAPTER 69 -- MAXIMIZING YOUR DOCTOR'S OFFICE VISIT

Except in life-threatening "911" conditions go to your family doctor whenever possible. He or she will be able to treat most conditions. He or she will know you and what you may be having trouble with instantly sometimes. And you will not have to pay a specialist two or three times as much for the same care.

Most physicians are often pressed for time. From a lot of personal experience I will tell you that the most carefully-constructed schedule can and will go awry unless everybody sticks to the one condition that they originally made the appointment for, and no emergencies occur. A laceration repair or a person with acute chest pain that could be a heart attack, or baby Huey with RSV, or little Susie with a bad asthmatic attack, all must go to someone else besides your doctor on that day if all is to go well for your own visit. When you make an appointment, it is very important for you to tell the person on the phone <u>everything</u> you want addressed that day. It is possible that they will squeeze you in for an acute illness only on that day; but if that happens you must be fair and not try to make the doctor also try to deal with your blood pressure, pap smear, or whatever, to save you the co-pay for another visit later in the month.

It is important, however, for you to be aware that you have every right to talk at least briefly about your condition face-to-face with your doctor after your pap smear or whatever is over and you are fully covered again with gown or clothing.

> *One of my elderly patients just a week before I'm writing this came in to our urgent care clinic with bruises all over her. She was taking an anticoagulant to prevent stroke that might be caused by her heart problem. Her prothrombin time was over 90! (normal therapeutic range for her condition is about 20 to 25!) She had listed both Warfarin and Coumadin among her medications. She said that she had been getting her prothrombin time done faithfully every week or two for the past three years, and she always was in the right range.*
>
> *I asked her daughter to go home and get her medicines. When she returned, I found that there was a bottle of Coumadin (the brand name for warfarin), along with a bottle, dated just two weeks previously, of "Warfarin." She was taking both of them and quickly poisoning herself with a double dose of anticoagulant!*
>
> *What had happened was that she had switched HMOs and thus had a new doctor. The new doctor had a copy of her records, lab tests, medications and all. But he wrote a prescription for the anticoagulant as "Warfarin" to satisfy her HMO's requirements for use of all generic drugs. Since she was on a different HMO, that also meant that she had to go to a different drugstore. So the new pharmacy had no record of previous prescriptions to compare for possible drug interactions -- or possible duplication of prescriptions. No one knew she still had a large supply of Coumadin and was faithfully continuing to take it in the same dose she had for the past two or three years.*
>
> *This lady was lucky. All she had was a lot of black and blue spots all over her body. An all-too-frequent result of massive anticoagulant overdose such as hers is a massive hemorrhagic stroke and death.*

Try to schedule your doctor's appointment as early in the morning as possible, because he or she will be less likely to have had to deal with emergencies throwing him or her behind schedule early on. Of course if your doctor has patients in the hospital or does surgery, anything can happen there. But at least the chances are better that you won't have to spend the whole morning in the office.

Included below in future editions will be a patient medical history, which you should copy and take with you to give to your doctor at the first visit. Many offices have you fill one out in the waiting room before you see the doctor, but filling one out <u>before</u> you go will let you ask members of your family for anything you might have forgotten. Also you may think of something else overnight that might be important. There may be something in your family tree that can predict what you may be facing in the future.

Many of us are using herbs and dietary supplements, some for somewhat obscure reasons (see the chapter on **Herbs and Dietary Supplements.**) Your doctor needs to know exactly what you are taking. This is especially important if you are possibly going to need surgery because some herbs can cause severe bleeding disorders. One of the problems with some of these is that often three or four herbs are combined into one pill with a name unrelated to the contents.

Bring <u>all</u> of the medications, herbs, and supplements you are or have been taking to the doctor's office with you for each visit. He may not ask for them each time, but if you have them, it could save your life.

So take all of your prescription medicines, diet supplements, and herbal remedies in a sack with you for each doctor's visit. Also it's a good idea to have a list of everything you are currently taking in your purse or wallet for quick reference in an emergency.

We physicians often have to be medical detectives in order to diagnose diseases that aren't straightforward. There are often as many as three or four conditions in our differential diagnosis with similar signs and symptoms. Any help you can give with an accurate description of your symptoms, as well as accurate and complete past, family and social histories can make a huge difference in your physician's ability to successfully diagnose and treat you. For example, if you have discomfort or pain, try to write down how it feels, what makes it worse, and what relieves it.

In a real life detective story, I had a lady patient several years ago who was born in India but moved to our country 20 or more years previously. She came to me complaining of intermittent spells of muscular pains, headaches, and spiking fevers of about two weeks' duration. This visit occurred during flu season, and I had seen several flu cases that day. Her story could have been consistent with a slightly unusual flu illness. But she didn't have much in the way of respiratory findings, and looked sicker than most flu victims her age (early 40s). So I asked if she had ever had a similar illness. "No"; had she been exposed to anyone with a similar illness? "No"; had she been traveling recently? "No". I went on, receiving no helpful replies. (continued on page 344)

> *Finally, as I was about to do a culture for flu, her companion reminded her that she had been back to India for 30 days and returned here three months ago. I asked her what part of India? "Northern"; did you see any mosquitoes? "No". Do people in northern India ever get malaria? "No". So much for the possibilities in the differential diagnosis.*
>
> *But I decided to get a malaria smear anyway because I knew we had a lab technician who was particularly good at reading exotic blood slides, and I just had a hunch. Bingo! Sure enough it was malaria. After two weeks on anti-malarial medicine, the fever was gone and she was well on the road to recovery. But without her companion's revelation the proper treatment might have waited too long.*

Malaria still has a high mortality rate in the third world where there are mosquitoes. As with other illnesses, unfortunately, the infective organism is developing resistance to the drugs that used to work. The only truly successful methods of prevention are the elimination of the stagnant pools of water where mosquitoes breed and staying indoors with small mesh screens during the hours from sunset to dawn.

Mosquito control is becoming increasingly important even here in the U. S. as our continent warms in part of the general warming. Mosquitoes are causing encephalitis in many areas of our country right now (West Nile Fever is getting the most publicity currently, and will soon be in every state.) Washington, D.C. was once a hotbed of yellow fever, along with New Orleans and most of the Deep South.

For each doctor's visit write down any questions you want answered or problems you want addressed before you get to the office. Then you can either read them yourself or give them to your doctor to glance through to facilitate getting the answers.

If you may be having a stressful procedure, or some possibly bad news at your doctor's office, take someone with you for comfort. That person may also be able to listen more objectively, as well as ask questions you might not think of.

When you need to talk to your doctor, sometimes you can have your questions relayed through the back office nurse or medical assistant. Sometimes that isn't adequate, and you must tell the back office person so. In some offices the person answering the phone can and will relay your request to the doctor. But in a large office that isn't going to happen. After a time or two you will know what it takes to get through to your doctor.

In general, I would always get the name of the back office person or persons when you first go to that office. Sometimes she will have on a nametag, and sometimes you will have to write her name down as she spells it for you. She will forever after be your ally in communications with your doctor. So ask to speak to her or her associate whenever you have to call the office for anything except an appointment.

And even for appointments, if you can't get one as soon as you think you need it, ask to talk to the nurse to explain the problem before giving up. She has the authority to go directly to the doctor to see if you can be squeezed into a busy schedule.

CHAPTER 70 -- MEDICAL ERRORS

Prevention of medical errors starts with you, the patient. Most medical errors can be prevented. Elsewhere in this book are suggestions for prevention in various areas. I may repeat some of those here just to be sure you remember them.

Quite a few of the malpractice cases that I review for both defendant insurance companies and plaintiff's attorneys would never have occurred if the patient had followed these suggestions.

First and perhaps most important is a thorough and accurate history of illnesses, medications to which you are truly allergic along with those which may have made you a little sick in one way or another, and any prescription, over-the-counter, and herbal medications which you are currently taking or have taken in the recent past. Bring all of your medications with you at your first visit to a new doctor. If you are elderly or taking a lot of medicines, bring them all to each visit.

Whenever the course of an illness, condition, post-operative surgery case or whatever, does not seem to be going as well as expected, you need to talk personally to your doctor, or to whomever is taking calls for him (or her). Even at three o'clock in the morning, if necessary.

Whenever you have <u>any</u> thought that something isn't as it should be for you or your family's health, call your doctor, or call 911, or go to the ER.

Most (but unfortunately not all) doctors *want* you to call at any hour, day or night if something looks like it is going wrong. Particularly a sudden change.

That said, please remember to use common sense, as pointed out in the chapter on **Sick Children**. Call early in the evening, or before the doctor's office closes if possible. Don't count on the office closing at a certain time -- if they get through with scheduled patients early for a change, they go home in most private practices.

In the case of surgery, be there when the surgical nurse discharges your spouse or other family member. Ask what symptoms to expect and how to deal with them. Ask what symptoms could be dangerous. Ask who will be on call in case you need to seek advice

346

and how to get hold of that doctor. Do not settle for talking to a Physician's Assistant, medical assistant, nurse or receptionist.

If you are having a problem during the day, and you get the runaround from office personnel, just get a ride from somebody and go directly to the office and wait there. I guarantee that they will fit you in!

Medication Errors

Medication Errors are high on the list of things that can go wrong.

When your doctor writes a prescription, make sure that you can read it. Even though you may not fully understand the words, be sure you fully understand what it is for. Be sure you know when and how to take it and that you are told and understand what possible side effects the medicine may cause.

When you receive your medication from the pharmacist, ask him to double check to confirm that it is the medicine and the dosage that your doctor prescribed.

(A word must be said here about generic drugs. They are very important in the lives of many of us because their cost is often less than half of that of a brand-name drug. However one must

One case as an illustration was a patient of mine whom I hadn't seen for awhile. On a Friday night he began to have, for the first time, chest pressure, which felt like someone was sitting on his chest, according to his daughter. He decided not to call his doctor but to wait until Monday and go into the office then.

Unfortunately, on Sunday morning his wife found him dead in bed. The autopsy showed that he died of a massive heart attack.

Even in this day and age, with all the very high tech capabilities we have for dealing with heart attacks, we might not have saved him for a few more years if he had called 911, or me, or gone directly to the hospital Emergency Room on Friday night. But we would have at least had a chance. If my patient wouldn't call me or the doctor on call for me, or 911, then his wife had some responsibility to take matters into her own hands and call herself.

be careful what drug company is making that generic drug. There are probably 100 or more companies making those medicines, but I really trust not more than 8 or 10 to have what they say they have in the tablet, and in the right strength. This is particularly important for drugs made in some foreign countries. Ask your druggist who makes the generic drugs that he is going to give you. Often it is a company that is a subsidiary of the brand name maker, such as Geneva. In a case like that you can feel pretty secure.)

Another case was a friend of mine who had had surgery by another physician whom I assisted. The surgeon caring for him was a very competent and caring man who always told his patients to call him at home if necessary. He sent my friend home to a nearby town only about thirty miles away. Once again it was a weekend. My friend got what was at first a mild nausea, which progressed to vomiting in a few hours. He continued to vomit for most of the weekend, but his wife never called his surgeon or me for advice or assistance. To make a long story short, he popped some internal stitches and had to be re-operated on Monday. His wife, for whatever reason, directly caused him to have to have that second operation, with its attendant risks and prolonged recovery. All she had to do was pick up the phone.

(My handwriting has been pretty legible ever since I got a D in penmanship in the eighth grade. I had a pretty good report card except for that, the only D I ever got. I was so embarrassed that I went home and practiced every day all summer. Ever since then my handwriting has been a whole lot better, unlike some doctors'.)

If a particular brand of a medicine is working well for you, question the druggist closely if a different-appearing tablet or capsule is in your bottle when you pick up your latest prescription. It is possible that you and your physician were talking about other things, and he didn't explain that there would be a change in medication.

In addition, since pharmacists are human, be sure you are getting the same drug every time your prescription is filled. I've had several occasions when my patient didn't get what I ordered. I have also had a lot of occasions when a pharmacist called me before filling a prescription I had written where something was obscure to him or her regarding the dose or what the prescription was to be used for. Sometimes the dose size was not entered. Or maybe my writing was less than legible.

Also on several occasions the pharmacist has picked up another drug from the list that was entered in the computer for that patient, prescribed by another doctor, that might cause a bad drug interaction.

The relationship between a physician and the pharmacists in town is a very important healthcare partnership, and a doctor does well to nurture it.

I remember one time that I had prescribed a drug that the patient was allergic to. The pharmacist, bless his heart, caught it. What had happened was that the patient had gone to another doctor for the previous illness, had had an allergic reaction for the first time with it, but had forgotten to tell me about it upon his return to my care. And since I had a clear list of the patient's drug allergies red-flagged on the front of the chart (and was probably in too much of a hurry that day), I didn't ask again about any known allergies to drugs. Thank goodness nothing happened. The pharmacist asked and my patient told her that she had this new allergy. She then called me, I just ordered a different medication, and the patient got well without further ado.

There is much to be said for always using the same druggist or pharmacy chain because they will have you in their computer for everything you are taking. Having made that statement, I will also hasten to add that you should call around to several drug stores for prices before getting an expensive prescription filled. I used to do this for some of my patients periodically and was amazed at the difference in prices for just brand name drugs.

And just because Pharmacy X has a lower price on Drug A than Pharmacy Y, does not mean that it has the lowest price on Drug B. You need to check on each really expensive drug with several sources. Check the Internet and AARP, too.

When generic drugs are factored into the mix, there is an even greater diversity. Also there is the issue of generic drugs in general.

Digoxin is an excellent case in point. Probably twenty or more years ago the FDA decided to test digoxin from each of the 16 or 18 drug companies that were producing what they claimed to be the 0.25 mg tablet. The results of that series of tests were a veritable horror story of the potential risks of generic drugs.

First, the tablets of only two companies, Burroughs Welcome (maker of Lanoxin) and Eli Lilly had the drug they said they had in the dose they said was in the pill. All but two of the other companies did have digoxin in their pills, but the doses varied from as little as 0.05 mg (which meant that the patients were receiving no benefit at all for the money spent for the medicine) to as much as 0.50 mg (meaning that over a period of time those patients were being poisoned! I have no doubt that many deaths resulted from that too high dose.) A few of the companies had a wide variation of the medication from tablet to tablet, so the results were totally unpredictable. Two companies actually had totally unidentifiable chemicals in their tablets!

As a result of those tests the FDA shut down the digoxin manufacturing of most of those generic companies. And the VA hospitals and HMOs, which always require their doctors to prescribe generic drugs if any are available, began to allow all doctors to always prescribe either Lanoxin or the Lilly brand. The FDA is so underfunded that it scares me to think what other horror stories there may be out there. I know that certain epileptic drugs fall into the same category with the VA and HMOs. There are now probably others that I haven't heard about.

Diagnostic Errors Are Very Close to Medication Errors in Frequency

One would think they would be higher on the list than they are.

Let me tell you how we physicians make our diagnoses. It's not all just our great skill and dexterity, as one of my colleagues used to joke.

When I was in medical school, we were told that there are three parts to making a correct diagnosis. First is the patient's history, which is worth 50% of the diagnostic process. Second is the physical examination by the doctor, which is worth 40% of the process. Third and last are the lab work and all the tests that may be ordered and completed, which are worth only 10% of the diagnostic process.

Even in this day and age, those percentages still are pretty close, I think. Obviously, there are cases where a diagnosis can't be reached until you, the poor (but lucky) patient has been to two or three large medical centers and had every test known to man before the life-saving diagnosis of Tsutsugamushi Fever is made, the proper medication is given, and you get well.

For every case like that there are literally hundreds where the doctor knows the diagnosis and how he is going to treat it by the time you finish your history. Hopefully he will do at least a focused physical exam to confirm what he thinks. But he knows, and he needs no lab tests at all. I'm sure I see a dozen patients a day who have that straightforward a diagnosis.

The very real fear of a lawsuit has driven up the cost of Medicine (not just drugs) to the consumer enormously. The lawyers are big on tests. If one isn't ordered that he or she or their hired consultants think might have shed some light on a tough situation, then the doctor may wind up in court, whether he deserves it or not. So we frequently order extra tests for straightforward conditions that weren't really needed just to cover our rear in the event of something going wrong.

Your History

Here is where you can really help your doctor in determining what is wrong with you. You can do that because you can access so many medical places on the Internet. Admittedly a lot of them have inaccurate information because they are not written by doctors or have been mis-transcribed by a stenographer from a doctor's dictation. But many are manned by prestigious medical schools and clinics and updated all the time. So you may have a good idea what may be wrong with you before you even go to the doctor.

Again, I can't stress how important your personally filled out and complete history is when you make your doctor's office visit.

When you have an emergency situation, it is easy to forget important parts of your past history, including even allergies to drugs from years ago that you have almost forgotten about. So it is a really good idea to keep a medical history in your files at home and update it every time you go to the doctor. Then just take a copy with you when you go on a trip, or go to the doctor or Emergency Room. They can make a copy of your original for their records.

Testing

(see also the chapter on **Lab Tests**)

Medicare virtually destroyed one of the best tools we had developed in the last twenty years. That was the blood profile. We used to be able to order a 35-test computerized lab panel for every complete physical exam and for every case where the diagnosis was not pretty clear. It was cheap, costing the patient less than $3.00 per test, where doing each test separately cost $5 to $35 each. Medicare, in their "wisdom" determined that they would not pay for any tests that were not accompanied by an actual diagnosis.

My Dad, when he had rabbit fever, knew that's what he had because he had seen the rabbit's diseased liver (and showed it to me -- that's another story we'll go into elsewhere in this book). He told his doctor and finally the Chief of Medicine at Indiana University Medical Center, and it probably saved his life because he had a rare form of the disease that was hard to recognize.

They wouldn't accept "possible" thyroid disease or "possible" anything else. Once the diagnosis was actually made, then they would cover the tests. But they wouldn't cover the computerized bundle of tests even though they might be cheaper as a bundle than as individual tests.

Medicare's attitude soon spilled over into the private insurance and HMO sectors. This put a big crimp in our ability to throw a bunch of tests at you and come up with a previously unsuspected diagnosis. The package deal, however, makes a lot of sense for those with unlimited funds. Right now in Phoenix, and at least several other big cities, there is a radiology group offering the general public full body scanning with all the latest high-tech stuff, for $1,500. No insurance will cover these, of course, first and most importantly because they aren't ordered by a doctor.

So the big panels are not used as much now. In order that your insurance, if any, will cover you, we just order what we think will confirm what we suspect you have. No exotic, out of the blue possibilities now.

If you have a test, be sure to call or go to the office and get the results. Your doctor probably has it set up so that he has to review and sign every lab and X-ray and consultation report that he receives. He probably also has it set up so that one of his assistants checks a report book daily and makes a phone call to the lab or wherever to see what is happening if a report hasn't arrived in a timely manner. Nevertheless when there are a few busy days in a row, as with a flu epidemic, or when a key person is out sick for a few days, things inevitably fall through the cracks. So find out about your test. No news is not necessarily good news.

Having Hospital Tests and Surgery

If you have to go into the hospital for surgery or some kind of a procedure, and if you have a choice, try to choose a hospital where a lot of those kinds of surgeries or procedures are done. The more familiar the hospital team is with what you are having done to you, the more likely all will go smoothly and turn out well.

> When I was an intern in South Bend, Indiana, we had a patient who had been operated on at another hospital for a tuberculous kidney. The only problem was that the surgeon took out the wrong kidney! We didn't have kidney transplants in those days, and of course the patient soon died. That is a situation that I have heard of, though with possibly different organs, several times in the years since. _So make darned sure that the area to be operated on is marked on your body to your satisfaction before anybody gives you any medicine to start putting you to sleep._

If you are having surgery, be sure your health care team agrees exactly on what needs to be and what will be done to exactly which part of your body. Always have your surgeon mark with indelible pen the site to be operated on before you ever are given any pre-operative medication. I can't _tell_ you how important that can be for you.

When you are discharged from the hospital, your doctor may be very busy. It is often said that the time actually spent with a patient in the hospital by a doctor may be measured in seconds rather than minutes. And the time spent treating the patient's chart exceeds the time spent face to face with the patients by a factor of ten -- or twenty.

I think this may not be quite accurate most of the time, but it has happened to me, both as a doctor and as a patient. So be prepared with questions as your time of discharge approaches.

Most of us have a set procedure, which we carefully follow when discharging a patient after surgery or illness. That procedure includes all the items below. BUT one of these areas might not be covered for some reason:

(1) Ask your doctor to thoroughly explain the treatment plan you will use at home, (2) review your medications, (3) be sure you have the proper prescriptions, and (4) tell you when to arrange a follow-up visit. (5) Ask him what he expects in the course of your condition. (6) Ask him what ill effects to especially watch for. (7) Ask him how to reach him or a covering doctor if things aren't going as expected. (8) Get the phone number.

Don't feel badly for making him spend so much time with you at the time of discharge. All insurance companies now allow an extra fee for the day of discharge treatment. And we _all_ want to get _everything_ right. But sometimes we need a little help from you to jog our memories, because our minds may still be on the last poor patient we saw before you, who isn't going to leave the hospital alive, or something similar.

When the nurse (I hope you will have a nurse -- they are few and far between nowadays), actually discharges you, she (or he) will bring you any prescriptions that your doctor may have written after he or she left you, perhaps some discharge medications from the hospital pharmacy to tide you over until you can have your prescriptions filled, perhaps some dressing materials for your home use in a surgical case, and instructions, often in writing, about your condition and aftercare. A lot of this will duplicate what your doctor has told you. *If there are conflicts, don't leave the hospital, no matter how much of a hurry you are in until those conflicts are actually resolved by the nurse contacting your doctor.

Speak up if you have questions or concerns that haven't been answered. It is not unusual for a person to think of something to ask after his or her doctor has left. Don't be afraid or shy about seeking more information from reliable sources.

Remember, you and your health team are just that -- a team. And what makes a team successful is coordination, cooperation, and a good understanding of what is going to happen. On a football team every player knows the plays. The quarterback may call the signals, but you are actually calling the plays yourself, after considering all the angles. Be sure you know the playbook by asking whatever questions you need for complete understanding. Only then should you tell the quarterback (your doctor) what play to proceed with.

CHAPTER 71 -- AIRPLANE TRAVEL TIPS

1) Wear earplugs in airplanes. 90 decibels of noise will cause hearing damage in the higher pitches if prolonged for very long. Most small planes have a noise level of more than 90 decibels.

Large airliners' noise levels vary from about 60 decibels to 85 decibels in some older models behind the engines. Noise exposure to 80 decibels for eight hours or more can produce demonstrable hearing loss; so people who fly a lot need ear protection. Besides the hearing factor, noise causes fatigue and headaches, and raises blood pressure a few points. Before I personally started wearing earplugs, I always used to notice a mild headache on arrival. No more.

2) Fluids such as water or juice should be consumed in as large quantities as possible. The air in planes is very dry and this contributes to insensible loss of water from the lungs. Avoid caffeine and minimize alcohol to your lowest comfort level. Both cause the kidneys to overwork and thus accentuate dehydration.

Do not drink water from the tap in an airplane. It is almost certainly contaminated with bad germs. Drink only bottled water or canned or bottled juice.

Actually it is a really good idea to take along your own bottled water, several quarts if you are on an overseas flight.

3) Take along an inflatable neck pillow that fits around three quarters of the neck.

4) Take a dark eyeshade.

5) Have your doctor give you a prescription for Ambien, 10 mg, for long transcontinental and transoceanic flights. Take one when you get on the plane, and awaken six or seven hours later with no lethargy or hangover. (Don't get started taking these very much at home or you will get hooked on them. But there is no such risk for travel, and I highly recommend them. Just don't take them with alcohol.)

6) When you are not sleeping, get up and walk around for a few minutes every hour. Stretching your legs helps the body in general as well as helping to prevent the development of blood clots in the legs.

7) If you are tall, remove the magazines and airsickness bag from the pouch on the back of the seat in front of you. That will net you an additional 1 to 1 1/2 inches of knee room -- a big plus on a long flight.

8) Refuse to allow a fat person in the seat next to you to raise the armrest. If the person insists, call a flight attendant and <u>politely</u> insist on your right to the full seat you have paid for. The attendant may make the arm be put down. You may be moved to another seat. The obese person may be moved to another seat. You may even be upgraded to first class, if they have an empty seat. Do not, under any circumstances, lose your temper or raise your voice.

9) Get an aisle seat when you make your reservation. And if your spouse is along, you might consider reserving aisle seats across from each other.

10) For flights of three hours or more, which is the time for communicable diseases to be dispersed in the air from an ill person to virtually everyone in the airplane, consider wearing a surgical mask to reduce the very real risk of taking an unwanted bug along on your vacation or return home. Another benefit of the mask is that you can dampen it with water to provide a little comforting humidity in your inspired air. For maximum effectiveness (an ill person sitting right next to you) change to a new mask every 30 minutes. For average effectiveness change it every hour.

This can be serious business. A couple of years ago a transcontinental traveler with active tuberculosis was found by health authorities to have infected *18* of his fellow passengers on the six plus hour flight.

11) If you yourself have a bad cold or anything potentially worse, by all means have a heart for your fellow travelers and wear a surgical mask yourself that you change every 30 minutes.

12) If worst comes to worst, if you are seated next to an obviously ill person before the plane takes off, call a flight attendant and <u>politely</u> say that you are very susceptible to illness and urgently request to be assigned to another seat. If you do this, be aware that you will have to take whatever is offered or stay where you are. If the change seems really bad, you could ask if there are any other options, then quickly make up your mind which is least bad. There is no doubt in my mind that you should avoid someone who is coughing or seems otherwise ill at all costs.

13) Try to time your long flights to arrive just before the evening meal. Then you can go right to bed and wake up the next day with very little jet lag. Flying across time zones affects your body in many ways, but the biggest thing is fatigue. The suggestions here will help the fatigue factor enormously, and greatly reduce the time it takes to acclimate your body.

14) That noted medical periodical, *The Wall Street Journal*, in their article "How Safe is Airline Water?" on November 1, 2002, printed the results of their survey of 14 airline flights, in which they took samples of water from the galleys and lavatories of each plane for laboratory analysis by good labs. The flights were a randomized sample all the way from Atlanta to Sydney, Australia. They were looking for possible disease-producing

contamination. And boy did they find it! Their idea to do this was triggered by some poorly publicized studies from Japan and The Netherlands in which E. coli and the Legionnaire's disease germ had been found. Apparently U.S. studies have had "mixed results." The WSJ samples produced "a long list of microscopic life you don't want to drink, from *Salmonella* and *Staphyloccus* to tiny insect eggs. Worse, contamination was the rule, not the exception."

Federal regulations require that the tanks of airplanes are supposed to contain drinkable water. Many, perhaps most, airlines dispense bottled water initially, but on long flights, when they run out of the bottled variety, they turn to the taps.

Lessons to be learned from these tests: When you drink water on an airplane, drink only that which is bottled. Bring your own bottled water, maybe several bottles, for overseas flights for use when the bottled water from the airlines runs out. Use bottled water for brushing your teeth, as you would in any third world country. Bring some disposable towelettes for washing your hands before eating.

CHAPTER 72 -- MUSCLE, BONE and JOINT INJURIES

The older we get, the less elastic our tissues are. Unfortunately that begins to happen at about age 19, or soon after we quit growing. I have stressed in this book the absolute need for you to exercise several times a week on an almost daily basis for your whole life. Now I'm going to tell you that certain types of exercise will be likely to produce injuries, even if you are usually careful. Mountain climbing, especially Mt. Everest, can be a very high-risk activity. Walking laps around your neighborhood or around the track at a local school when the weather is fine, or riding a stationary bike at home should all be very low risk activities. But I have seen injuries that occurred with all of them. Those occurrences are called accidents, and we all know that most accidents occur at or near home.

Swimming laps is one of the two or three best aerobic activities.

Running or jogging are very good, as is cross-country skiing.

Bowling and softball are not aerobic activities. Neither is golf, unless you walk the course and pull or carry your bag. Then it is aerobic for short periods of time.

To help prevent muscle and tendon strains (tendons attach the muscles to the bones that you want to move and are actually a part of the muscle, while ligaments tie the bones together) and ligament sprains here are a few suggestions that will reduce the frequency of injuries considerably.

1. Stretch, warm up for 5 minutes, then stretch again. Get a stretching book and read it. Be careful to be gentle when you stretch. Also keep a constant pull on the area being stretched. Don't bounce or you may actually tear the muscle by stimulating a contraction.

2. At the conclusion of your exercise, stretch again.

3. Always start gradually whenever you are doing a new exercise. Then slowly increase the amount of time that you do that exercise so that your muscles and ligaments can gradually get stronger from day-to-day.

4. Cross training, that is, doing a different exercise on alternate days, is a great idea because it gives your tissues the chance to recover between sessions of that particular exercise.

5. If something becomes sore during your activity, stop and stretch that area again. Then try a little more activity. If it remains sore, then stop that activity and go do something else for the rest of the day.

6. If you have a sore spot at the end of your workout, put some ice on it for 15 minutes after you do your stretching. The next day do something different that doesn't involve that particular area of your body.

7. If the same sore spot is there for two or three days in a row, give that area a rest for a week or so. When you come back to it, start with shorter time and less intensity.

Ankle Sprains

Start gentle range of motion exercises the next day. It takes three weeks for the injured ligaments to knit firmly, but longer for proper rehab to make your ankle as strong as it was before the injury. A good exercise is just balancing yourself on the injured foot whenever you talk on the telephone for as long as you talk. Another is rising up on your toes and rocking back on your heels with your toes up off the ground, gradually increasing the number of repetitions until you reach 100 in a row. When you get to 100, then start again, this time by putting the balls of your feet up on a one-inch board to rise up, then coming back off the board onto your heels. Again work up to 100, before moving on to a two-inch board and again working up to 100. If you like, you can just do them on stair steps instead of boards. By the time you get to 100 on the two-inch board you will be well, or all but well.

Knee Injuries

Knee rehabilitation after surgery or a bad sprain is usually inadequate due to insurance limitations unless the person is an athlete. Muscle atrophy begins immediately after an injury, so rehabilitation should too. There are a number of activities that can be done at home, such as riding a stationary bicycle, doing straight leg raises (you can do this while still swollen, with the brace on), doing quadriceps exercises with knee extensions, and hamstring curls. Do _something_ every day. The worse the injury, the longer it takes for full-strength recovery. An ACL repair, for example, takes a full year for even the best-conditioned and most highly motivated athletes.

Weekend Athletes

People who exercise only once or twice a week cannot maintain their conditioning level. You must exercise at least three times per week just to maintain your current level. To improve your current level, you must exercise at least four times each week.

These athletes are more susceptible to injury. For that reason it is especially important to gently stretch and warm up before participating, quit before you are really tired, then warm down and again wind up with gentle stretching. If any area is a little sore afterwards, put some ice on it for 15 to 20 minutes.

These suggestions will greatly reduce the number of injuries that I see on Mondays.

Overtraining

For more complete coverage of this important subject, see the chapter on **Exercise.** Prevention is the best medicine. For example, after a heart attack I have my patients start walking 50 to 100 steps the first day and increase by 10 steps each day. The most extreme example I know of was a man who followed this approach and climbed a 14,000-foot mountain three years after his myocardial infarction!

Briefly, increase your training gradually to allow the muscle fibers to grow and strengthen themselves, along with giving your blood vessels time to grow along with the muscles. (This works for the heart as well as other muscles.) For all training never increase your particular activity total effort more than 10% per week. Do cross training, using different muscles on alternate days. Wear different shoes on alternate days.

Avoid shin splints by running on softer ground whenever possible. Put Spenco insoles in your shoes for cushioning.

Work-Related Injuries

25% of all work-related injuries are backs. Most back injuries occur in people who are in relatively poor physical condition, and/or use poor body mechanics for lifting. See the chapter on **Back Injuries** for a complete discussion of this very common problem.

More work-related injuries occur on Mondays and Fridays (or the day before a holiday) than any other times. The reasons for these seem to be that on Mondays, people are still tired, hung-over, or thinking about the weekend's activities, while on Fridays our minds wander, and our concentration tends to be on what we are going to do on our days off. Also, on Fridays we may be tired from lots of overtime. The most dangerous hours are the first hour on Monday and the last hour on Friday.

Workers compensation in all states pays for all medical and surgical expenses for work-related injuries. This includes all special tests, drugs, supplies, and equipment, as well as specialist care, if needed, and physical therapy. Many of these must be approved by the insurance carrier before we can order them. In addition, the insurance carrier is required to pay a percentage of the employee's regular wages if the employee is unable to work for a prolonged period of time. But the first thing is to get the needed documentation taken care of by the employee and the employer, so that the insurance company will have no choice but to accept the case as work-related. Some insurance companies are deliberately slow about giving this approval, and you may need assistance from your human resources person where you work. Sometimes you may need a lawyer.

Exhaust every possible appeal avenue before you go that route unless you have an oil well somewhere.

Coverage varies considerably from state to state. In one state that I am familiar with the employee doesn't start receiving money until he or she has been off work for five consecutive days. In another state where I have practiced, it is three days.

At the end of the initial time off, paperwork is filled out by the employer and the attending physician. Then those papers are processed, and in a few weeks (plan on 5-6 weeks) your checks begin to come in. Unfortunately, those checks are usually for much less than your normal wages. In Arizona, the state I am most familiar with, the injured person receives only about 2/3 of his base salary. This doesn't include the weekly overtime pay that many of us come to depend on. So the money you bring in if you are off work completely is just subsistence pay, something you can barely live on.

Advice: When you get overtime pay, don't plan on always getting it. Take it and put most of it in a savings account. Most of all, <u>never</u> buy something new and plan to use your overtime to make the payments for it!

Most physicians who see very many of this type of injury are well aware that many studies have shown that workers who return immediately to some kind of modified duty at the work place will recover faster from almost *any* injury than someone who just sits around the house.

There are a number of reasons for this. One, of course is the economic one where the injured person continues to have a weekly paycheck, and thus does not fall into a depressed state from lack of money to pay the bills.

Another is also a mental thing, where you are under foot with your spouse at home, and bickering may occur that disturbs your mental health.

Another is that continued physical activity of <u>any</u> amount will help prevent the muscle and other tissue atrophy (atrophy means the muscles shrivel up and get weak), which slows down recovery and makes for a longer rehab time. Not only that but making the muscles actively move reduces spasm and therefore reduces pain. Couch potatoes don't get well as fast as those who are physically and mentally active.

Smokers take twice as long to recover from even simple injuries, mainly because the injured tissues don't get enough oxygen for rapid healing.

The opposite of the fourth paragraph is that some people who aren't supposed to do a particular physical activity (or their spouses) find chores they have been putting off around the house, some of which may not be what their doctor or physical therapist have in mind for their rehab program.

> *One recent patient of mine had sore and swollen knees. He was supposed to give them some rest. Well, he felt so much better in three days that he decided he could put on the new roof, which he had been putting off, over the weekend before he saw me again on Monday. He hauled the asphalt shingles up the ladder all by himself, squatted and knelt down all day for two days, and guess what? When he saw me on Monday, he said, "Gee, I'm not any better." After a little discussion, the story came out, bit by bit. So I sent him back to regular duty, figuring that he would strain his knees a whole lot less at work than at home.*

Computer-Related Injuries

Many of these involve repetitive stress as well as improper keyboard-monitor-mouse-chair ergonomics (or just relationships to your body mechanics).

<u>Sore neck</u>. Probably your monitor is not at the proper level, and the material you are reading from is not either. The monitor should be at eye level, and the material you are reading from should be close enough to eye level so that you don't have to move anything but your eyes when inputting on the keyboard. You especially don't want to have to tilt your head back and forth all day.

<u>Sore shoulders, arms, elbows, forearms, wrists, and hands.</u> These are especially related to your posture at the keyboard. Usually, you aren't sitting properly.

You should be sitting so that your elbows bend at right angles (90 degrees) as the hands work on the keyboard. For this you may have to raise or lower your keyboard.

The wrists should be supported with a slightly spongy support, and there should be a similar smaller padded mouse support attached to the mouse pad. 3-M makes the best of these that I have seen, but there are lots on the market.

You should also be able to rest your elbows on the arms of your chair without disturbing the 90-degree angle.

<u>Sore back.</u> Ideally you should be sitting upright with your back supported in the small of your back with a small lumbar support. If you are slouching, or your chair doesn't give enough support, you might try a small pillow in the small of your back, or get one that you can strap to the chair from a physical therapy supply store. Or just roll up a towel and put a couple of rubber bands around it to hold the roll.

Sometimes putting one or both of your feet on a footrest will cause the hips to bend just enough to change your lumbar angle and relieve the strain.

<u>Numbness in legs or feet.</u> This may be caused by too much pressure on the blood vessels of your legs from two or three possible causes: the angle of flexion of the hips, same for the knees, or pressure on the thighs just above the knees. Again, a footrest might be helpful, or a chair with the front part of it sloping downward a little.

<u>Sore bottom.</u> This is caused by too much pressure on the portion of the posterior pelvic bones called the ischial (is-key-al) tuberosities. We all know what those are, especially of us with pretty bony behinds. The way to relieve that is to transfer much of your weight to the backs of your thighs. So ideally you should have a soft enough chair that supports at least the top 6 or 8 inches of the backs of your thighs as well as your bottom end. Just be sure it doesn't go far enough out to press on the blood vessels behind the knees, as noted above. A swivel chair that tilts may be a good solution because you can then easily change positions when you notice a hot spot developing.

The perfect workstation chair is not easily found! I once spent over two hours checking out all the chairs in a business furniture warehouse before I found one that would fit the measurements I took from my receptionist. I'm happy to report that she loved it.

CHAPTER 73 -- NOSEBLEEDS

Most nosebleeds come from damaged blood vessels in the wall (septum) between the two nostrils in a little triangular area. This is where crusts tend to form more than other areas, and that is also where a person can pick the crusts off with fingernails. Unfortunately the fingernails are a dangerous weapon where delicate tissues such as skin and mucous membranes are concerned, and they often damage the membranes of the nose and cause some bleeding. Most of the time it stops right away, but sometimes it can be severe. I have had two or three patients with nosebleeds who wound up needing blood transfusions, but their bleeding was from arteries farther back in the nose.

Bleeding can also start from a sneeze, or from a blow to the nasal area, either in a fight or in a game (more often basketball than football since face masks began to be required). Or it can start in the middle of the night while you are sleeping for no apparent reason.

High blood pressure can be a cause, where the nose begins to bleed as kind of a safety valve, perhaps, when the BP is too high. Better there than inside the head, where bleeding causes a stroke! These bleeds tend to be arterial, and much harder to stop.

Dry air, especially in the middle of winter in cold country, makes the membranes crack open, often breaking a blood vessel along the way.

So we see that there are a number of common conditions that can make your nose bleed: Dry air, picking crusts off the septum, high blood pressure, a blow, a sneeze. People who take aspirin are more prone to these, as well as someone on anticoagulants, and people with serious blood diseases. Infections may cause enough local irritation, but I can't recall even one person I have ever seen for a serious nosebleed who had an infection as the cause.

Treatment consists of finding a way to stop the bleeding, then trying to correct the underlying cause, if it can be easily identified. *You can save a lot of money here.

Sometimes you are bleeding from both nostrils. What is happening in that case is the blood is running around the back of the nose to the other side too. Believe me, unless there has been a blow to the nose, only one side is bleeding. You can more easily identify which side by blowing your nose and spitting out what blood has gone down the back of the throat. Then lean forward and see which side bleeds more, then take it from there with the suggestions below.

First, when your nose begins to bleed, take your thumb and one finger and squeeze the soft part of your nose tightly together so as to press on the blood vessel that is bleeding. If you are doing it right, it will be a little uncomfortable. Do this at first for at least 5 minutes. Most bleeding stops by then because most people's blood will clot within that time if they aren't on aspirin. If 5 minutes doesn't do it, then blow your nose gently to get all the clot out, put some Kleenex, folded to about four layers, inside your nose, and this time press on it for 15 minutes by the clock. You can then leave the Kleenex in place for several hours, if you want to. This will take care of probably 99% of nosebleeds and is about all you can do for yourself. But that is really quite a lot.

Then take care of whatever applies to you from the list above: put moisture into the air of your house, particularly your bedroom because you spend probably more time there than all the others put together. Put some Vaseline or other ointment onto the crusty areas inside the nose several times a day. Get your blood pressure under control. Don't blow your nose so hard, or not at all. Instead, when you sneeze, open your mouth and let most of the pressure of the sneeze go out your mouth. Stop taking aspirin. If you are on Coumadin or another anticoagulant, you have to consult with your doctor.

Do not mess around with putting ice on the back of your neck, for Pete's sake. That isn't where the problem is! I don't know how many people have told me that they have done that, but it's been a lot! If you want to use ice, feel free to apply it to the nose itself, but not to some remote area.

If that doesn't stop it, then it is time to see a doctor. Don't wait until you have donated a couple of pints of blood to the bathroom sink! Also, but perhaps less quickly, see him if the nosebleeds come back, a few times if not bleeding very much each time, or as soon as possible if it bleeds pretty heavily each time.

Here is what your doctor can do: He can usually identify the source of the bleeding. Once the source vessel is known, he can cauterize it, usually with a silver nitrate stick. That stings a little, but not much.

For a pesky pumping artery that won't stop with the silver nitrate stick and pressure, he may have to anesthetize the nose with some pontocaine solution or something similar. Sometimes we will mix the pontocaine with some 4% cocaine, which really shrinks the blood vessels and that combination almost always works.

If that doesn't stop it, then electrocautery must often be used, while suction is applied to the bleeder. We like to hold that back as long as we can, because the cautery on a really bad bleeder can burn the thin underlying tissue and the cartilage of the septum, leaving a hole between the two nostrils that can be troublesome in the future.

If nothing has worked to that point, then we pack the nose tightly with cotton or other packing material soaked in the pontocaine-cocaine mixture, sometimes two dozen or more pieces of cotton. Then we leave them in place for one or two days, depending on whether some blood continues to seep from the packed side. Believe me, if you have to have your nose packed, you will need some pain medication until the packing comes out, because it is a miserable feeling.

The worst cases for stopping the bleeding are those where the bleeder is in the back of the nose. I'm glad to be able to say that I have had only three or four of those to deal with. What we do there is put a thin rubber tube with a balloon on the end of it back through the bleeding side until we can see it at the back of the throat, then inflate the balloon and pull from the front while putting the finger into the back of the mouth to push it up firmly behind the soft palate and thoroughly block the back of the nose. Then we pack it as above from the front, but using about four times as much packing. You may wind up with an overnight stay in the hospital with a blood count in the morning to be sure you haven't lost too much.

Nosebleeds are a very common problem. The opportunity for saving lots of money (as well as many red blood cells) is something you can seize the next time someone you know and love has one.

CHAPTER 74 -- OBESITY

Obesity is the new (old) nutritional disease. It is important to talk about it here because it is a deadly disease, as well as one that greatly interferes with the obese person's quality of life.

It is an undesirable condition of the human body which afflicts more than 35% of us. And that number is rapidly growing. Estimates suggest that more than 50% of us are at least somewhat overweight. Researchers tell us that obesity starts in infancy when the fat cells produced by overeating are first formed. Feeding an infant foods containing empty calories, such as mashed potatoes, and sweets of all kinds (candy, cookies, cakes, pies, and anything else you can think of) contributes the most to the early obesity.

In 2000, the most recent fully cost-analyzed year we have full figures for, the medical cost of treating obesity-related ailments amounted to $117 billion, which closely approaches the medical costs of treating the number one killer in the world, tobacco use, at $130 billion. Approximately 300,000 people died as a direct result of obesity and its complications, compared to 500,000 for tobacco.

It is no coincidence that this obesity epidemic is also causing an epidemic of Type II diabetes (see the chapter on **Diabetes** for a more extensive discussion). And Type II diabetes, which used to occur only in older people, at least past 35 or 40, and was also called "mature onset diabetes," is now showing up in younger and younger people.

I know of cases in 5- and 7-year-old children! These are children are morbidly obese and weigh at least twice as much as they should for their ages.

Hypertension, arthritis, back injuries, stroke, heart attack, diabetes, pulmonary emboli (blood clots in the lungs), and injuries from falls are just a few of the conditions caused or aggravated by being too fat.

Obesity strongly contributes to poor outcomes in many conditions, such as surgery, where the thick layers of fat often make an impossible situation for even the best surgeons in the world during the operation and increase the risk of pulmonary embolism (blood clots in the lungs), heart complications, poor wound healing, and slow recovery post op. Hospitals spend an average of $396 more per obese patient for outpatient and in-hospital care.

Whereas both obesity and smoking by the primary user are preventable, obesity at least does not have a direct effect on anything but the financial health of others in the family. Second hand smoke from family smokers, however, also damages the health of those around them, with somewhat over 60,000 people killed by second hand (or side stream) smoke exposure in 2001, the last year with fully-reported figures. 1999 had about 50,000 such deaths, so the loss is rising.

Older people worry that they will "look old" if they lose weight so that their skin sags. That certainly does happen in many cases (especially in smokers and people who have spent a

I helped (actually I was third assistant and just held a retractor until my hands went to sleep) at surgery for removal of the gall bladder of a morbidly obese woman when I was a senior in medical school. It took the senior resident (who had done two or three hundred of these procedures by that time) a little over six hours to complete that operation. In stark contrast, I was the only assistant when a surgeon friend of mine in Flagstaff, Arizona removed the gall bladder of a woman of normal weight in 10 minutes by the clock from the first incision until the last staple was in place, in the early 1990's, a year or so before everyone started doing them laparoscopically. Obviously the surgeon and his assistant had had a few more of these procedures under our belts by the time we did the second case, but the biggest difference was that we didn't have to dig through ten to twelve inches of fat to even find the gall bladder.

lot of time out in the sun unprotected by sun blocks) but much less than expected. Particularly if the weight loss is combined with mild to moderate exercises that tone up your underlying muscles on an ongoing basis. And your friendly neighborhood plastic surgeon will be happy to remove the excess skin, for a hefty fee.

So, to avoid (or at least reduce) the sagging skin of later years, lose the weight while your skin is still elastic, certainly before age 50, stop the use of tobacco, and protect your skin from ultraviolet rays (see the chapter on **Skin**). Then you can reduce the urge to have cosmetic plastic surgery, none of which is ever covered by health insurance.

How can you tell whether you are overweight (besides looking in the mirror with your eyes wide open), obese, or morbidly obese?

There are two measurements, which you can do yourself (remember this is all about how to be your *own* doctor). The first is the body mass index (BMI), which you will hear about over and over until something else replaces it in 20 years or so. Weigh yourself (in pounds, as we usually do in the USA), divide that figure by your height in inches squared, and multiply by 703. So some one who weighs 264 lbs and is 5 feet 3 inches (63 inches) in stocking feet will divide 264 by 3969 (63" × 63") and then multiply that answer by 703. (Or, weight in pounds divided by height in inches, then divided again by height in inches, then multiplied by 703 = BMI.) In this extreme example, which happens to be a woman I saw for a pre-employment exam last week, the BMI is 46.76, which is definitely morbidly obese. We consider a BMI of 25 or more as "overweight" and a BMI of 30 or more as "obese." There is still some discussion as to where morbid obesity begins, but most of us are comfortable calling it a BMI of 40 or more. Some just say that anyone more than 100 lbs over normal body weight is morbidly obese. That is probably true most of the time (except possibly in pro football players), but using the BMI is a little more scientific. Just looking at someone in an undressed state, including yourself in the mirror, is also probably accurate if you aren't in some kind of a denial state.

The other method of accurately measuring obesity is just measuring yourself around the waist at the level of the navel (belly button, umbilicus). <u>A man who measures more than 40 inches or a woman who measures more than 35 inches is obese</u> and subject to an increased risk of obesity-related health conditions. One of these is <u>Type 2 diabetes</u>, with which the waist measurement is <u>highly</u> correlated (see the chapter on **Diabetes**). Another is <u>high blood pressure</u>, where the loss of just two inches results in a 15 to 20 point reduction in the blood pressure in many cases (see the **Hypertension** chapter). Big bellies, with not much fat elsewhere, are often the result of too many simple or refined carbohydrates, such as sweets and alcohol, rather than just too many calories in general. These carbs are just empty calories and should always be avoided in losing weight or just maintaining a normal weight.

Begin to prevent obesity in infancy. A fat baby is more likely to become a fat adult. Don't mistakenly think that your "success" as a mother is measured by how plump your baby is. Breast fed babies tend to be leaner than bottle babies till about 1 1/2 years of age. Avoid sweets at all times early in life. Food can have emotional aspects, but don't treat your child like a dolphin by rewarding him or her with food for every trick. At least one study suggests that breast-feeding may provide protection against obesity lasting even into adolescence and beyond.

Fat infants can still be undernourished in important areas of nutrition. The one that comes to my mind first is the chubby little guy who eats a lot of mashed potatoes and doesn't get enough protein and iron to build red blood cells. So he develops iron deficiency anemia. I've seen <u>a lot</u> of those kids.

Breast fed kiddies need to have their mothers be sure to take vitamin K supplements during the first three months of life to help prevent hemorrhagic disease of the newborn.

Vegetarian breast feeding mothers need to be sure to include foods in their diets that are fortified with vitamin B-12.

A lot of our vitamin D, which is responsible for proper bone growth (a deficiency results in rickets -- malformed bones), comes from cow's milk fortified with it. It also comes from a chemical in our skins called ergosterol, which converts to vitamin D upon exposure of the skin to the sun's rays.

So if you are breast feeding and also using a sun-block on your child's exposed skin, as I firmly believe you should, I recommend giving a vitamin supplement that includes Vitamin D, 300 International Units per day for babies up to 6 months, and 400 International Units per day for babies from 6 to 12 months.

> *In Phoenix, Arizona, this year, the health department reports that some cases of rickets have been reported. This seems very strange in the Valley of the Sun until you realize that Phoenix also has a very high rate of skin cancer. What is happening is that parents are putting sun block on their children to prevent skin cancer later in life, and blocking the ultraviolet rays also prevents the conversion of ergosterol to Vitamin D.*

Further, iron supplements may occasionally be needed in breast-fed tykes after about 6 months, particularly if meat is not a part of their diets by then. Fer-in-Sol drops or syrup are the best on the market for this purpose, I believe. Have your child's blood count checked at or before 6 months just to be sure.

A fluoride supplement to prevent dental cavities should begin by age 6 months and continue until about age 16 years after all teeth are in. This can be in your city's water supply or in chewable vitamins or drops. If your family drinks only bottled water, then you must use the pills or drops.

In fat kids, we want to carefully avoid pushing them too far in the other direction, with resulting anorexia nervosa or bulimia. Therefore it is best and probably sufficient to get them on a healthy diet with no snacks so as to prevent further weight gain, start exercising, limit TV, computers, and video games, and let them grow into their present weight. The healthy diet means reduced carbohydrates and fats. They need protein for growth, so if they are allowed a snack, make sure it includes some protein, like non-fat milk and maybe a leftover chicken leg, for example.

We parents should take a look at ourselves and set an example for our kids by living a healthy lifestyle in weight management through healthy eating and regular exercise.

I've seen many family groups walking or bicycling around our neighborhoods every evening, usually after supper. These new motorized scooters should be avoided -- no exercise. The ones where the kids have to push are the way to go. Make your kids walk to and from school if at all possible.

Lobby your schools to include physical education classes several times a week, preferably daily, from kindergarten through all four years of high school. PE is <u>not</u> team sports. Team sports are good exercise for those whose strength and coordination allows them to be competitive.

A good PE program teaches skills in all *kinds* of physical activities. A kid who is blind, for example, may learn skills that will enable him to be the second blind person to climb Mt. Everest (it's too late to be the first -- he did the climb in May, 2001). A fat kid whose feet hurt when he tries to run may find that he is a natural swimmer. And so on.

Get your kids into summer Parks and Recreation camps in your town. Most are free or very inexpensive.

For those of you who are overachievers and expect your kids to be so also, fine. I had a mother like that, and, bless her heart, I don't regret much of what she made me do. BUT make sure you give your kids some totally unstructured free time (away from TV, computers, and video games) where they can do whatever they want to. Be sure, also, that the young violinist gets at least 30 minutes of physical activity each day. Same for the kid that reads six books a week, like I used to do. My problem with my mother's agenda was that it exercised my brain but not my body. So I was a sissy when it came to games at school. My dad was a fine athlete, but his work schedule didn't allow him to be home for outdoor activities much when I was in grade school. There was a war going on, and he was needed to make parachutes, with lots of overtime work. PE was what rescued me and helped turn me into a pretty well balanced person in regard to "a sound mind in a sound body."

Strive for a healthy weight all your life. To do that you must combine good dietary habits with increased physical activities. These must become permanent lifestyle changes. I'm the first to admit that having donuts, birthday cakes, and other goodies around the office several days each week requires enormous will-power (or *won't*-power) to resist. For me, taking the first bite is fatal. So what I do is weigh myself several times a week at the same time of day, with same amount of clothes on. If (actually *when*) I gain 5 pounds, I go on a diet. There was a time when I weighed 30 pounds more than I do now. I have found that it is a *lot* easier to lose 5 pounds than 30. So I try to avoid the first bite of the cake, or whatever, or limit myself to just half of one when I do give in (you know as well as I do that I almost never stop with just half of a donut!) Believe me, I know the problems very well.

Prevention of obesity is most successful if begun in infancy. The new use of the Body Mass Index will be useful here, but only if the parents <u>care</u>.

The Guaranteed Weight Loss Diets for correction of your obesity are fully explained and spelled out in the chapter on **Losing Weight** and are guaranteed to help you lose serious weight. Be sure to fully read that chapter before starting on your **weight-loss-for-life program**.

CHAPTER 75 -- OSTEOPOROSIS

Osteoporosis is the brittle bones condition, mostly of post-menopause and old age, but also of women who stop menstruating prematurely, such as distance runners and those on thyroid supplements -- who may still be menstruating but still need extra calcium daily -- and people with other risk factors noted below.

In the past, almost half of all women have been affected by this condition in their lifetimes, more than cervical, uterine, and breast cancers all put together. The disease causes thinning of bones through loss of calcium and is responsible for the loss of height and stooped shoulders in older women because of collapse of the vertebrae in their spines. Improving the old person's appearance and posture is important, but the fragility of the bones in the rest of the body can turn even a small fall into a disaster.

Fractured hips almost never happen if there is no osteoporosis. We have all known at least one older person who died of complications after breaking a hip in a fall, usually around her own house. My impression is that perhaps 50% of older people who break their hips die soon after. As we get older our bones lose some or a lot of their calcium unless we take steps to prevent that from happening. Because of the very high morbidity and mortality associated with hip fractures, it is urgent that we try to prevent them.

Osteoporosis is a silent condition, and most people don't know they have it until a bone breaks. Then you lose your ability and freedom to move around, along with your independence and possibly your life.

Warning signals that osteoporosis may be occurring:

1. You are thinner than normal, this may be caused by eating disorders, such as anorexia nervosa or bulimia. If so, get help from your physician.

2. You are shorter than you used to be. This is particularly evident in older people who may lose height through collapse of vertebrae in the spine, which have been weakened by loss of calcium.

3. One of your bones breaks too easily.

4. You have a chronic backache.

5. You have thyroid abnormalities, especially those requiring medication.

Osteoporosis happens more in women than men (about 75% of cases are in women), especially older women after menopause, and especially if the woman does not take hormone replacement therapy, specifically estrogen, along with calcium supplements.

How can we diagnose this condition? Previously the diagnosis was made only after enough calcium had been lost to make the bones look like eggshells on X-rays. In the past six years we have been able to measure bone density directly with a really great machine, which is now available in the radiology departments of most hospitals. The other good news is that many, if not most insurances, including Medicare, will cover a bone density screening test at this time. Now being shown at medical meetings are some smaller portable machines, which may soon also be available in your own doctor's office.

> *I have had a few small fractures in my very active life, but no big bones in spite of some fair amount of trauma. Ligaments and tendons are another matter! I attribute this to a considerable degree to the fact that my dad bought a cow when I started growing fast at about age twelve. So instead of water when I was thirsty, I drank milk, about a gallon a day for several years, according to my dad. I don't advocate everybody buying a cow (I'm not sure how that would play in Peoria, or New York City), but a lot of milk and/or calcium supplement is a very good idea, especially when kids start their last big growth spurt. Always remember that girls start that spurt about two years before boys.*

Drug treatment of this condition has been available for less than ten years, and new medicines are coming. But treatment with medicine doesn't get you fully back to where you were before. The best approach by far, as with so many other conditions, is prevention. It is important to know that the foundation for strong bones is laid in childhood and adolescence. As young folks we deposit much more calcium into our bones than we withdraw until about age twenty, when we reach our peak bone mass. Starting about age twenty-eight we begin to lose more calcium than we store. If we have taken in a lot of calcium when we are young, then we will have more to withdraw as we get older, before we have to be concerned with osteoporosis.

Since this condition is so predominant in women, we will address their situation first.

Abnormally low levels of estrogen are at the root of most osteoporosis in women. Anything that stops menstruation will also cause calcium to be withdrawn from your bones and not replaced fully. This is true of female athletes who train so hard that their menstrual cycle is disturbed, with periods often stopping completely.

We used to think that no harm was done since menses began again within a month or two after training levels had been reduced, and pregnancy was still possible after the menstrual cycle resumed. But then some smart person invented the bone densitometer, which measures how dense or strong ones bones are. And when we in medicine get a new toy, we always try it out in every way possible. When it was used on female athletes, it was found that their bones weren't as strong after several months of no periods. And, worse, they never quite recovered to their original strength.

So now we who treat athletes simply add estrogen in a cyclic fashion to the routine of lady athletes whose periods have gone away. This prevents the bone calcium loss, and can be stopped when the athlete is no longer competing at such high levels. It is a good idea to also add a calcium supplement to the several supplements that truly dedicated athletes take daily. If you are one, then I suggest 1,000 to 1,500 mg of elemental calcium daily -- 1,000 if you drink milk with meals, and 1,500 if you don't drink milk. There are, of course, other foods which contain calcium. Read about them in any nutrition book, especially if you are unable to drink milk.

Calcium is necessary for strong bones, and any diet that is deficient in it will also lead eventually to osteoporosis.

There are many factors other than estrogen which adversely affect bone metabolism. The following is a list of other factors that increase the risk of developing osteoporosis, which in many cases can apply to men as well as women:

1. Smoking. Yet another reason to avoid this dangerous and potentially lethal combination of toxic chemicals.

2. Use of steroid medications for more than short periods of time. Those who take thyroid medication or oral cortisone (or other members of the cortisone family, such as dexamethasone or prednisone for asthma, arthritis, and other less common conditions) tend to have lower calcium levels and are at higher risk for osteoporosis.

3. Use of thyroid replacement hormones, especially in higher dosages. These must be monitored by at least annual TSH blood tests. And take supplemental calcium.

4. Use of thiazide diuretics, hydrochlorthiazide being the one most commonly used currently for high blood pressure, tends to reduce your calcium levels.

5. Milk intolerance, such that you can't drink it and thus lose a valuable source of calcium.

6. Presence of Irritable Bowel Syndrome -- I have no personal experience with this aspect of IBS, but it is well documented as a potential problem.

7. Being treated for endometriosis with hormones that prevent you from having periods for several months at a time.

8. History of kidney stones/abnormal calcium metabolism. I must caution those who have already had a kidney stone known to be composed of a calcium compound to talk to their doctors about how to get in the necessary daily amount of calcium without incurring the risk of additional stone formation. Each case is unique to that individual, and I can't address every case here. However, I can tell you that preventing kidney stones depends upon keeping the urine dilute enough to prevent crystals from appearing. We

can often see them under the microscope when doing a urinalysis on urine that is very concentrated.

How do you know whether you are drinking enough? Easily. If your urine is dark yellow, you are a little dehydrated (which can cause a number of other problems besides kidney stones), and thus need more water-containing fluids. If your urine is very light yellow or colorless, then almost certainly you are getting enough water.

Usually three quarts of water per day will assure you of enough dilute urine output to prevent kidney stones even when you are taking calcium supplements. This number changes in hot weather and depends upon how active you are physically. If you are hiking in the Grand Canyon in June, for example, then you need at least one quart of water per hour. Also if you are playing football in August almost anywhere in the country, but especially in Phoenix, Arizona, then you need upwards from a gallon of water per two hours of practice.

Drinks with caffeine or alcohol in them do not help your hydration because they stimulate the kidneys to put out more fluid than you take in; so you are a net loser of body fluids in those cases. Don't take salt tablets very much in the summer. They can cause cramps and other problems because they are so concentrated. What you need is water. Drinks like Gatorade provide some sodium and potassium to replenish those lost in sweat. Salty foods are good idea too. Also juices are terrific for these purposes. But as salt is lost in sweat, the sweat becomes more dilute in salt as our bodies try to conserve what we need. Water, first and foremost. No matter if cold or warm. Just wet. (See the chapter on **Heat Injuries** for more on this.)

9. Female athletes who train so hard that they don't menstruate, as described above.

10. Excessive alcohol intake.

I had an alcoholic in my office yesterday who has cirrhosis of the liver and may soon die from his alcoholism. Along with his abnormal liver function tests he had a quite low blood calcium level. This is causing him some severe muscle cramps, and could soon cause a dangerous heart irregularity.

11. Eating a diet which is low in calcium, especially after about age 50.

12. Osteoporosis is also more likely to occur in women with menopause before age 47, and also in younger women who have had their ovaries surgically removed and haven't started taking estrogen immediately after the surgery.

13. Inactive lifestyle with little or no regular exercise, particularly weight-bearing activities, at any age.

14. A small, thin frame, especially when combined with a lack of physical activity.

15. Eating disorders, such as anorexia or bulimia.

16. Family history of osteoporosis, numerous broken bones, or spinal curvature below the neck in old age (the so-called dowager's hump). I am not aware that scoliosis, which begins in the teenage years, causes any increased risk.

How do we prevent, and how do we treat this disease?

First is to be sure that you have adequate calcium in your diet daily. Aim for 1,500 mg of elemental calcium daily your whole life, but especially after age 40 or so. A glass of milk may contain up to 300 mg of calcium. Calcium supplements, preferably with vitamin D added, come in sizes from 200 to 1,000 mg tablets. Some of those tablets may be hard to swallow, especially for older people. Tums has chewable tablets, and Viactiv is a delicious soft chocolate calcium candy, which also contains 20 calories each, by the way. A diet that includes plenty of green leafy vegetables is also important.

> *I can still remember the ridiculous statements by nutritionists as recently as 15 to 20 years ago to the effect that adults don't need milk. That has been proved to be one of the biggest hunks of baloney in medicine for a long time. I have always advised my adult patients to drink milk, but to use reduced fat, even skim milk, if possible. Now I recommend milk daily, if you can drink it, plus supplemental calcium for all those over 40.*

An analysis by a well-known testing laboratory five or six years ago found that only two of the dozens of calcium preparations were fully absorbed by the body in the test subjects. Those were Tums and OsCal. New ones are coming out every year, so there may be others that achieve full absorption now.

Second, take estrogen, if you can, starting in the pre-menopausal years before your own ovarian hormone levels fall significantly. Don't wait even a single year or you will have lost bone mass that can never be replaced. In other words, start estrogen while you are still menstruating. (You might get an idea of when you may stop your menses by asking your mother when she stopped having periods.) A blood test called an FSH (for follicle-stimulating hormone) should be done once a year along with your PAP smear starting in your early 40s, and when it gets abnormally high, that means it's time to start estrogen replacement.

Third, do some weight-bearing active exercise at least three days per week. Apparently swimming, even though it is one of the two or three best cardiovascular exercises, does not afford as much osteoporosis protection as we previously thought. House cleaning certainly helps the brittle bones situation, along with some other onerous things.

Men get considerable protection from their male hormone, testosterone. Since most men still produce testosterone to much more advanced ages (along with healthy sperm in many cases) than women produce estrogen, they are at a much lower risk of developing osteoporosis. Still, it can and does happen. So, men, take your calcium, and do your weight-bearing exercise. Some men begin to lose testicular function beginning in their 50s, with resulting less testosterone. You can get an idea that this may be happening to you if your balls start to feel sort of mushy and also if you start having sexual problems of one type or another.

A blood test will tell you whether you might need testosterone replacement. If you do, then it is even more important to have your prostate checked every year, along with a PSA, because it isn't a good idea to take testosterone if you ever develop prostate cancer. (But it doesn't <u>cause</u> prostate cancer.)

A program consisting of milk, calcium supplements, and a nutritious diet that includes plenty of green leafy vegetables, plus at least 30 minutes of weight-bearing exercise daily will help you build and maintain strong bones, thus greatly reducing the risk of developing osteoporosis. Hormone replacement therapy will help prevent any further bone density loss. These are true for both men *and* women.

CHAPTER 76 -- PHYSICIAN EXTENDERS

Physician "extenders" include Physician Assistants (PAs), Registered Certified Nurse Practitioners (CNPs), midwives, etc. The nurse practitioners have the most extensive training and are allowed the most freedom of practice with minimal supervision in most states.

Always remember these medical people may be very nice and sound very knowledgeable, but they are not doctors. They do have medical training, but it is very superficial compared to a doctor's. Never hesitate to ask the extender to allow you to consult with his or her supervising physician. Most will be happy to oblige.

I have worked with PAs many days each year for over five years. Mostly we work together seamlessly as a team. I am required to review and sign off on all of the PAs' charts every day in our clinics.

And for a year and a half I have been involved with teaching PA students from a local medical school when they rotate through our clinics. I have also helped in the teaching programs for medical students and residents for three years. It is all on-the-job training in our clinics (as it was for our medical corpsmen in the Air Force), and many of the PA students are bright enough that I wish they could go on to medical school. The ones I have been fortunate enough to work with have almost all done good jobs and weren't afraid to ask questions. By the way, having to have correct answers for their questions has made me personally a better doctor.

By the time the students get to our clinics, they have had a very concentrated training course in general medicine. They then get to see patients with the physicians and discuss anything interesting or puzzling. After a year of this they take a national exam, become licensed in the state where they want to practice, and find a job. The good ones are snapped up pretty quickly, and they get some more O-J-T with their new employers, gradually becoming more and more proficient in that type of practice. In Arizona the PAs are required to have a supervising physician who is supposed to review their patients with them several times each month.

I've been involved recently in the review of a malpractice case where the extender never once consulted his supervising physician, nor even any other physician in his office, about ongoing treatment of a medical problem, and another case where the extender consulted her supervising physician after each patient visit. In both of these cases, as you might suspect since I am referring to them here, things turned out badly for the patient.

In the first case the extender made the correct diagnosis but made bad mistakes in his treatment recommendations. He never consulted the supervising physician, and he allowed the patient to call him "doctor" even though she knew better. She liked the extender a lot, much better than she liked his supervising physician. Obviously the extender had an ego problem, and this interfered with his seeking the advice that he needed to arrange for his patient's best treatment. See page 379 for the second case.

Treatment by one of these professionals normally will be very similar to being treated by a physician. Most are dedicated to our profession and seek advice from their supervising or other physician seamlessly and constantly, much as physicians often discuss cases among ourselves. For the most part you can feel comfortable with their care.

If you ever have a condition that doesn't clear up after just one or two office visits however, always ask to see the supervising physician on your next visit. Also, for any ongoing long-term condition, such as diabetes, hypertension, high cholesterol, or obesity, always ask the person who schedules appointments to allow you to see a physician on every second or third visit, no matter how good your relationship is with the extender.

I'm painfully aware that physicians also can and do fall in into the ego trap. We're supposed to be perfect, and sometimes make the mistake of thinking that we are.

> *In the second case the extender consulted her supervising physician after each visit of the patient, and he initialed the chart. The two of them together agreed after just two visits that the patient had a bad condition and they needed help. They subsequently referred her to five different specialists for various bad conditions. This extender and her physician did all right things, and so did all five specialists; but things turned out just as badly for this one as for the first case above.*
>
> *In the first case consultation with his supervising physician would have saved the patient. The second patient had the benefit of all that modern medicine can offer and got just as bad a result. I want to mention these cases to illustrate what we all know: some things can't be cured, but those that can deserve to be given the best possible chance.*

And we all die. **But our goal as physicians or physician extenders is always the same: to help people live a normal life span with as good health as possible without pain or suffering, either mental or physical.**

Physician extenders allow a physician to take care of more patients, at less cost than hiring another physician. This is a very important consideration for a doctor who has a lot of HMO patients on capitation. (See the chapter on **HMOs.**) You will see more and more of them as time goes on. Just be aware that they are not doctors.

CHAPTER 77 -- THE PLACEBO EFFECT

Let me tell you about the placebo effect, which is well known to all doctors. <u>A placebo medication works because the person thinks it is going to work</u>. This gives us a little hint of how powerful suggestions are to our minds. Hypnosis is a good example. Most of us have seen or heard of the very unusual, even fantastic things that people can do under hypnosis. I have successfully hypnotized quite a few people, and I will tell you here and now that it <u>works</u>.

If your doctor tells you that a new drug is going to make you get well, between 20 and 40% of you will proceed to get well, no matter whether it is a sugar pill or the latest and best drug on the market for the condition. So when a new drug is being tested to see whether it is really beneficial, the placebo effect is cancelled out by doing what is called a double blind, cross-over study, in which neither the patient nor the doctor know whether the patient is being given the real drug or a "sugar pill" (placebo) that is identical in appearance to the active drug. The patients are assigned randomly, and ideally are matched as to age, sex, and economic status, along with other aspects of their lives that may be pertinent. The bottles have only numbers plus instructions as to how to take them on the labels.

The doses are taken by the first group of patients for a certain amount of time, with careful monitoring of signs and symptoms, along with appropriate lab tests. At the end of the first study period, which may be even as much as a year or more, the roles are reversed, and those who got the active drug at first begin to take the placebo, while the other group begins to take the active drug. Again the patients are monitored carefully to see if their condition is improved, getting worse, developing side effects, whatever, and only the computer knows that a change has taken place.

It is a well-established fact that a certain percentage of people, up to as high as 40% or more, will get better on the placebo. That is our powerful minds at work. ***Feelings are facts!** We'll talk more about that elsewhere. But for now just be aware that what you feel is real for you personally, if for no one else. And what you feel has an enormous effect on how your mind and body respond to all kinds of things.

To illustrate: A competitor in any activity who feels that he is going to win has a much greater chance of doing so than someone who has a different feeling. They may have each trained and prepared physically in an identical manner. Their skills may be similar. But one person will win because of his mental preparation that led him to believe that he would win. And feeling that you are going to win causes things to happen in your mind and body that make it happen, over and over and over.

When I was at the U.S. Olympic Training Center for mental training one Labor Day weekend, we were taught that winning begins with high self-esteem. We were taught various things to enhance that feeling in ourselves that we won't go into here because that would take another whole book.

Suffice it to say that each of us is a unique individual, though with different capabilities in many different areas of our beings. It is absolutely wrong for <u>any</u> of us to compare ourselves unfavorably to someone else. It almost a certainty that <u>each of us</u> has the potential to be better than most other people in the world at doing <u>something</u>. It may not be in what our parents have in mind. And we may have to fail a few times before we find what we do best. (Look how many times Abe Lincoln failed before he was elected president.)

Very few people wind up doing for life what they started out to do. Sometimes we don't ever figure out what we do best, and that is sad. Sometimes we get stuck in an economic situation that is hard to get out of. If you are such a case, go to night school, trade school, or junior college. If you are a single parent, trade baby-sitting nights with a friend or friends so you can get the additional education. It is estimated that your lifetime earnings increase by at least $100,000 for every year of post high school education.

So skip the cokes and beer and tobacco to save money for additional education. I worked my way through medical school; so I know what I'm talking about. Exercise daily for twenty to thirty minutes every day (ideally at least 30), even if it is just sprinting around doing the household chores without stopping. That will clear the brain, make you a more confident person, and also make your body function more efficiently. Plus a <u>lot</u> of other good stuff discussed in the chapter on **Exercise.**

If you feel good about yourself, the placebo effect is more powerful for all of your activities. Let it flow!

CHAPTER 78 -- POOL SAFETY

Do not use air-filled swimming aids (such as "water wings") or inflatable toys and rafts instead of life jackets where such might be needed.

If you have a home swimming pool:

1. Install a four-sided isolation pool fence with self-closing and self-latching gates around the pool. The fence should be <u>at least</u> five feet tall and should completely separate the pool from the house and the play area of the yard.

2. Prevent children from having direct access to a swimming pool. The parents in the anecdote on page 383 now have a padlocked gate with a combination lock, because a keyed lock key could probably not be kept hidden successfully from their bright little girl.

3. Install a telephone near the pool and post the emergency number 911 in an easy-to-see place.

Teach your kids what 911 means and how to use it. Tell them they can say anything they want to into the phone, or just scream "help!" and then <u>leave the phone off the hook.</u> Tell them that someone will come.

4. Please be aware that swimming programs for infants and toddlers will <u>not</u> prevent them from drowning. You alone can protect your kids. Don't get a false sense of security from these programs.

The American Academy of Pediatrics made some strong statements about these programs for little ones last year:

Children younger than four years are generally not developmentally ready for formal swimming lessons. Their parents may be ready, but they, almost certainly, are not.

Swimming programs for infants and toddlers should not be promoted as a way to decrease their risk of drowning.

Parents should <u>not</u> feel their child is safe from drowning after participation in such programs.

5. Water wings and other non-life vest flotation devices will not only <u>not</u> keep your little one from drowning, but may actually hold them underwater if they get reversed so that the flotation device is on top of the water.

Do not think for a minute that just having a high fence around the pool will prevent a motivated child's access. Two of our friends have a 2-1/2-year-old little girl whom they had found within the pool enclosure with the gate closed on two separate occasions. The little girl pretended not to know what they were talking about when they asked her how she got in. Needless to say they were pretty scared about the danger and mounted a secret spy operation to see how she did it. She was way too short to reach the latch, which was mounted at the top of a six foot gate.

Here's what her mother saw her do. The little girl pulled and pushed their beautiful large Golden Retriever until it was standing still beside the gate. Then she climbed up onto the dog's back, and, while balancing herself by leaning slightly against the gate, stood up on its back in her little bare feet. Then she stood on her tiptoes to just reach the latch and open it. She then climbed down off the dog, opened the gate, walked through it, turned, and closed it. Then she walked over and sat at the pool's edge and dangled her dainty little toes in the water.

This young lady is already an accomplished problem solver at age 2 1/2. Think what those parents are facing when she becomes a teenager! But don't pity the long-suffering family pet, which was probably proud of being an accessory to the "crime."

Adults should always be within an arm's length of infants and toddlers when they are in and around the water to provide "touch supervision" (and instant protection).

All swimming programs should include information on the mental and physical limitations of infants and toddlers, the inherent risks of water (even small amounts), strategies for prevention of drowning, and the role of adults in keeping kids safe around the water.

That is the goal of this chapter.

CHAPTER 79 -- PREGNANCY

Selecting Your OB Doctor

First, try to find out whether your state board of medical licensure has any information about all doctors you are considering, particularly whether any disciplinary action has been taken against any of them. A lot of this information can now be accessed on the Internet. In particular you need to know whether he or she has ever had a complaint for malpractice and alcohol or other drug abuse. Stay away from one of those.

The last thing you want is someone under the influence delivering your baby.

If you get to the hospital and smell alcohol on the breath of your doctor, <u>immediately</u> tell the nurse that you do not want him or her to deliver your baby. Bad stuff can happen unexpectedly at the time of delivery, and your doctor must have a totally clear head to be prepared to deal with it (or as clear as his or her head can be at three o'clock in the morning). I don't care how great your relationship with that doctor; don't let him deliver your baby.

The worst of the bad stuff that can happen is uterine hemorrhage. I have successfully treated several dozen cases of postpartum bleeding, only eight of which progressed far enough to be called hemorrhage.

Those eight were saved from possible death by my experience with the patient of one of the staff OB doctors in the hospital where I interned in South Bend, Indiana. That patient literally bled to death despite heroic efforts by at least half of the OB staff, along with the house staff (including me). I was the house officer for the hospital that night and was called frantically to the OB floor by the night nurse. I walked into the room and found the patient in shock and lying in a bed full of blood, which was not clotting (she had used up all of her clotting factor trying to stop the bleeding). I quickly ordered several pints of type O negative blood (universal donor) and all the fibrinogen (clotting factor) we had in the hospital. Unfortunately that was only 3 grams. I got blood going into all four extremities and gave the fibrinogen. Her doctor soon arrived, and within minutes half of the whole OB department was at hand. She continued to bleed.

The priority then was to get more fibrinogen and blood from the other hospital across town. Unfortunately they also had only 3 grams, and the same lab person was on call for their hospital as for ours. Thus another lab tech had to be called from home at 1:00 AM. It took 45 minutes to get the additional fibrinogen and blood.

Meanwhile her heart stopped. I had a scalpel in my hand from doing the "cut downs" on the large veins to allow massive blood replacement; so I asked if we should try open heart massage. I got a quick "yes" from the entire staff; so I opened her chest rapidly and massaged her heart. It quickly resumed beating in less that a minute. Within only a few more minutes we had blood, both from St. Joe's and from our walking blood bank of volunteers, and the anesthesiologist began to get a measurable blood pressure.

Since it wouldn't stop bleeding, the decision was made to remove her uterus, and the two best GYN surgeons on the staff quickly accomplished that. With the removal of the uterus, the massive bleeding stopped. The chest and abdominal wounds were closed, and I went off duty (I was supposed to go off at midnight, but a little overtime work was not uncommon). When I returned to work the next day, I learned that she had finally died during the night. At autopsy there was found 3000 cc of blood in the abdomen and 2000 cc in the chest cavity, more than the total for a normal whole body. Due to the lack of clotting factor, she had just kept on bleeding internally. Since the bleeding couldn't be seen, the level of concern was not as great, the rapidity of whole blood replacement was reduced, and this time when her heart stopped, it stayed stopped. The baby survived, and perhaps may read this book.

I gained heart-rending experience from this case that enabled me to save all of the other eight cases of post-delivery uterine hemorrhage that I encountered during my OB career of about 1100 deliveries. First and foremost, I made sure that every hospital in which I practiced from then on always had at least 10 grams of fibrinogen on hand at all times. That alone saved seven of the eight.

The eighth case should have died. The lessons I learned in South Bend five years before were what saved her.

She was a lady with twins in her first pregnancy, who was within a week of full term in Warsaw, Indiana. I had just arrived home from a house call (yes I really did make house calls, a lot of them) when my wife ran out to meet me and told me that the nurse in the OB department had just called to tell me that my patient was in labor, but that she was having some mild vaginal bleeding and she could not hear a heartbeat! Since I was well aware that twin pregnancies have a very high risk of premature separation of the placenta (abruptio placentae), I told my wife to call the hospital back and order a blood type and cross-match, and an IV started with an 18 gauge needle.

We lived across Pike Lake from downtown Warsaw, but three miles around. So I broke every traffic law except overtime parking and was there in five minutes. When I walked in, she looked pale and shocky. The uterus was tender and there was no heartbeat. Her cervix was fully dilated, and the baby's head was ready for delivery. In the delivery room I administered a saddle block anesthetic and prepped and draped her for the delivery. As I delivered the first baby, it was just like removing the plug from a dike and letting in the ocean! Immediately the bucket was full of blood, and the floor was covered with it. The baby was dead. So was the second one, which I delivered two minutes later.

At that point our very sharp lab tech walked in with two pints of whole blood and the statement that the blood he had drawn for the cross-match had not clotted. He showed me the tube. She had bled so much that all of her clotting factor had been used up.

Things happened very quickly then. My good surgical friend, G.H., walked in and asked if he could help (a classic understatement, if I ever heard one). I asked him to start blood in all four extremities while I packed the uterus. I ordered that we immediately give all 10 grams of fibrinogen in the hospital and get more from Ft. Wayne, 45 miles away. The lab tech had already activated the walking blood bank, and we ordered more blood also to be brought from Ft. Wayne.

The State Police had the blood and fibrinogen there in a lot less than an hour. (It must have been fun for them to be able to drive fast without chasing bad guys for a change.) I sent them a letter of commendation later but never got the name of the officer who did as much to save this lady's life as any of us.

I had learned in the tragedy in South Bend that packing the uterus as tightly as possible to press on the bleeding open blood vessels is the only thing that will have a chance of working. My surgical friend and I had each done many hysterectomies, but I knew that was not an option. So I packed it, gave massive doses of IV pitocin (it makes the uterus contract), and blood and fibrinogen – 16 units of blood and 19 grams of fibrinogen later she stopped bleeding.

A couple of days later she developed lower nephron nephrosis of the kidneys from the shock, and her kidneys shut down. We sent her down to the I U Medical Center in Indianapolis for dialysis. Her kidneys healed themselves in 10 days, and she was physically completely well. Mentally was another matter. It took a long time for her to smile again. But she did smile when I delivered a lovely child for her younger sister a year later.

The lady in South Bend did not die in vain. Her death made it possible for at least one life, and maybe more, to be saved from the same fate. If she had not died, I would not have had the knowledge to save the lady in Warsaw. And I would not have made sure that the hospitals where I delivered the other seven women with hemorrhage whom I successfully treated with up to 8 grams of fibrinogen were adequately stocked with that necessary clotting factor. So one or more of them also might have died.

At present we no longer use fibrinogen, but rather fresh frozen plasma, which provides improved clotting and other benefits. The thing you must do when you are pregnant is to ask your OB doctor to make sure that the hospital where you will deliver has adequate stores of this product, just in case you might need it.

This brings up another important thing. There seem to be a trend toward home delivery by midwives right now. Partly this may be due to economic factors. Or just the desire to have more control of your surroundings.

In Vienna in the days of Dr. Ignatz Semmelweiss, the man who discovered the cause of childbed fever, women did not want to be delivered in the hospital – for good reason – 50% died of infection. No more. A hospital is, by far, the safest place to deliver today.

For whatever reasons, <u>do not, under any circumstances, allow a delivery at home.</u> Even the most experienced of midwives are unprepared for post delivery hemorrhage. It is sudden and almost always totally unpredictable. Probably at least 75% of those cases above would have died if delivered at home by even a full OB doctor, much more likely if performed by a much lesser-trained midwife.

Foods, Supplements, and Medications in Pregnancy

Calcium and iron supplements, plus a healthy diet, are essential in all pregnant women.

Taking folic acid supplements for a couple of months before trying to become pregnant will greatly reduce the risk of neural tube defects (such as spina bifida), and other congenital malformations in your baby if the folic acid is taken along with a multivitamin supplement.

A new study now indicates that women who take medications which antagonize folic acid just before and during the early weeks of pregnancy appear to increase the risk of neural tube defects, facial clefts (hare lip and cleft palate), along with abnormalities of the heart, blood vessels, kidneys, and bladder.

The medications to avoid include trimethaprim (Bactrim or Septra taken for urinary tract infections, as well as some respiratory infections), triamterene (Dyazide taken usually for swelling and high blood pressure), sulfasalazine (Azulfidine taken usually only for ulcerative colitis), phenytoin (Dilantin taken mostly for epilepsy), and Phenobarbital, primidone, and carbamazepine (all of which are taken mostly for seizures).

Swordfish and mackerel have the highest concentrations of mercury in their bodies of all fish, apparently no matter where they are caught. Better avoid eating them during pregnancy and breast feeding.

Smoking and Pregnancy

Several good medical studies suggest that harm to the fetus may occur from even infrequent passive smoke exposure. The risk of miscarriage is greatly increased in the first 3 months of the pregnancy with <u>any</u> kind of smoke exposure. <u>Any</u> young woman who works <u>anywhere</u> in a place where smoking is allowed is being exposed to that risk right now if she is pregnant. The risk is there even before she has missed a period and becomes aware that she may be pregnant. So she has an increased risk even if she quits her job the day she misses her first period. So try to find another job before you stop using contraception.

> *The worst smoker I ever had as a pregnant patient smoked three packs of cigarettes daily throughout her pregnancy. I tried every trick I could think of to get her to at least cut down. She totally ignored me. I tried to enlist her husband as an ally, but he was of no help. He smoked two packs a day himself. She finally a delivered an underweight (4 lbs 12 oz) but full term baby with mental retardation that was apparent within a few days after birth and got progressively worse as time passed. She left my care within a month or two after delivery; so I don't know where the child is today. Probably in an institution if still alive.*
>
> *If I had the same patient today, I would try to have the court send her to jail for child abuse until after the delivery and not let her smoke in jail. But that happened thirty years ago, and child abuse by tobacco was not so well documented then as it is now. I knew the poor baby would be a bad case. I didn't suspect just how bad it would be.*

If you smoke, you must stop as long as possible before you become pregnant. The bad effects on your baby are the same as those from second hand smoke, but affect your baby to a greater degree. Stop smoking before you stop using contraception.

Several studies have shown that passive smoke exposure by a pregnant woman for as little as 2 hours per day will double the risk of having a low birth weight baby, with its many complications.

An even more important drug to totally avoid is alcohol, in any form. It is the number one cause of mental retardation in our country today. Do not take even one drink of beer, wine, or a mixed drink of any kind on New Year's Eve or any other time if you want your baby to be normal. Do not take any cough medicine that has alcohol in it. Read the labels and ask the pharmacist. Tell him you are pregnant so that he or she will check for any possible harm to the baby before dispensing your medicine. Also do not drink alcohol the whole time you are breast-feeding.

My experience with the OB case described above suggests that combining smoking with alcohol, as so often happens in our culture, is a double whammy to the brains of little fetuses and babies. Stay away from both.

Being a good girl during pregnancy will save you many thousands of dollars in medical costs for the child if it is born abnormal. In addition, it will save incalculable anguish and guilt feelings for the rest of your life. It may also save your marriage, as your husband will never forgive you, at least deep inside if you did something that even might have caused damage to the baby. If somehow the baby is abnormal in spite of all your precautions, then you will be able to deal with it without guilt or blame.

Again, I can't stress too strongly that you should <u>never</u> take any medicine or supplement without the express approval of your OB doctor. In the present day it is increasingly common for women to have a family doctor for most problems, but a different OB doctor for pregnancy. If your family doctor does not deliver babies himself, it is unlikely that he will know all the latest drugs to avoid in pregnancy. So clear <u>all</u> medications, prescription, herbal, or otherwise with your OB doctor before starting to take it.

Never take a sauna or a bath in a jaccuzi if pregnant. Both provide too much warmth for safety, and the jaccuzi increases the risk of infection developing up in the vagina and uterus.

If you have a cat, never change or come anywhere near the kitty litter box. The risk of getting toxoplasmosis, a very dangerous disease in pregnancy, is too great.

After Delivery

Every woman wants to regain her flat tummy as soon as possible after delivery, but most doctors seem reluctant to help you do that. Your abdominal muscles have been severely stretched by the baby, and they will return to the way they were before you became pregnant only by making the muscles work. Start doing tummy exercises the day after the baby was born. Just lie flat on your back and, with the knees straight, raise first one leg up to 45 degrees, hold for a few seconds, then slowly let it down. Repeat that 10 times. Do the same thing with the other leg. Rest awhile. Repeat that three to four times the first day.

The second day increase the number of repetitions by one or two for each set. Work up to where you're doing at least 30 in a row with each leg by itself at least twice a day. When you get to that stage, then it's time to add something else. Now do the straight leg lift with first one leg and then the other and then both legs together. Again gradually work up to where you're doing 30 repetitions of each at least twice a day.

When you get to that stage, then it's time to add crunches after you finish your straight leg raising each time. As you may know, you put your feet flat on the floor with your knees bent about 45 degrees and your hands on top of your head. Then simply raise your head and shoulders a few inches off the floor while you pull your knees a few inches toward your head. Start with four or five and gradually increase the number you do by one every day. But don't overdo this or your stomach muscles will get sore and give you an excuse to stop.

No one should have to motivate you; but I promise you that your husband or significant other will give you a lot of positive feedback as your stomach gets flatter and flatter. Do these exercises faithfully, every day, and I promise you that you'll have a flat abdomen in less than three months.

If you developed severe stretch marks during your pregnancy, there will always be some extra skin in the lower part of your abdomen, no matter how flat it is otherwise.

These are your badges of valor for being a mother and bringing a new life into the world. No man in his right mind will hold them against you.

Weight Loss After Pregnancy

One of the highest risk factors for long-term obesity in women is excessive weight gain during pregnancy. The most important part of this is prevention.

Limit yourself to a weight gain of about two pounds per month early in the pregnancy, and three pounds toward the end. If you were underweight to start with, you can gain perhaps three or four pounds more; while if you were overweight in the beginning, you should gain three or four pounds less.

Obese women should gain no more than about 13 or 14 pounds in the whole nine months. I had several obese women who, with good nutrition and exercise within their capabilities, actually had a net weight loss during their pregnancies. I watched them pretty carefully because I knew we were stretching the envelope, and they all delivered normal healthy babies.

Exercise daily, right up until you go into labor if possible.

With resumption of normal activity and eating habits, most of your weight gained during pregnancy will be lost within three months, and then there will be further steady loss for another three months. Some highly motivated individuals will lose faster. This chapter is devoted to some of those who are less motivated.

Mothers who breast feed their little ones and try to follow the "recommended daily requirements for lactating women" of 2,500 calories per day will almost certainly find themselves unable to lose any weight at that level. Part of this is due to the fact that a lot of women who lactate don't get very much exercise. Therefore they should eat no more than 2,000 calories worth of food per day.

> One of the main goals of this book is to promote good health through natural methods. Here we want all women, who can, to breast feed their infants for as long as possible, perhaps even a year. We also want those mothers to exercise, because exercise serves many important functions for us, not just as an aid to weight loss. We also want these mothers to recover from the obesity that all too often accompanies pregnancy as soon as possible.

One small recent study of overweight breast-feeding women produced the good news that you can have all of the above. By lowering daily calories by 500, and exercising for 45 minutes four days per week, these women lost an average of one pound per week between one month and 3 months after delivery. Their weight loss did not affect the normal growth of their babies as compared to the babies of a control group of mothers who did not restrict their calories, and did not exercise during the same time period.

So mothers, breast feed your little ones, eat less, and exercise for 30 minutes a day. And enjoy life more!

CHAPTER 80 -- PROSTATE ENLARGEMENT

Benign Prostatic Hypertrophy (BPH)

It is estimated that 80% of men past age 80 have this condition of the prostate. My own experience has been that probably 60%+ of the prostates I examine after about age 55 are at least a little bit enlarged. Others may be enlarged in a part of the gland beyond the reach of my finger. We can feel and evaluate by that method only the posterior 1/3 of the gland, which butts up against the front of the thin rectal wall. We feel for this every time we do a rectal exam. The front part of the gland surrounds the tube (urethra) that leads from the bladder to the outside through the penis. If this part of the gland is enlarged, then you may develop symptoms long before a rectal exam can notice enlargement to the finger's touch.

Not everyone with an enlarged prostate has symptoms. The symptoms that send men to their doctors are almost all related to their urine functions. One of the earliest symptoms is having to get up in the middle of the night to urinate. We call that nocturia. The next thing you may notice is that your stream is not as strong as it used to be. Then you may have to go to the bathroom a little more often. Next you may feel some urgency to get to a toilet because you can't hold it as long as before. On the other hand, as the urethra becomes more obstructed, you may have trouble starting the stream, and then have to strain a little to void. You may feel that you haven't completely emptied your bladder (and you probably haven't). Finally you may find that you can't void at all, and that requires a trip, usually in the middle of the night, to your doctor's office or the Emergency Room. (Most Urgent Care facilities are not set up to deal adequately with this situation.)

If the enlarged prostate gland prevents the bladder from emptying completely when you urinate and if there are any bacteria left in the bladder after urination, they may grow and multiply and cause an infection. All men with BPH should have a urinalysis at least once a year to watch for infection in the urinary tract. These can be silent and may not produce symptoms until they have become fairly severe.

As you begin to have prostate symptoms or at about age 50, you should begin a regular annual visit for a rectal examination, a urinalysis, and a PSA blood test to screen for early prostate cancer. Other tests may include catheterization for residual urine in the bladder after you empty your bladder as completely as possible (more than one oz of urine left is significant, and more than four ounces needs pretty active treatment.) Urinary flow rate and flow pressure tests are also helpful to your doctor in determining how to proceed.

If the obstruction becomes severe enough over a long period of time, the urine can back up into the kidneys and cause damage there in the form of hydronephrosis and high blood pressure. This is one of the few causes of hypertension that can be actually cured -- by the surgery to relieve the prostatic obstruction. See below.

Black men and men of any race with a family history of prostate cancer are at much higher risk of cancer, and these men should have their first exam at age 45. Perhaps your doctor will decide that you won't need to be checked again until 50, but follow his advice.

Your doctor may have you fill out a BPH Symptom Score sheet developed by the American Urological Association. The form assigns numbers from 0 to 5 to the amount of the above-listed symptoms you have, and active treatment is not needed until the score reaches a certain number, usually above 7.

Besides the actual enlargement of the prostate, these symptoms can be produced or aggravated by certain medications taken for other conditions. These include so-called anticholinergic drugs taken for depression (tricyclics, such as amitriptyline), or intestinal tract spasms in conditions like Irritable Bowel Syndrome (IBS), ulcerative colitis, peptic ulcer disease, or just diarrhea. Certain narcotics do the same thing, as do some diuretics and common cold remedies with decongestants in them. First-generation antihistamines for allergies, such as benadryl and chlorpheniramine (Chlortrimeton) are also causes of symptoms, especially if there is already some prostatic enlargement. Men whose BPH Symptom Scores are 15 to 20 or more should avoid all of these classes of drugs. If you take them, your urine may shut down completely until they are out of your system.

Medical treatment is usually deferred until the symptom score becomes high enough to be noticed as possibly interfering with the quality of life.

Medications include so-called complementary herbs, particularly **saw palmetto** (Serenoa repens), which inhibits an enzyme that may be responsible for the enlargement. This is used in a dose of 160 mg. twice a day. It is probably just as effective as the much more expensive drug **Proscar**, but less effective than the next drugs, which are Alpha-blockers, such as **Hytrin or Cardura**. Other plants used elsewhere in the world but not standardized or even studied very much so far include **African plum**, **South African star grass**, **stinging nettle**, and **rye pollen**. See the chapter on **Herbal Remedies** for more on herbs.

Medications such as **Flomax**, **Hytrin**, and **Cardura** may be taken to help contract the muscles of the prostate to make it smaller. These cause an immediate shrinkage of the prostate size by their direct effects on the muscles of the gland. The so-called non-selective ones include three used for control of high blood pressure (Cardura, Hytrin, and Minipress -- **prazosin** in the cheaper generic form, but it needs multiple doses). Use of these may cause dizziness, fatigue, drop in blood pressure on standing up, and general weakness in up to 10% of men with normal blood pressures. These effects can be greatly reduced by taking the medicine at bedtime, starting at a very low dose, and increasing the dose slowly so that you have a chance to get used to it.

There is just one so-called selective alpha-blocker, Flomax, and it is pretty expensive.

Proscar works by slowly reducing the level of dihydrotestosterone in the blood by up to 90%. This causes some prostates to shrink and thus reduce the symptoms of blockage of the urinary tract caused by the large size of the prostate over a period of up to 6 months. This drug is more likely to be effective if your PSA test is above 4.0 and your gland is large. It may produce unwelcome sexual side effects, including lack of desire, impotence, and problems with ejaculation.

A newer one that is part of the same family as Proscar is **Duagen**, with the same sexual side effects. I don't know yet whether it will be more effective than Proscar or saw palmetto. The drug company would like for us to think so.

Surgical Treatments

Surgical treatments include, from most to least side effects:

Suprapubic or retropubic prostatectomy with improvement in 98% of patients but lots of side effects: bleeding, incontinence, and loss of all sexual functions being the most troublesome.

Transurethral resection (TURP) through the penis, with improvement in 88%, and complications consisting of inability to void, clot retention in the bladder, infection, retrograde ejaculation in 70%, impotence in up to 30%, incontinence to some degree in 7%.

And, a new one, transurethral incision of the prostate (TUIP) through the penis, in which only one or two incisions are made in the prostate capsule to reduce its constricting effect. TUIP is an outpatient procedure that is especially good for younger men who want to continue to be sexually active and possibly father more children. There is much less bleeding and much less risk of impotence. No long-term follow-up studies are available yet, as it is too new.

Next is a nonsurgical outpatient procedure called transurethral microwave thermotherapy (TUMT) that takes about an hour. A microwave antenna is placed inside a urethral catheter and positioned in the urethra at the level of the prostate. The microwave is turned on to produce deep rapid heating of the gland, while a cooling system protects adjacent tissues that are not intended to be treated.

No major complications have been reported so far. Retreatment has been required in two years in about 7.5% of cases.

Next are destruction of the prostate by laser as transurethral vaporization of the prostate (TUVP), or electrode as transurethral electrovaporization of the prostate (TVP), and transurethral needle ablation of the prostate (TUNA). These are all relatively new, and I can't tell you much about them. They aren't offered everywhere because generally only doctors training at centers where they have been developed are able to do them. Some look promising.

Tune in later in the next edition of this book.

CHAPTER 81 -- PROTECTING YOUR CHILDREN

Supervision of small children -- who by nature are impulsive and quick -- is a full-time job. It requires one's <u>full</u> attention, particularly if the child is playing in a driveway or on a sidewalk near traffic, or around a swimming pool, ocean, lake, river, or stream -- or Morning Glory Pool in Yellowstone National Park (where a toddler fell in many years ago and was scalded to death). When in doubt of your ability to focus your concentration, put your toddler in a chest harness on a leash, one of those that extend and contract like we use in walking dogs.

Talking on a cell phone, carrying on a conversation with another adult, reading a book or magazine, running into the house "for just a minute" -- as in answering an insistently ringing phone that may well be a telemarketer -- are distractions that can lead to tragedy in the blink of an eye.

Phones are intrusive. They seldom ring at a really good time for you. You <u>don't have to answer it</u> if it is not totally convenient at that moment. That's what answering machines are for. What if the answering machine picks up, and it is someone you really want to talk to on the other end? <u>Don't answer it until you bring your child out of harm's way!</u>

Like it or not, <u>being a parent is a full-time job</u>. Take turns being in charge of watching the kids when others are around. But be sure the parent in charge at the time knows it is his or her turn to be fully alert.

At picnics and outings with friends who also have kids, let each parent take a 10 or 15 minute turn at caring for the kids. <u>Do not, however, let anyone who has had even one alcoholic drink be in charge of the children.</u>

Do not let the older kids run off somewhere out of sight. Inevitably one of the little ones will follow and may get into trouble. Have a buddy system where each child pairs up with another when you call them together, perhaps with a whistle, which you should do every 10 or 15 minutes. If one child is missing, then a search can be instituted right away instead of at the end of the outing. Perhaps the missing one just went to the bathroom, but you have to find out frequently.

It's almost impossible to anticipate all the things your kids can get into. Sometimes the problems are related, at least in part, to their perception of reality. They see people in cartoons getting knocked around, falling off cliffs, and so on, as Wily Coyote does, then getting up and shaking themselves off before running on as good as new. Most young children believe everything they see on TV or have read to them in comics.

Teach Your Kids Constantly

1. Tell your children about the dos and don'ts of safety, security and self-defense.

2. Tell them that most people are good but some people are not.

3. Tell them that there are ways they can tell when someone is not good.

4. Tell them that no matter what anybody tells them, they can and should, always come and tell you when something has happened that made them feel uncomfortable. And do not get mad at them if they do, even though you will be mad at the perpetrator. It will confuse the child, and she may not want to tell you next time.

> *We bought my older son a Superman suit for Halloween when he was about three. Unfortunately, he then thought that he could fly like Superman and jumped off our second story balcony to do so. Fortunately for his present-day patients there had been a lot of rain recently and the ground was softer than normal.*
> So he sustained only a concussion, and after a day in bed he was fine. *Had it been concrete below him when he jumped, it might have been a different story. I have been told that now all the super hero costumes come with a tag on them that says something like "just because you have this costume on doesn't mean you can really fly." Of course a three year old might have a little trouble reading it, but I guess it has happened to others as well as my son.*

5. Tell them they should immediately run away from someone whose words and actions make them feel strange or afraid and then tell their parents or teacher.

6. If someone is trying to take them somewhere against their well, they should yell as loudly as they can, "this is not my Mommy/Daddy!," and run or struggle as much as they can while they keep yelling.

7. Make up a code word with your children to be used when you can't pick them up and need to send someone else. They need to ask the pick-up person what the code word is. If the person can't say it, then the child should run away and get to safety.

8. Change the code word after it has been told to anyone outside your family.

Then there was the time when I was in the Air Force when I got an almost hysterical call at the Base from my wife telling me that our two-year-old daughter had just eaten a giant cockroach outside our trailer door. Mom found only the legs sticking out of her mouth. That time there was more damage to mother (her mental state) than daughter (none). I think we may have decided that she might need a little more protein in her diet.

9. If in danger, they should run to a safe place where there are lots of other people. Someone will help them.

10. Tell them to throw down what ever they are carrying if they need to run faster, that they will not get in trouble if they do.

11. All children should memorize their parents' first and last names, their addresses and their telephone numbers including work numbers. In our grade school when I was a child, our teacher taught us a little song about what to do. I hope that song, or one like it, is still around in every school.

12. Children should be taught to <u>never</u> take rides from strangers.

13. Children should never go with someone who offers them money or anything else to get in their car.

14. They should never go with someone who wants to help them look for a lost pet, nor with someone who wants help in looking for a lost pet.

15. They should never go with someone who says, "we caught your friend stealing and we will arrest you if you don't come with us."

16. They should never go with someone who says, "your mother has been hurt and we're here to take you to the hospital."

17. Teach them the difference between good and bad touches. Anytime someone touches them where their bathing suits are worn, they should run, yell, and always tell their parents about it.

18. They should be told it's not their fault if someone does this, that you love them and they did the right thing by telling you.

19. If you child is molested, get counseling for your child. And for yourself.

20. Tell your children to report to you anybody who does a bad touch

When my children went with us as pre-schoolers to Yellowstone National Park we put harnesses on them and a leash to keep them from venturing off the paths and possibly falling into one of the pools of boiling water. Same thing when we went to the Grand Canyon. Speaking of which, it seemed every year that I lived here in Flagstaff, there was a report from the Canyon where someone climbed over a rail to get a better view or to take a picture and fell a thousand feet to his death. This happened to the college student daughter of a close doctor friend of mine.

even if that person tells them, "you'll get in trouble if you do," or "let's keep this our secret," or "I'll hurt your puppy, brother, sister, or family if you tell."

These Are Important Even for Older Children:

21. Never go out alone.

22. Always tell an adult where you are going and when you will be back.

23. Say "no" if you feel threatened. Get away from the person or situation that is making you feel this way.

Kids (and adults too) must always wear protective helmets when riding on or with someone on a bicycle. (Don't even <u>consider</u> letting your child of <u>any</u> age ride a motorcycle or an ATV until old enough for a drivers' license.)

There is a problem with bike helmets for kids. The August 2003 edition of *Pediatrics* reported that a pediatrician had done a study of 479 patients and their siblings involving whether their bike helmets fit properly and thus provided the expected protection for fragile heads in children from ages 4 through 18 years.

Only 4% of the helmets were in good shape and fit right, according to the article. Most of the problems involved poor fitting. 52% of the helmets were too high on the forehead; too much front-to-back movement in 52%; and the straps were too loose in 33%.

The article's author, Dr. Gregory W. Parkinson, recommended a three-stage fitting process which he calls "MVP": M for moving the helmet down to less than two finger breadths above the eyebrows for forehead protection; V for the position of the two side straps, which should be snug in a V shape on both sides of the ears; and P for pulling the chin strap snug.

Never leave your child in the car alone in the summer, especially where I live, in Arizona. A baby can die in just a few minutes, and an older child can become overheated to the point of needing IV fluids, also in just a few minutes. Better yet, never leave your child alone in a car. Period. Never mind that it is a pain in the rear to get the child in and out of the safety seat. If your child is always with you, it will be safe. Believe that, even if you have heard of exceptions.

Missing children can be identified even years later by their dental record, which is actually better than fingerprints. Also by their DNA. An easy, inexpensive way to make your own dental records for your children is to take a 1/2 inch thick piece of styrofoam the size of each child's mouth and have them bite into it moderately. This gives you not only a dental record, but also a sample of DNA from the child's saliva. To complete the ID kit for your child, put a recent color photo along with the styrofoam into a Ziploc bag and store it in a safe place. Include a note with any birthmarks or other identifying information. Then you will have something that will be of great value to the police if something should happen to your child. Update the photo every 6 months. Be sure it is a full face picture.

Do not let children have alcohol at any time until legal age. Many studies have shown that the younger the child is exposed to alcohol, the more likely it is to become an alcoholic when older. I'm not even sure medicinal alcohol, as in cough medicine, is a good idea.

Babies

Never sleep with your baby in your bed with you. There have been many cases where the infant somehow slipped down under the covers and suffocated. That happened to a baby that I personally delivered. I was sad about that for many months.

Use of Walkers. In 1999 about 8,800 children were treated in hospital ERs for injuries caused by the use of infant walkers. By far a huge majority of these also involved stairs, as in pushing the walker to the edge and then falling down the stairs. Most of the injuries were fractures and head injuries. How many more less severe accidents there were that were treated at home, family doctor's office, or urgent care facility can only be guessed at. But there were probably a lot more than 8,800.

Most walkers are used with the idea of getting the child to walk sooner. Although this may seem logical, a number of studies have conclusively shown that those who use walkers show sitting, crawling, and walking capability <u>later</u> than those who do not use walkers.

Preventing walker-related injuries. I highly recommend <u>never</u> starting to use one.

If you feel you must use the one that great aunt Tammie gave you for a birth present, then do the following things: first, watch the child just as though you were at the swimming pool.

Second, make whatever changes in the household structure that you must, such as stair and/or door gates, to ensure that falls won't occur.

Third, try to get or exchange for a walker that is more than three feet wide and thus won't pass through standard three-foot wide doors. Or, with heavy duty strapping tape, tape a couple of lengths of cutoff broomstick handles to front and back of the walker. This, of course means that anything on the coffee table is at risk, but it does help keep the child in the same room with you -- perhaps.

You won't always be able to protect your children. By their very nature they try very hard to do anything they can to get away from parental control. But keep trying anyway. Do the <u>best</u> you can.

CHAPTER 82 -- PULMONARY EMBOLISM

Pulmonary embolisms (blood clots in the lungs) kill or incapacitate thousands of people each year. The mechanism is very simple: due to the fact that there is very low blood pressure in the deep veins of the legs (the vessels that return the blood to the heart, you recall) they partly need the assistance of the squeezing action of the surrounding muscles of the calf and thigh to push the deoxygenated blood uphill to the heart.

When you sit or stand almost perfectly still for a long time (in as in a military review, where someone always seems to pass out because too much blood has pooled in the legs to allow the brain to continue to receive its full share) the blood just sits there in the veins without moving. After awhile in certain individuals a clot will form in that unmoving blood.

This clot will usually get larger and larger, sometimes extending all the way from the foot to inside the lower abdomen before medical intervention is sought. Swelling of the foot and ankle on the affected side begins to occur when the clot extends above the knee, and when swelling reaches the thigh, the clot is already up into the abdominal blood vessels.

*<u>See your doctor.</u> **If you notice new swelling of just one foot and ankle for no apparent reason, see a doctor immediately. It could be deep venous thrombosis (DVT), and you need to find out right away before a piece of the clot breaks off and passes up into the heart and lungs.**

There are basically two types of DVT: (1) those where there is a lot of associated inflammation and therefore tenderness of the vein, and (2) those where there is little or no deep vein inflammation. Number (1) is much less dangerous because the inflammatory reaction tends to attach the clot to the vein wall and keep it in place.

But in number (2) there is nothing to prevent a clot varying in size from that of a sesame seed all the way up to a cylinder of thick gelatinous material several inches long from breaking lose and traveling up the inferior vena cava to the right side of the heart and on out into the lungs. That event quickly and totally stops the body's ability to transport oxygen to the tissues. A man who is walking with his daughter in the hospital hall while recovering from surgery starts to say something and instead suddenly crumples to the floor, dead. CPR is of no avail in such cases.

It is important for you to know that having a blood clot under the skin or in a muscle anywhere is not in itself at all dangerous. It will definitely be sore if caused by a bump or bruise. The only danger that bruises or blood clots under the skin represent is that of something wrong with your blood clotting mechanism if there was no trauma. Usually in those cases there will soon be <u>several</u> areas of "bruising" where there was nothing to explain them. (See the chapter on **Drugs in the Elderly** for an example.) The only clots that you have to worry about are those in the blood vessels.

Treating and being treated for DVT is a pain in the rear; and many doctors who are very good in other areas miss some of the subtle tricks needed to produce the best possible outcomes. I studied under an internationally renowned vascular surgeon who made sure that his students learned all the tricks. First, you need medical assistance to stop further clotting from occurring (after you have a diagnostic procedure, such as an ultrasound, that gives you a positive diagnosis). This almost always means hospitalization while you are started on anticoagulants, usually heparin and coumadin. When the coumadin level in the blood reaches the therapeutic range in three days or so, if all else is okay, you can go home.

Here's where this book will prove its worth. Treatment must be done <u>exactly</u> as outlined here to be sure of the best possible result.

(1) Anticoagulation usually must go on for at least six months, with <u>frequent prothrombin clotting time (pro time) determinations</u>, which measure your blood's ability to clot. These are very important. <u>Do them faithfully</u>. If you don't, the clot could become active again. Or your blood's ability to clot could become too impaired, and <u>you could have a hemorrhagic stroke and die</u>. Normally you should have a prothrombin time every two weeks after your dose has stabilized. In some people once a month is often enough, but I have personally seen two people who had been on the monthly schedule, with no change for <u>several</u> months, suddenly get into trouble for no apparent reason. I recommend every two weeks now, and I always will, more often if the pro time isn't stable. <u>You can't take herbs when you are on this treatment.</u>

(2) You must wear elastic stockings (not "supp hose") from your toes to as high as your doctor recommends -- at least knee length -- 23 hours a day.

(3) You must elevate the leg higher than the heart all night and as many hours as possible each day for at least the first several weeks.

(4) You must elevate the leg at work, while watching TV, while waiting in the doctor's office, etc. When traveling, don't be the driver. Sit in the back of the vehicle with your leg up on the seat. Stop the car every 30 minutes and get out and walk for two or three minutes.

(5) At all times when you are awake, pretend that you have ants in your shoes and keep wiggling your toes and moving your ankles. This will make the muscles in your leg contract and keep squeezing the blood up toward the heart.

(6) When you are not in bed, you must never stand totally still nor sit with your legs hanging down. When you are up, you must be constantly moving your feet, toes, and legs to promote circulation. You are either up and walking, or you are down with your foot elevated while wiggling your toes and moving your foot up and down. Never sit with your foot on the floor (no "dangling").

The clotted veins usually develop some permanent valve damage; so you may need to wear elastic stockings for the rest of your life. But if you pay full attention to these instructions, you will have the best possible chance to get completely well.

Be aware that Coumadin and Warfarin are different names for the same drug. Coumadin is the brand name, while Warfarin is the generic name.

Prevention of Blood Clots in Everyday Life

Traveling for long hours in airplanes, for example, from the Orient back to the United States for 12 or 14 hours, puts one at higher risk for developing blood clot in your leg. The dehydration* that occurs from lack of fluid intake thickens the blood to make it more likely to clot. Caffeine and alcohol intake actually act to *increase* the tendency to dehydration by causing hyperactivity of the kidneys, so stay away from them on a long trip. And sitting for long hours with the legs dependent lets the blood just sit down in your legs without moving, waiting to clot. England's Heathrow Airport reported recently that several hundred travelers each year are diagnosed there with DVT.

> *Recently an elderly patient of mine was given a new prescription for Warfarin at a new drugstore contracted with her new HMO, while she continued to refill her Coumadin at the old drugstore. She got into serious overdose problems within two weeks with a prothrombin time of 92 seconds (normal therapeutic level is about 22-24) and bruises all over her body but, fortunately, did not have the severe stroke that she was headed for when we discovered the mistake.*

(1) Since clots occur more often after a long ride of more than an hour in some form of transportation (and especially after a twelve to fourteen hour airplane flight to the Orient), you should wiggle your toes, move your ankles, and tighten your calf and thigh muscles about every five minutes throughout the trip. Besides preventing blood clots, you will find that you feel more refreshed when you arrive at your destination. If possible, get up or get out and walk around for at least a minute or two every hour. If you are in an auto, stop at a safe place about every hour and walk around for a couple of minutes. Rise up on your toes and rock back on your heels many times every time you are up.

(2) Taking aspirin before starting the trip is also a good idea, particularly if you're in a higher risk group, as in smokers.

(3) And drinking lots of fluids which do <u>not</u> contain caffeine or alcohol will help prevent the dehydration which causes the blood to thicken, making it more likely to clot. If you are flying coach, you will not be offered *any* fluids, much less extra water, more often than about every two hours, and then only about 4 ounces at a time. So it is best to take along a couple of containers of bottled water for personal use in addition to that provided on the plane. Also, don't hesitate to make a pest of yourself by turning on the cabin attendant light for your seat and asking for water several times. If the "fasten seat belt sign" is off, then take the opportunity to walk around and go back to the flight attendants to make your request for water in person. Or juice. Or 7-Up. Or anything that doesn't contain caffeine or alcohol.

(4) Older people especially, and those at higher risk for blood clots, such as smokers and those with recent injuries or surgery, would be better protected if they would add knee-length elastic stockings to the above suggestions for the duration of the flight. Do not use full-length stockings because your knees will be bent almost all the time, and the kinking of the stockings behind the knees will interfere with the circulation enough to actually *increase* the risk.

The collapse and death of Emma Christoffersen, a healthy, physically fit 28 year old woman, from pulmonary embolus immediately after a Sydney, Australia to London, England flight in September 2000 has *finally* alerted the airline industry abroad to the risks that we physicians have been aware of for years. As a result several foreign international carriers have included warnings in their in-flight pamphlets, along with suggestions for in-flight exercises for prevention. Emirates Airlines of Dubai has even started handing out inflatable footpads to increase blood circulation in the legs of their passengers by allowing them to exercise in their seats. There appears to be some movement toward preventive education in some U.S. carriers soon also.

All the suggestions above apply equally to long bus and auto trips. But in those modes there are many more opportunities to actually get out for rest stops. They don't, however, provide beverages on call, so take bottles of water with you.

(5)If you smoke, stop.

(6)If you take estrogen for hormone replacement therapy or in a birth control formula, your risk of developing a blood clot some time is increased. If you also smoke, your risk increases enormously. At this time most of us feel that anyone over 35 who smokes should not be on birth control pills, nor be given estrogen hormone replacement therapy. For sure <u>you should take a baby aspirin every day to provide as much protection as possible</u>, in addition to these suggestions.

Prevention After Surgery

There is considerable risk of developing blood clots in the legs after surgery, especially if the surgery lasts more than an hour. For this reason (and others) your surgeon will tell the nurses to get you out of bed very soon after the procedure. And you may have elastic stockings on your legs. And you may (and should) be urged to wiggle your toes and stretch and flex your legs a lot to promote circulation in them.

There is a recent movement toward the use of low molecular weight heparin during the first day or two days after certain surgical procedures. There is also some discussion about starting to use it in most surgical procedures. This can be tricky. We want our blood to clot completely at the surgical site before we do anything to affect our clotting capability. But when the risk of bleeding at the operation site is past, then we want the extra clotting tendency to go away.

The reason that blood clots occur after surgery is that part of our bodies' defense mechanism involves making the blood clot quicker and easier all over the body after even a small wound to the skin. That helps to prevent us from bleeding to death (as people with hemophilia sometimes do) when we have a bad laceration.

A person having a second surgical procedure within a short time after the first one has a much greater risk of developing deep vein thrombosis. If you or a member of your family is about to have a second operation, be sure to talk to the surgeon about doing something to actively prevent deep venous thrombosis from occurring. It can occur within an hour or two after surgery the second time around. I have reason to believe that giving long-acting heparin (Loxitane or enoxaparin) is now absolutely essential in second surgery situations.

Prevention in a Full Leg Cast

Wiggle your toes constantly. Pretend you have ants in your cast and that you are trying to get them out. Elevate your leg as high as you can as often as you can. Never sit with the leg just hanging down and doing nothing.

Prevention if You Have Congestive Heart Failure

Don't give up just because your heart is failing. I had one wonderful lady who lived a little more than 20 years with heart failure! Your ankles and feet tend to swell, and the circulation is sluggish. But the same things work here too: Elevate your feet as high as, or higher than, your heart as often as possible. Walk around within your limitations several times an hour if possible. If you are attached to an oxygen tank, ask for ten or twelve feet of tubing so that you can at least walk around in one room a lot. Wiggle your toes a lot when you are sitting or lying down. Watch for a sudden marked increase in the swelling of one leg but not the other. That could mean a clot is forming in the more swollen leg. Take your aspirin.

Following these suggestions will <u>greatly</u> reduce your risk of ever having a deep vein thrombosis and improve your rapid and full recovery chances if you do get one.

CHAPTER 83 -- RAPE

Treatment and Possible Ways to Prevent it

I'm not an authority on rape, but I've taken care of far too many women who have been raped to not have some pretty strong ideas.

Many men become sexually aroused by the mere sight of a naked or almost naked woman. Most of the men who haven't had too much to drink at a topless bar have a continuous erection while the dancers are on stage.

Wearing mini skirts without panty hose to work may be sending the wrong message to the men there. Unless, of course, you are advertising your wares to two or three guys you would like to go out and maybe have sex with. In other words, examine your motives before wearing clothes that may be sexually provocative, whether it be to work, at a bar, or on a date.

But mentally ill rapists even rape old women, so it's not just the mini skirts.

Date Rape

My wife, a former school teacher, tells me that most girls enjoy flirtation and think that it begins and ends with verbal and light physical "teasing" or just appealing behavior. They only want to attract the interest of the guy. But men read this behavior as "she's hot" or "she wants it." As they say, men are from Mars; women are from Venus. Date rape is often the ultimate breakdown in communication between the sexes.

Most girls learn very early the things that turn men on. They read magazines; they talk with their girlfriends; and they practice their wiles on boys. Practicing your wiles on boys may be fairly safe if the boys are young and inexperienced. Doing the same with an older boy who may want to be sexually active can lead to date rape. If your glances and your clothes and your body language suggest that you want sex, then many boys and men won't want to stop when you suddenly say "no." Most but not all boys and men are taught to respect a girl's wishes when she says "no." (And you are allowed to say "no" at any time, no matter how far foreplay has progressed.)

Other boys and men, especially those who have been sexually active in the past and those who are used to having their own way, and those who have had several drinks, may force themselves upon you. This is called date rape.

Many, if not most, date rapes are planned ahead of time. Girls, don't leave your drink unattended while you go to the ladies room or dance, especially with a new guy you don't know very well. Date rape drugs have a way of finding themselves into your drinks if you are inattentive. And always limit yourself to one alcoholic drink. You begin to lose control of yourself with more than one. If you feel sick, ask the waitress for help. Don't leave with that new boyfriend. Go home in a cab -- the people at the bar can call one for you. Or call 911.

It is best that you get acquainted in a safe environment with a guy you are going to go out with. A Coke or brunch after church would seem to be a really ideal situation. Unfortunately, not very many relationships start with that kind of idealistic condition. The next best thing is a lunch date or a Coke after work with both of you bringing your own transportation. A double date with another girl you know pretty well and trust is usually good. Always take at least enough money with you on a date to be able to pay for your half of a meal and a long cab ride home. Don't wear sexually provocative clothes unless that's what you have in mind. Don't allow the guy to touch you in any kind of a suggestive way, or even repeatedly touch or stroke your bare skin.

Non-Date Rape

This can happen at any time, in any place, but mainly if you are alone. Obviously trying to walk home alone late at night when you can't get a cab is asking for trouble. At the very least, you may be robbed. We read all the time about what can happen at the very worst! How ironic if you successfully fend off a date rape, only to be then in a situation where even worse can happen. Call 911.

Also carry a container of MACE. If your local laws don't allow you to do that, move somewhere else.

I can't tell you how important it is for all women to take a course in self- defense. They aren't very expensive, especially when you consider the peace of mind that the course empowers you with. These courses should, and usually do, include teaching you how to avoid potentially dangerous situations. Martial arts courses are not for everyone, but I guarantee you will learn something useful even if you are never in a dangerous predicament. Prevention is the best medicine.

In many states, Arizona is one, a private citizen can take a course, learn to shoot and get a concealed carry permit for a gun. The courses require you to pass a written exam on the law and teach you when you are legally allowed to defend yourself with deadly force. They often include a chapter on the historical right to bear arms conferred by the

Second Amendment to the U. S. Constitution. The final exam is always a trip to a shooting range where you are required to demonstrate that you can properly handle a firearm and hit a man-sized target at 5 to 20 feet with the weapon that you plan to carry.

I have <u>several</u> lady friends who have these cards and do carry small handguns under certain circumstances. The favorite weapons are the Lady Smith and the Smith and Wesson Model 60. Both of these are .38 caliber pistols for self defense which are heavy duty enough to stop a thug but small enough to carry in a handbag or fanny pack or in a strap-on holster under your dress. They are 5-shot revolvers. Glock has a small lightweight semi-automatic (it fires one shot each time you pull the trigger) which holds ten rounds and seems to be very reliable. My experience with guns is quite extensive, and I have seen jams occurring in semi-automatics at every one of the hundreds of pistol matches I have attended. For women, I believe that the simplest gun is best. With the revolvers about all you have to do is point and pull the trigger. <u>But never point a gun at anyone unless you feel that your life is in danger and you want to kill him.</u>

Paxton Quigley has a great little book on the subject of self-protection for women. It is available, not

An attractive fifty-year-old lady I know in Phoenix was going home from the Symphony, walking alone down a side street to where her car was parked. it was a night when the Phoenix Suns were in town, so the downtown parking was at a premium. A friend whom she had expected would be with her had begged off at the last minute. As she walked, a car with three men in it drove slowly by. Then it speeded up and turned the next corner. She didn't like the glances directed at her by the men and increased her pace. The car came up behind her again and she heard suggestive remarks being made about her. Again the car sped away around the corner. It circled the block one more time, drove past her and stopped. This is one cool lady! Without breaking stride, she reached into her purse and pulled out her Lady Smith, making sure it was visible to the occupants. The next sounds she heard were, "Oh, shit, she's got a gun!" then the screeching of tires and, "Fuck you, lady!" as they drove off.

She told me later that she now even more firmly believes in the bumper sticker frequently seen here in the West, "Nobody ever raped a Smith and Wesson." She was scared, but she had mentally prepared herself for just such a situation by taking a self-defense class and thinking through several possible scenarios. The first thing her class taught her was how to stay away from possibly dangerous conditions. The next time she has to compete with basketball and/or baseball fans for parking places, she will get there much earlier, before the parking barns are full.

surprisingly, at most gun shows, but can be ordered by any bookstore for you. It costs about $11.00 and will be worth many times that to you in peace of mind, if nothing else. **The book is** *Not An Easy Target, Paxton Quigley's Self-Protection for Women.* **A Fireside book published by Simon & Schuster.**

I would not ever hesitate to kill a rapist. Don't think of it as killing another human being. Those people are sub-human. I firmly believe they do not belong in our society and deserve to live far less than the animals killed by the thousands at the stockyards every day so that we can eat.

If a man bent on sexual assault catches you, you must use your wits to stay alive. You don't want to be raped, but you will survive and, with professional help, get well. Rapists are often killers.

Never allow him to get you into a car without screaming, fighting, kicking, biting. Getting into a vehicle can literally be fatal. Scratching doesn't accomplish much as a deterrent, but getting some of his skin under your fingernails will set him up for a conviction based on DNA match if he is caught. Also it makes him easier to recognize by the police when they are out searching for suspects.

An elbow to the nose can break it easily and will probably end the fight. A knee or your heel to the testicles (the best angle is from below) will put him down if you really hit them squarely. You rarely will be as strong as he is, but you can do a lot of damage when your adrenalin is pumping.

You must use your wits! First and foremost, scream! And keep screaming.

> *Be aware that many people won't do <u>anything</u> to help. There was a case in the courtyard of a New York City apartment complex several years ago, where a poor young girl was being attacked by a man with a knife. She screamed and screamed and fought until she bled to death over a long period of time. It was summer, and everyone had their windows open, but no one even called the police until her cries stopped! I haven't liked New York very much ever since. I grew up in a small town in Indiana, and I guarantee you that girl would have received help very quickly there. Probably someone would have grabbed his or her gun from the closet and shot him. Same thing in Arizona. In New York shooting him would just get the shooter put in jail probably.*
> *It occurs to me that New Yorkers may have an entirely different approach to helping others since September 11, 2001. No one in the Midwest, or anywhere else, could have done any better in any way than the good people of New York did at that time!*

One girl talked a rapist out of it when she insisted that he wear a condom. Another told the attacker that she was HIV positive. Another started crying and curled up in a ball and sucked her thumb. Another asked him what his mother or sister would think of his conduct. Would he rape them? Another just kept screaming.

I'm sure that many women have died resisting. Usually the man is bigger and stronger and will ultimately have his way with you unless you can talk him out of it, or scream for help until someone hears you and tries to help.

If you have been raped, you will feel very ashamed and helpless. Just remember, it isn't your fault. <u>You are not a bad person because you have been raped. It is not your fault!</u> Be angry! That is the most normal and healthy reaction. Find help any way you can: call 911 and tell them you have just been raped.

Go to an Emergency Room, within a couple of hours if possible. Don't wait till the next day. Certain things need to be done by the doctor as soon as she can get to you in the ER. The ER doctor will take a semen sample from your vagina, as well as comb your pubic hair for any loose hairs that might have come from your attacker. He or she will give you a prescription for the "morning after pill" to keep you from getting pregnant. It actually is two pills which need to be started within 24 hours of intercourse to be the most effective, but will still have a pretty good probability of success out to 72 hours. Taking an anti nausea pill with them, such as compazine or meclizine, to reduce the nausea that the hormone sometimes causes is a good idea, and the doctor should think of that. If not, remind him.

See your family doctor or gynecologist as soon as possible for follow-up, the next day if possible. Tell the receptionist that you have been raped and need to see the doctor that day. Don't take no for an answer and they will almost certainly squeeze you in. You will need support and <u>several sessions with a good psychologist or a caring doctor</u> to help you through it. If you don't get professional help, you will likely not be a whole person the rest of your life. The mental scars will always be there, but the psychologist will help you to work through it and put it permanently behind you.

> *If they catch the man who did this to you, you must be prepared to testify against him. Be tough! Make sure he isn't allowed to stay free and do the same to other girls. His attorney may make all kinds of insinuations about you at the trial. She (it will almost always be a woman, to try to show the jury that he is such a good guy that a woman is defending him) may try to persuade the jury that, because you may have had sex with other guys, you are therefore a whore and it's your fault. Just remember that even whores have the right to say no. And tell her that!*

She will go through your life as far back as she can to look for any little thing she can find to divert the jury, as, for example in the Kobe Bryant case in Colorado, where the fact that the victim was treated for depression was brought up in a derogatory way to be used against her. Of course the defense attorney failed to mention that being raped might make her depressed for the rest of her life!

The most important thing is to survive. <u>Then you must seek his punishment.</u>

CHAPTER 84 -- RESISTING INFECTION

Resisting is different from *avoiding* infection. Avoiding infection involves staying away from germs, while resisting involves our bodies' defense mechanisms after we have been exposed. Avoidance is a good plan when possible, especially when a flu or SARS epidemic is going on. As a general rule try to avoid allowing people with obvious respiratory symptoms to get any closer than three feet away from you. Move, when possible, if there is someone coughing behind or beside you in a theater or other gathering.

Wash your hands a lot, several times a day -- particularly before meals and after going to the restroom. If you get a small scrape on the skin, wash it right away and leave it open to the air.

Flush your nostrils with eight or ten squirts of a saline nose spray, then blow it all out after every time you have been out in a crowd during cold and flu season, also after an airplane flight. ***Save money by mixing your own spray solution, 1/8 to 1/4 teaspoonful of table salt to 8 oz water.**

Resisting the germs already in our bodies is a job for our immune systems. The immune system works the hardest when we sleep. One hour of sleep before midnight is worth two hours after midnight. Hundreds of my patients have told me that they became ill after one or two nights of shortage of sleep. The antibodies that kill germs work best during the sleeping hours. The antibodies are in the white blood cells and travel to infection sites in the blood stream. White blood cells come in several types, some directed more towards bacteria and others more towards viruses. Lymph glands filter out infectious agents so that they won't spread to the rest of the body. The liver, spleen, and bone marrow all play their parts in the immune system.

Resisting germs also involves trying to eliminate them from our bodies before they set up shop and cause an infection.

The way our respiratory system works to resist infection is pretty easy and effective when functioning normally. In simple terms, the mucous membranes secrete a thin fluid that is intended to wash foreign material, such as air pollution particles (including tobacco smoke), bacteria (larger) and viruses (smaller), off the surfaces clear down to and out of the alveoli (the last little air sacs of the lungs, you remember from our anatomy lesson, where oxygen passes from the lungs into the bloodstream and waste carbon dioxide passes from the blood into the lungs, to be breathed out).

The surfaces of the air tubes in the lungs have tiny hair-like structures called cilia. They move rhythmically in waves, causing the mucous to flow up toward the top of the trachea, where it flows over the edge and down the esophagus into the stomach. In the stomach the bacteria are usually are killed by the hydrochloric acid in the digestive juices. Or, if the quantities are larger at times, then a cough is stimulated and the material is coughed up. So a healthy mucous membrane is continuously washing itself.

This mechanism breaks down when the mucosa is swollen and inflamed, as in acute infection or chronic irritation from noxious agents such as tobacco smoke.

Just one puff of a cigarette paralyzes your natural airway resistance for eight hours. Smoking one whole cigarette paralyzes your natural resistance for twenty-four hours.

Alcohol in any amount also inhibits your body's resistance to infection by poisoning the immune system a little, especially the liver. So at the very least, avoid alcohol (except, perhaps, in the cough syrup) whenever you have any kind of infection.

One of the major illnesses of alcoholics in the inner cities is tuberculosis, (and drug resistance is becoming an increasing problem.) One of the first things we look for in a wino who comes to the hospital is active tuberculosis. Their immune systems are virtually non-existent. Same thing for smokers with respiratory illnesses. The natural cleansing mechanisms of the lungs are chronically paralyzed, so they harbor disease-producing germs at all times, just waiting for the overall immune system to be weakened by a virus, lack of sleep, too much alcohol at holiday parties (or otherwise), getting chilled, etc. Then, instead of throwing off the virus and getting well, the smoker adds one or more of the bacterial colonies to the mix, and thus multiple antibiotics often will be needed because some of these bacteria have developed antibiotic resistance.

As tobacco exacts its toll on the lungs, the mucous membranes become thicker, so that less mucous is produced. What is produced is thicker and doesn't flow and cleanse as easily. The third nail in the coffin is that just one puff of a cigar or cigarette causes paralysis of the little cilia for eight hours, while a whole cigarette paralyzes them for twenty-four hours. Thus the lungs of smokers never properly cleanse themselves. Secretions, often laden with germs, build up in the little alveolar sacs. The walls of the sacs break down by the hundreds and thousands, and infections occur over and over.

Eventually emphysema (also known as COPD) results, with its constant shortness of breath, buildup of carbon dioxide in the blood and large pockets of dried secretions blocking any air exchange of carbon dioxide and oxygen. The death is a horrible one. For several years the person will be on oxygen constantly, with a walk-around bottle when leaving home and an oxygen concentrator (much cheaper than oxygen tanks) at home.

Near the end the person will be on life support in the hospital. <u>This is a very expensive terminal illness.</u>

Stopping smoking personally in time, as well as avoiding second hand exposure, will prevent this terrible condition.

*100 percent of asthmatic or formerly asthmatic people who smoke will eventually get emphysema (COPD).

Resisting urinary tract infections involves most simply being sure that you drink enough fluids to make you urinate every two hours and thus flush out bacteria that may be accumulating in the bladder before they can burrow into the bladder wall. There are special instructions for women in the chapter on **Urinary Tract Infections.**

Exercise definitely helps one to resist infection, and to throw off infections more quickly when they do occur. The mechanism isn't totally clear, but there are some good educated guesses as to why. One is that the normal slight rise in body temperature that occurs with exercise kills germs. Another is that every tissue in your body is made more healthy by exercise.

One caution is that you shouldn't run or do any more than just some mild exercise without getting tired when you have a fever of 100 degrees or more. There have been cases reported of myocarditis in people who exercised too much while feverish. So listen to your body, not the mind that is telling you about all the conditioning that you are losing. Go for a little walk, but forget about running or playing ball for awhile.

> *In one malpractice case that I was recently asked to consult on, the patient was a 30-plus-year smoker whose doctors had repeatedly told him, to no avail, to quit smoking. When he died of overwhelming sepsis within three days after the onset of an infection, cultures from his lungs revealed Klebsiella, Pneumococcus and Staph aureus. Any one of these could have been enough to kill him with the weakened state of his lungs. There was no malpractice. He never had a chance.*

CHAPTER 85 -- SAVING MONEY ON DRUGS

There are numerous ways that we Americans are seeking ways to save money on prescription drugs. If you have read the chapter on **Herbal Remedies**, then you have already started to save, mainly by drastically reducing your use of potentially dangerous herbal products.

We ask our friends who are going abroad to buy us a supply of the more expensive drugs we are using while they are on foreign shores. We go to Mexico, where whole small cities are devoted to helping Americans save money on their drug and dental bills. We do the same in Canada, where the drugs are likely to be safe, unlike off-brand medications in Mexico. We get on the Internet and order meds from New Zealand, where again they are likely to be safe.

If you do order from a foreign country, you are allowed to order or obtain only a three-month supply at a time. In Algodones, Mexico the American INS personnel will send you back into Mexico if you are too blatant about importing large quantities. We are not talking about illegal narcotics here, but regular drugs that require a prescription in the U.S. but not in other countries.

If you obtain drugs from foreign sources, especially third world countries such as Mexico, it is safe and prudent to get only brand-name drugs made by U.S. companies and in the same packages that they appear in here. The bottles should be sealed and not re-packaged.

Drug companies in this country are putting a lot of pressure on the FDA (Food and Drug Administration) to prevent states and individuals from obtaining medications elsewhere. The chief reason has nothing to do with safety but is because they drug companies charge more here than in any other country in the world. Safety does enter into the equation because the FDA does keep out drugs which have not met their stringent rules for demonstrating that they work, that the pills have in them what the package says they have, and that the drug won't cause babies to be born without arms (remember the terrible thalidomide problem of 45 years ago that the FDA saved our country from?).

The drug companies do have a point because it costs more to bring a new drug to the market here than in most other countries. So they probably should be allowed to charge more, but more within reason than now.

I am probably not one who can objectively assess present day prices of *any* kind because I grew up during the latter part of the Great Depression. While my own family survived well due to the hard work of both of my parents, I had many young friends who often did not have enough to eat, nor a warm sweater in winter.

I believe that the cost of Medicine is high, in some instances obscenely high. That's part of the reason for my writing this book. I believe that governmental interference plays a large part in that high cost. The cost of medical education is astronomical (see the chapter on **Doctors' Fees**). I know young physician colleagues who are as much as $150,000 in debt as they start their practices. Yet their fees are tightly restricted by the HMOs and their friends on the Federal Trade Commission (FTC).

What can you personally do to combat these high costs? We've already mentioned a few above. Here are some more.

1. Request a trial on a generic drug before being put on a brand name medicine that is still on patent. We now have good generic drugs available for 90% or more of all medical conditions. Almost all physicians are more than a little sympathetic to the plight of our patients as far as drugs are concerned. We will oblige you any way we can.

2. Ask your physician if any free samples are available for that medicine. If so, then he or she will give you at least enough to get started and thus defray some expense.

3. Explore drug prices on the Internet: on www.google.com, type in the name of your drug. Google will then list all the online pharmacies that handle that drug. You must write notes for each site. Some advertise "lowest prices on the Net" but charge for shipping and handling, while others don't. Some advertise a three month supply for $xx, while others advertise a one month supply for a much lower price.

4. Buy drugs from cities and states that don't charge sales taxes on them. Most don't by now.

5. If you are over 50, you can join AARP and become eligible for reduced rates from their pharmacy

6. The price of different sizes of many drugs is the same, or almost the same price. A partial list of these drugs, recently compiled by one of my longtime pharmacist friends, follows below. Some are in pill form and are scored for easy cutting in half. Some are in pill form but not scored; however most pharmacies carry inexpensive little pill cutters to help you cut more accurately.

The point is: if you can tell your doctor that larger sizes are available for about the same price, he or she can and will order the larger size for you and thus save you up to 50% on your cost for that particular drug. Sometimes the drug has a special coating on it and should not be cut. In that case, maybe a non-coated form is available. For example,

Viagra comes in 25mg, 50 mg, and 100 mg size tablets. All cost from $8 to $10 apiece. Cutting them in quarters, as a lot of my patients are able to get adequate benefit from, reduces the price to pretty cheap lovemaking.

Drug	Scored?	Use
Accupril 10, 20, 40 mg	not scored	high blood pressure
Actose 30 mg	not scored	diabetes
Amaryl	scored	diabetes
Benical	not	colds and flu
Bextra 10, 20 mg	not	arthritis
Cefzil 500 mg	not	antibiotic
Coreg 6.25 mg, 12.5 mg, 25 mg	not	heart
Diovan 160 mg, 320 mg	not	high blood pressure
Effexor 75 mg	scored	mental health
Fosamax 10 mg	not	osteoporosis
Lipitor 20 mg, 40 mg	not	high cholesterol
Levoxyl (all sizes)	scored	thyroid deficiency
Lotensin 20 mg, 40 mg	not	high blood pressure
Lotensin HCT 20/25	scored	high blood pressure
Menest 0.625 mg, 1.25 mg, 2.5 mg	not	estrogen replacement
Monopril 20 mg, 40 mg	not	high blood pressure
Norvasc 5 mg, 10 mg	not	high blood pressure
Risperdol 0.5 mg, 1, 2, 3, 4 mg	not	mental health
Synthroids (all)	scored	thyroid deficiency
Viagra 25, 50, 100 mg	not	erectile dysfunction
Valtrex 500 mg, 1000 mg	not	herpes viruses
Vioxx	not	arthritis

Drug	Scored?	Use
Zocor 10, 20, 40 mg	not	high cholesterol
Zofran 8 mg	not	vomiting, post-op
Zoloft 50mg, 100 mg	scored	mental health

I hope that these suggestions will help to save you many times what this book cost.

CHAPTER 86 -- SEDUCTION

Girls, if you don't want to be seduced, don't wear mini-skirts, don't wear blouses that expose your shapely shoulders, and don't go to a topless bar. If you <u>do</u> want to be seduced, a topless bar is a great place to start. Try to limit the alcohol consumption of you and your boyfriend to one drink apiece, with an absolute maximum of two, or the seduction won't be as much fun. (Also if you're driving, you may not make it safely home.) Be sure to use a condom plus one other method of birth control. Bring your own Trojan ultra-thin lubricated condom just in case he doesn't have one.

Seducing your husband. Fixing him a big meal is <u>not</u> a good way to start. Rent a sexy video. Sit together on the sofa while you watch it, and explore his body gently as you sit there, particularly touching bare skin. Kiss him on his neck. Lick his ear. Loosen his collar. Lean your breast against his arm. Put his hand on your thigh. Maybe have a soft rug on the floor and possibly some Kleenex nearby in case you each decide to make love right there in front of the TV. A pornographic video is guaranteed to produce your desired result.

One, possibly two, alcoholic drinks may enhance the seduction. More than two is almost guaranteed to make the experience less pleasurable and occasionally disastrous. The guy might be unable to get it up, or the girl might pass out as soon as she lies down. Either thing might end a promising relationship before it is well started.

CHAPTER 87 -- SEXUALITY AND EMOTIONAL INTIMACY

To be fully human we need to be connected. Humans experience connectedness through sexual intimacy and through bonding emotionally. Don't ever let *anyone,* not your spouse, son, daughter, church, or Aunt Susie, tell you that "you shouldn't have those feelings" or "act your age" or "have some dignity" or "just accept the cards you're dealt" or any of the other putdowns that people use to rob you of your humanity.

Physical and mental health need these components, and people who don't get enough of them die prematurely. It may not be dramatic, but they just slowly wither away. There is an overcast of sadness that defeats the most arduous efforts of the doctor and other caregivers.

In babies it is called "failure to thrive." Babies who never get stroked, talked to, sung to, cuddled, or held quite literally die. Doctors and nurses have been well aware of this as long as I've been alive, and probably a lot longer. When I was on the pediatric wards as a medical student, it was common to see this order on a little baby's chart: "TLC t.i.d." Freely translated that meant "give this little tyke Tender Loving Care three times a day. Hold it and stroke it, and talk to it and sing to it for a while at least three times a day."

And in young people and adults the lack of strokes or warm fuzzies is every bit as toxic. "A hug a day keeps the doctor away."

The benefits of sexuality -- and here we mean the whole range of sensual activity such as touching, stroking, massage, sexually stimulating and erotic activity (foreplay) and all forms and variations of sexual behavior leading to orgasm and afterglow -- are profound and measurable. The blood circulation improves, the sinuses clear. Endorphins surge through the body, and the stimulation of the limbic region of the brain enhances feelings of well-being and happiness. This is truly cheap psychological therapy. Self image is improved, and mental outlook is more positive. Zest for life, that twinkle in the eye, is so important in physical health.

Emotional intimacy is wonderful when experienced with another human being, and is the foundation for our feelings of wholeness and wellness. However, the needs of a human for intimacy are so strong that a dog, cat, or other pet can indeed often mean the difference between a person's wanting to live and not wanting to live. Even a goldfish or turtle can have this amazing influence on our outlook and happiness.

It is the feeling of being connected to another living creature which brings us this satisfaction.

Don't ever let anyone tell you that you shouldn't try to find another mate after the death of a long time companion. Don't pay attention to such phrases as, "one should be enough," or "you're too old to start over," or "they'd just be after your money." Don't buy into the falsehoods that you are too unattractive, overweight, physically impaired, or whatever 'logical' things people say to deter you from forging emotional bonds.

Go with your heart.

CHAPTER 88 -- SEXUAL PROBLEMS IN WOMEN

The National Institutes of Health now recognizes **female sexual dysfunction** (which by informed estimates affects 43% of American women) as a disease. For doctors to establish a diagnosis of this condition, a woman must be personally distressed by one or more of four recognized components of dysfunction: decreased sexual desire (low libido), decreased sexual arousal, pain during intercourse, and personal difficulty in achieving or inability to achieve orgasm. This means that Medicare, Medicaid and other insurance programs will now pay for treatment of this condition.

With the huge success of Viagra for impotence in men, there is now a search for treatments to help women also.

I have prescribed small doses of testosterone successfully for years, but it must be combined with an adequate amount of estrogen produced by your own ovaries or by estrogen supplements that you take. The testosterone works mainly by stimulating a slight growth response in your clitoris, the seat of most arousal responses.

When I was in the Air Force I worked a lot in the GYN Clinic and was even acting Chief of the department for a short time. One day the wife of one of our wing commanders came in because she loved her husband but was having much trouble with arousal. She appeared to be still producing enough of her own estrogen; so I started her on a small dose of testosterone. About three weeks later her husband stopped at my table at the Officers' Club. I commented that he looked tired; and he laughed and thanked me profusely. It seems that he wasn't getting much sleep while making up for lost time!

Any married couple knows that the female sexual response is much more complicated than the relatively simple effect of male arousal (although male arousal certainly can be reduced under certain circumstances, such as putting cold cream on your face every night before going to bed, and changing the subject when your significant other is making what he hopes are sexual overtures. Cold cream won't prevent wrinkles, but it will definitely prevent meaningful sexual activity.)

Sex therapists who are studying the sexual response in women are finding that a large number of women don't fit the standard sexual response model, which includes desire and sexual fantasies, followed by arousal, orgasm, and afterglow.

Lack of desire is the most common form of female sexual dysfunction, and there are a variety of causes. These include emotional causes such as stress, fatigue, relationship problems, or depression. Fear of pregnancy is also a common cause, so be sure you have a good method of contraception if pregnancy is not desired by either of you. See the chapter on **Contraception**.

It is important to have a good blood supply available to your pelvic organs for you to fully enjoy the experience of making love. Smoking, diabetes, high cholesterol, heart disease, a heavy meal, and anything else that can reduce the circulation to your pelvis, may interfere with the sensitivity of the vagina and clitoris and thus stifle your enjoyment.

Too much alcohol or any one of a long list of common medications may chemically interfere with your libido. The classes of medications that may have an unpleasant effect on your love life include antihistamines (for allergies), especially the older OTC ones, anticonvulsants, antidepressants, beta blockers used in high blood pressure, and a few oral contraceptives.

Physical problems include fatigue, but also hormonal changes in menopause, lack of physical conditioning, or the above medication side effects, same as in men.

Fear of interruption by the kids when making love is a common turnoff. One very successful suggestion I have used all my career is to put a lock on your bedroom door and use it when you feel romantic. Do not, under any circumstances, allow your kids to see you making love. It may seem self-evident, but I had a three-year old patient who came upon her parents in the throes of lovemaking and was very scared. "Daddy was trying to kill Mommie," she told me.

After the kids are old enough that they no longer need Mommie or Daddy in the middle of the night, then if you can have a room, such as a den or office or bathroom between your bedroom and that of the closest child, by all means do so.

There are many for whom desire does not initiate sexual arousal. Indeed, desire is a difficult subject because it has nothing to do with a woman's genital area. Some women feel that desire is an interest in experiencing the sexual part of their being. It has much more to do with the mind and emotions than with the body. Arousal now is being paid particular attention to because of the possibility of doing something about it with medication.

Identifying arousal in women is much more difficult, obviously, than in men. Complicating that is the fact that many women do not know when and whether they are physically aroused. Getting wet is certainly a very good indication of arousal.

A lot more in women is mental than in men. <u>Feeling safe and secure in the arms of a gentle lover goes a long way toward producing sexual feelings in women</u>. Studies are now being done at many clinics around the country to find out whether medications may be of value. Finding a medication similar to Viagra for women would be hugely profitable for one or more drug companies, and all women can benefit.

> *A patient of mine with three pre-school children had a husband whom she loved very much. He was a good husband and father, always remembering even the smallest excuse for a thoughtful gift to her. But he wanted sex every night, just like when they were first married. She was unable to be aroused most of the time and had no desire at all. Their marriage was foundering.*
>
> *This exhausted woman didn't need romance. She needed help. I had a couple of marriage counseling sessions with both of them. I suggested that instead of bringing her romantic gifts, her husband should assume responsibility for the kids for a few hours every evening. He could take them to the park, fix them supper, bathe them and put them to bed while Mom read a book or luxuriated in a hot tub. He agreed to do this, and guess what? In two weeks her desire, as well as her ability to become erotically aroused had returned. They had compromised on making love three nights a week. Her husband was very happy with the three nights a week because, he told me, "those three nights are like a honeymoon again!"*

CHAPTER 89 -- SEXUALITY IN OLDER WOMEN

Women past menopause, many of whom may have been widowed or possibly have not otherwise had a close relationship with a man for several years, may be faced with a new relationship in which both people desire to become sexually active. This has become a joke in Sun City West in Arizona, where the local police receive several complaints every month of residents necking or going further in the local parks, golf course, etc. All I have to say about those folks about whom the complaints are being made is "more power to them!"

As I said in the chapter on **Sexual Problems in Women**, it is very important to have a good blood supply available to your pelvic organs for you to fully enjoy the experience of making love. Smoking, diabetes, high cholesterol, heart disease, a heavy meal, and anything else that can reduce your circulation may interfere with the sensitivity of the vagina and clitoris and thus stifle your enjoyment.

Improving your general physical conditioning through stopping smoking if you do, losing weight if you need to, and a daily exercise program of at least 30 minutes within the limitations imposed by any possible medical problems will go a long way toward helping with all of these conditions.

There are some things that one must consider about intercourse at advanced ages. First, it can be <u>very</u> satisfactory. But in women who have been on little or no estrogen replacement therapy, lubrication can be a problem. If your doctor doesn't want to put you on estrogen at your advanced age, he or she can and should let you use an estrogen cream on the vulva and up in the vagina on a daily basis. Within two weeks there will be a very marked improvement in your ability to lubricate when sexually aroused, while the tissues (skin and mucous membranes) which may have shriveled up become thicker and healthier and more responsive to sexual stimulation. So if you are starting a relationship that you think could lead to serious sexual activity, see your doctor for some hormones and other possible suggestions.

I have always noticed that older women who come to me for advice about sexual activity in later life mostly act as though they are doing something naughty and are a little embarrassed at the mere suggestion that there might be sex after sixty, or seventy, or eighty! I always say "go for it!"

Second, in case lubrication is still a problem, or the hormones haven't had enough time to work adequately on the delicate membranes, I suggest the use of a lubricant such as K-Y Jelly. It is non-staining, water soluble, and I've never heard of anyone being allergic to it. Just have your consort put a little on his fingers and gently apply it to the appropriate surfaces, especially the clitoris. Vaseline, of course, is an old standby and there are others, but K-Y is currently the best. For what it is worth, it also has a pleasant odor and taste.

> *And in case someone else might wonder about what a couple of my older lady patients asked (you may have wondered if younger also), there is no bad effect whatsoever from swallowing semen and sperm, and swallowing it will never make you pregnant. Nor will it make you gain weight. It is 100% protein.*

Obviously you don't have to use anything to prevent pregnancy from occurring. However, I must caution you that the fastest growing (percentage-wise) segment of the population with AIDS is the one of people over 65 years of age. This is not large in numbers, but it is a risk that one should consider. In other words, use a lubricated condom.

Other sexually-transmitted diseases are possible but less likely to occur than in younger age groups. I suggest you both read the chapter here on **Safe Sex**.

Don't let a well-meaning relative stick you in a females-only retirement or assisted-living facility. You will be much happier and do better mentally and physically in the more stimulating environment and activities provided by a mixed-sex facility. This will be much better even if you are no longer sexually active, from the genital standpoint.

CHAPTER 90 -- SEXUALLY TRANSMITTED DISEASES (STDs)

These are diseases which may be transmitted from person to person by anal or vaginal intercourse. They include AIDS, Chancroid, Chlamydia, Gonorrhea, Granuloma inguinale, Hepatitis B and C, Herpes genitalis, Human papilloma virus (which all too often causes cancer of the cervix in women), Syphilis (which has been around for thousands of years – mummies have been found with typical organ changes caused by tertiary syphilis!), and Trichomonas.

Yeast infections (monilia or candida) in women are not considered STDs, even though they are occasionally transmitted to male consorts who have not been circumcised. These organisms are everywhere in our environment, especially in moist climates, usually come from the woman's own skin or intestinal tract, and are most likely to flare up after use of a broad spectrum antibiotic (meaning most of the antibiotics we now use), which kills the good germs in the vagina that normally keep yeast in check.

Yeast vaginitis is also more common in pregnancy, in those on oral contraceptives, and in diabetes, particularly if poorly controlled. It is more likely to flare up during menstruation in susceptible women.

Treatment is sometimes frustrating because the organisms have developed resistance to many of the anti-yeast drugs. The best treatment at this time (also the most expensive, unfortunately) is Diflucan, one dose of 150 mg. I routinely prescribe it whenever I prescribe an antibiotic for women who tell me that they get the yeast problems whenever they take antibiotics. It is important in these cases to use a vaginal 'conazole cream for at least some relief until a couple of days after your last dose of a regularly-acting antibiotic, so that it is out of your system, before you take the Diflucan. If you take it while the antibiotic is still in there killing germs, you will just have wasted your money.

Another little trick is to douche with acidophilus or Lactinex, the contents of 4 or 5 capsules in 8 oz of warm water, twice a day, starting before you start getting the symptoms. You can do this during your periods and other times when you know that you may get a flare-up.

Men who are uncircumcised, and have a significant other with yeast problems must carefully pull the foreskin all the way back and wash with regular soap and water at least twice daily. Pulling the foreskin all the way back when urinating and drying the end of the penis with toilet paper will help in prevention, as yeast requires moisture to grow.

Use of one of the 'conazole vaginal creams after you are infected is usually much more effective in men than in women. For some men circumcision is the only permanent cure, and it must be one that removes at least 90% of the foreskin so that the organ can be free of moisture except during intercourse.

> *A cardinal rule is: if you have, or have reason to believe that you could have, one STD, then you should be tested for all of them that you can. That basically means a vaginal smear in women, including a Pap (these will look for Human papilloma virus, trichomonas, and occasionally herpes), and genetic probe tests for Chlamydia and Gonorrhea taken from the urethras of both men and women, along with a VDRL or RPR blood tests for syphilis (I prefer VDRL) and HIV blood test.*

Syphilis

Syphilis was under pretty good control for years. The reason was not just education about prevention, but also due to blood tests for syphilis being required as part of pre-employment physicals, any admission to the hospital, and even before you could get a wedding license. In Indiana they were still requiring a physical exam of both man and woman for possible venereal disease (that's what STDs were called then), along with the blood test for syphilis when I practiced there in 1966. After the results of the blood test came back, usually in three days (the basis for the so-called three day wait after the marriage license was applied for), we physicians would fill out the form from the county marriage license bureau certifying that the couple was either free of any venereal disease or had been adequately treated for any found. They would then go over to the courthouse, pay their three dollars for the license, and then be married.

The state of Nevada did not at that time require a three-day wait, and I'm not even sure they required a blood test –certainly not a physical exam. So Las Vegas capitalized on that with wedding chapels where you could (still can, I believe) just walk in and get married by a justice of the peace or whoever was empowered to marry people in that state.

Careful follow-up of all contacts of a person that tested positive for syphilis by county health departments all over the country ensured that more than 99% of all cases were treated very quickly. So Syphilis almost disappeared – for awhile. Now it is coming back in all its virulence.

Syphilis is a more hardy germ and is much more contagious than AIDS. It is caused by a germ called a spirochete, which quickly burrows into the skin and mucous membranes of those who even touch a drop of the fluid secreted in the sore on the skin that is the mark of the primary type of infection. You really can get this from a toilet seat.

AIDS, on the other hand (see the chapter on **AIDS**), dies quickly when left alone on a dry surface and will not infect healthy unbroken skin.

Syphilis kills as surely as AIDS if untreated, but over a much longer period of time in most cases. The primary lesion is a sore, usually on the penis or vagina, but I have seen it on nose, ear, and finger. After a time, it goes underground for months or years, then emerges usually as a rash that is hard to diagnose. Secondary syphilis again lasts a few weeks or months, then again becomes dormant as far as obvious symptoms are concerned for up to several years. When it again emerges as Tertiary syphilis, it can attack every organ in the body, including brain, bone and heart, and is deadly.

Syphilis, however, unlike AIDS, can be quickly and surely killed by a single shot of penicillin, or another antibiotic if one is allergic to penicillin.

Because we haven't seen much syphilis for a long time, many younger doctors have never seen a case. I recently had a classic case of primary syphilis with the chancre on the penis that looks like the crater of a small volcano after the fluid stops being secreted. The fluid is among the most contagious of all diseases, and a dark field examination of it under the microscope reveals a lake just teeming with spirochetes.

He had been seen by two health professionals who had failed to make the correct diagnosis. Penicillin cured him.

Because all STDs are required by law to be reported confidentially to the health department, He was interviewed by the health officer, who had to do a lot of detective work to find all of his contacts over the past three months for treatment.

Chancroid

Chancroid is caused by Hemophilus ducreyei and involves painful ulcers in the genital tissues, along with abscesses of the inguinal lymph nodes. Culture is difficult, and it easily may be confused with syphilis and genital herpes until the typical large abscesses appear. It disappeared for thirty years, then re-emerged in the 1980s. Once again it is under pretty good control. It is highly correlated with associated AIDS infection in other countries. Syphilis, HIV, and herpes, along with Chlamydia and gonorrhea, must be also tested for if you have this condition.

Chlamydia

Chlamydia in men usually begins with burning on urination, along with a discharge from the penis that may be clear or have some pus mixed with it. Gonorrhea usually has a lot worse discharge that is thick with pus. Symptoms in a chlamydial infection begin from 7 to 28 days after sexual exposure. They may be more apparent in the morning, when the tube may be glued shut with secretions, The opening may be a little red or occasionally severely inflamed, with a thick discharge more like gonorrhea.

Inflammation in the anus and rectum may be present after anal sex, while the throat may be red and sore after oral sex. Complications include lingering infections in all the tubes up to and including the prostate. Treatment of a case of gonorrhea in a man may be followed by the above symptoms a few days later, and the man thinks the GC is coming back. Not so. The new symptoms are Chlamydia, which has a longer incubation period than GC and is not killed by the same antibiotics that kill GC. For this reason most doctors will automatically treat someone with gonorrhea also with a drug that will kill any associated Chlamydia at the same time. <u>If your doctor doesn't think of this, then you must save yourself time and money by requesting treatment for both.</u>

Women often have little or no symptoms, but are susceptible to sterility with this infection as well as with gonorrhea. They may have a mild vaginal discharge, burning on urination, frequent urination, pelvic pain, and painful intercourse in advanced cases. Symptoms around the rectum may occur in women, along with throat infections. They may get infections in their Fallopian tubes, which leads to infertility, ectopic pregnancy from scarring in the tubes, and chronic pelvic pain. Symptoms of tubal infections are usually less severe than in gonorrhea.

Treatment is Zithromax 1000 mg in one dose (the most expensive approach, but also the most likely to be effective because you can't forget doses), doxycycline, 100 mg twice a day for 7 days (the cheapest way), or erythromycin 500 mg 4 times daily for 7 days (good but sometimes upsetting to the stomach).

With all of these diseases, you must be tested again in 6 weeks or so for possible relapses, and in 3 months for syphilis, which may have been just incubating but not yet positive when tested for initially. AIDS is similar in the need to test again in 3 months if possibly exposed.

Genital Herpes

Genital herpes (Herpes genitalis) is a life sentence. It usually appears first as a cluster of little blisters, which may or may not be painful. It can easily be controlled for months at a time with antiviral medications such as acyclovir, famcyclovir, or valcyclovir, but the organisms go dormant inside the genital nerves for the rest of your life. It is the most common ulcerative sexual disease in developed countries.

It can be a painful condition, particularly in the sensitive genital tissues of women, but it is actually dangerous only to newborns, who can die from it. For this reason any pregnant woman with an active case of genital herpes at time for delivery must have a caesarean section to prevent the baby from exposure to the infecting fluid.

Genital Warts

Genital warts, caused by human papilloma viruses, are little growths on the skin or delicate mucous membranes of the genital areas of men and women. They are highly contagious, and often grow around the base of the penis where a condom hasn't covered the skin. They often come in clusters, particularly around the anus in homosexual men. Incubation from time of exposure to appearance varies from 1-6 months. They must be differentiated from the flat-topped warts of secondary syphilis by a blood test for syphilis at the first appearance, and three months later.

In women with cervical warts, which often can be seen only with a culposcope (a microscope with a light on the end of it) HPV types 16 and 18 may cause cervical dysplasia and even cancer of the cervix. Women with one or both of these types must have a PAP smear or culposcopic exam every six months. Their sex partners also should be followed up carefully. There are several different treatments, none of which can be sure to afford permanent cure. Podophyllin, Efudex, electrocautery, laser, cryotherapy, or surgical excision under local or general anesthesia, along with a number of other locally-applied medications, are all being used with about the same degree of success.

Gonorrhea

Gonorrhea is caused by the gonococcus, and thus is often referred to as simply GC. Another common name is "the clap." For some unknown reason some people call it "a strain." In women with tubal infections it may be called "pus tubes." It used to be considered the most common STD; but since better testing for chlamydia came along, it has moved into second place. The most important problem with GC is the severe pelvic inflammatory disease (P.I.D.) it causes in women.

Women with this condition can come to medical care with severe pelvic pain, accompanied by fevers to 104° or more, and all the symptoms of peritonitis. It can be challenging to decide whether such a patient needs surgery for some other condition or not. We don't want to operate on someone with acute P.I.D., although they almost all will eventually need to have the uterus, tubes, and ovaries removed.

Because of the scarring caused by infection, the eggs can't get all the way down the Fallopian tubes to the uterus to implant if fertilization occurs. (The sperm are much smaller and so can get through going upstream.) So the eggs may implant in the wall of the tube. Or implant in the abdomen without ever reaching the tube. This is what we call an ectopic pregnancy, and they can be very bad if they continue to grow long enough to break apart and cause severe internal hemorrhage. I have seen several of these, and operated on a couple myself.

Symptoms in men begin 2 to 14 days after sexual exposure, usually with burning on urination, and a very yellow, thick discharge from the penis. This may be as far as it goes because most men instantly suspect what they have and come in for treatment. If left untreated long enough, however it can spread to the prostate and produce a very sick man, with high fevers and prostatic pain like the women with P.I.D.

Women and gay men often have GC in the rectum, with the more severe cases being in the men. GC in the throat from oral sex is usually mild, but may result in typical strep throat signs and symptoms.

Gonorrheal arthritis results from infections that aren't treated before they spread to the blood stream and fall out in the little blood vessels in joints. There are numerous other less likely complications that I haven't seen and won't discuss here. One that my partner saw involved the liver too, and looked like a gall bladder attack.

The diagnosis is made easily now by genetic probe, taking a sample of the discharge with a tiny cotton applicator, along with testing for Chlamydia on the same sample. Some labs now offer diagnosis from a urine specimen.

Treatment has become more difficult because of emerging resistant strains from improper use of antibiotics, along with rapid spread of these resistant strains around the world with air travel.

Ceftriaxone (Rocephin) 125 mg by a single injection is currently the best treatment. Several other antibiotics have been developed to cope adequately with resistant strains -- so far. All treatment for GC must be accompanied by either Zithromax, 1000 mg (1 gram) in one dose (expensive), or doxycycline 100 mg twice a day for 7 days (cheap). Pregnant women should not take either of these but instead take erythromycin 500 mg 4 times a day for 7 days. Women with P.I.D. almost always need to be in the hospital until the fever subsides, and they, obviously, need higher and longer doses of Rocephin.

Hepatitis B and Hepatitis C

Hepatitis B and Hepatitis C are fully covered in the chapter on **Liver Diseases.** They are caused by exchange of body fluids and are classed as "blood-borne pathogens," but are present in most of the body's other fluids as well.

Lymphogranuloma venereum and Granuloma inguinale

Lymphogranuloma venereum and Granuloma inguinale are mostly found in tropical climates and rarely in the U. S. Go to CDC.gov if you really think you might have one of them.

Trichomonas

Trichomonas is a little one-celled creature that swims around in the bladders and vaginas of those infected with it. It may cause a little burning on urination in both men and women.

Women usually have an irritating, frothy and bubbly, heavy vaginal discharge, and the diagnosis is made by doing a vaginal smear and seeing the little critters swimming around in the saline drop, or by doing a Pap smear and having the lab report Trich. The diagnosis is seldom made in a man until his sexual partner calls and tells him that she is infected, and that he needs to be treated also, although some have a little discharge in the morning.

The best treatment is Flagyl (metronidazole) 2,000 mg in one dose for women, or 500 mg three times a day for 10 days. Men may get well on the same single dose, but we still mostly treat them with 500 mg twice day for 7 days. This drug makes things taste like metal, and will make you very sick if you drink <u>any</u> alcohol within 48 hours of your last dose.

Prevention is the best policy in STDs. "Safe sex or no sex." At the risk of being thought an old fuddy-duddy or a member of the far right moral minority, I would like to point out that <u>avoiding sex before marriage has a lot going for it.</u> For sure stay away from sex with someone you pick up at a bar (or someone who picks <u>you</u> up). Limit your sexual activity to good friends whom you trust. And always use a condom!

CHAPTER 91 -- SKIN DAMAGE

Skin Damage from the Sun

(a) How to minimize it: 1. Avoid being out in the sun from 10:00 AM to 2:00 PM. (10:00 to 4:00 in the middle of summer). Wear a sun block with the higher SPF (sun protective factor) number the better whenever you will be out in the sun any time. Some dermatologists are recommending only SPF 15 and reapplying it every two hours, but I believe that the higher the better, preferably over 40. Coppertone has some with SPF 45 that I highly recommend. There are several other good ones on the market. Rub it in well at least 15-20 minutes before going out into the sunlight. Some of these cause skin allergies, and you have to look around until you find one that doesn't bother you. Some new formulas are coming on the market, with reportedly fewer dermatitis effects.

(b) Here's what happens if you don't protect yourself, starting from infancy: as you get older you develop such premalignant lesions as actinic keratoses; skin cancers such as basal cell carcinoma, squamous cell carcinoma, and malignant melanoma; and premature aging of the skin with thinning, wrinkles, and sagging. The bad effects from the sun don't go away when your tan goes away in the fall. They add onto each season's dose every year, and all too soon undesirable things begin to happen to the exposed parts of your skin. I've had a number of patients coming in with skin cancers on their backs who swore that they hadn't lain out in the sun to get a "healthy tan" for at least 20 years. But those beautiful tans every summer were like a time bomb which eventually does its damage. The worst future damage occurs when you get a sunburn.

Radiation from the sun spans wavelengths from 270 to 5000 nm. Visible light is from 400 to 800 nm. It can be separated into the colors of the rainbow by passing a beam of white light through a prism. The radiation in the visible light spectrum is poorly absorbed by the ozone layer. Therefore most of it reaches the earth's surface. Most of the damage to the skin is caused by the ultraviolet wavelengths, from 200 to 400 nm.

Ultraviolet A (usually referred to as UVA, 320 to 400 nm) is familiar to us as black light, the purple color seen when all other wavelengths are filtered out. Two uses that you may be familiar with are to detect the eggs of head lice and to look for scorpions in and around your house at night. It may also be used in clean rooms to kill certain types of germs. UVA, like visible light, is poorly absorbed by the ozone layer and so is at full strength when it reaches your skin. This longer wavelength is the one mostly responsible for premature aging (A is for aging, otherwise known as photoaging), wrinkling, and leather-like appearance of the skin in some individuals; or severe thinning of the epidermis, irregular color changes, and spider veins in others. It can penetrate the skin more deeply and thus damage the tissues which maintain the elasticity and general health of the skin (melanocytes, collagen, and elastin). It doesn't contribute very much to the redness of a sunburn.

Ultraviolet B (UVB, 298 to 320 nm) overlaps UVA somewhat but is absorbed to a considerable degree by the ozone layer. Enough to cause trouble, however, still reaches our skins. UVB is responsible for most of the effects of sunburn (think B for sunburn) on the superficial layers (the keratinocytes) of the skin and the cell damage that results in the three skin cancers: basal cell, squamous cell, and malignant melanoma. This is why we are very concerned about the ongoing loss of the ozone layer above our Earth. The loss is caused by fluorocarbons (chemicals used in the propellants for aerosols and the refrigerant in car air conditioners, for example). UVB is much more dangerous at high altitude, where there is less atmosphere to filter it out. There is a big hole in the ozone layer over the North Pole that is getting larger.

The UVB is very important in the conversion of ergosterol to vitamin D in the skin especially if vitamin D intake in the diet is poor. Vitamin D as you already know, or will learn elsewhere in this book, is very important in the development of strong bones. But exposure of just a small patch of your skin to the sun for a few minutes each day (as in going from your house to your job, or walking your dog) provides all the vitamin D you need. If you drink a glass of milk or take a multivitamin pill each day, you will also get all the vitamin D you need.

In Arizona recently there have been some cases of rickets reported recently in kids of middle and upper class families. The parents have been so conscientious about applying sunblock to their little ones that they aren't getting any UVB exposure to provide vitamin D. So if you live in the Valley of the Sun, use sun block on your kids, but give them vitamin supplements that include vitamin D.

Ultraviolet C (UVC, 200 to 290 nm) is well absorbed by atmospheric ozone, so relatively little reaches our skin. Most of our exposure to UVC comes from halogen light bulbs. This wavelength plays a part in the development of sunburn and helps stimulate a protective thickening of the surface of the skin after a lot of exposure, as does UVB. It is not usually a significant cause of skin problems,

Infrared (wavelengths above 800 nm) is felt as heat. It can be used to cook. The military uses infrared detectors to locate the enemy at night because all warm-blooded creatures produce heat, which can be measured if the instrument is sensitive enough.

The way we tell, most often, when it's time to get out of the sun on a hot day is by how warm our skin feels. The problem with this is that the blood vessels in our skin dilate as the skin attempts to cool down from the heat of the sun. The infrared rays of the sun are absorbed by the water droplets in clouds; so on a cloudy day there isn't much heating effect. UVA and UVB, however, are not absorbed very much by clouds; therefore the heat of the sun on your skin will not tell you when you've had too much of the damaging wavelengths exposure. When you are at high altitude, the protective effect of the atmosphere is reduced rapidly the higher you go as the air gets thinner and less capable of filtering out UVA and UVB rays. Also the total thickness of the atmosphere that the rays must travel through is reduced the higher you go. This is also true when the sun is directly overhead. Therefore it's a good idea to stay out of the sun between the hours of 10 AM to 3 PM no matter where you are. The layer of the atmosphere between the earth and the sun is thinnest around the equator. So the latitudes between the Tropic of Capricorn and the Tropic of Cancer produce the most skin cancers. Airplane pilots will tell you that the air is less dense on hot humid days; and, as a result, they have more trouble getting their planes off the ground. The ultraviolet effects are likewise magnified on those days because the thinner air doesn't filter out as much UV.

Tanning

UV light causes both an immediate and a delayed protective response. Immediate pigment darkening occurs but fades within minutes after exposure. The delayed-onset and longer-lasting tanning effect begins in two to three days after UV exposure. Cells in the skin that contain melanin increase their production of that chemical and pass the pigment to the superficial layers of the skin. This tan may last for a few weeks or more, depending on further exposure to UV. Darker skins contain more melanin and thus provide more natural protection against UV. Thus people with blond or red hair, who also have fairer skin, are much more likely to develop skin cancers than those with darker hair and skin under the same conditions of exposure.

Those of you who are active outdoors can afford yourself quite a bit of protection from UVA and UVB, if you have decided that you can't live without a tan, by putting on a SPF 15 sun blocker each time you are out, especially when swimming. (Be sure to wear one that is water resistant or you will have to put it on each time you get out of the water).

For those of you who spend a lot of time out on the water, as in fishing, please be aware that you get a double dose of ultraviolet rays because they are reflected up off the water as the light is.

Be aware that the sunrays reflect off of almost everything. I got a mild sunburn on my face when I graduated from medical school on June 13 in Indiana. (13 is my lucky number -- my daughter was born on the 13th, and the best shooting score I ever had when I was on the U. S. shooting team was on target 13). I was out in the stadium for about 1-1/2 hours, always facing away from the sun, most of that time with the black robe of one of my fellow graduates about 2 feet in front of me. Still I got a sunburn that required some cream to relieve it.

> *One of my fisherman patients, by the time he retired and moved away, had had 57 skin cancers removed by me and his previous doctors. He had three at one time on his lower lip so that I had to remove the whole lower lip and build him a new one with plastic surgery. He fished every spare minute of his life, as far as I could tell.*
>
> *We used Efudex on his exposed areas twice a year to kill early cancer cells, used a sun protective cream even under his shirts in summer (always long-sleeved), had his wife make him a white mask to wear that covered everything but his eyes and his nostrils, and had him wear one of the cowboy hats with the super wide brims like they use in Wyoming. With this program we were able to slow down the rate of new cancers to one a year.*

Tanning Salons

In spite of all the negative medical articles about them, they still flourish, even in the Southwest. Avoid them like the plague, because most of them emit large quantities of UVA and UVB, thus escalating your risk of developing skin cancer.

Photosensitivity

Many skin diseases such as lupus erythematosus are triggered or aggravated by exposure to the sun. This can also be produced by certain medications, such as tetracycline antibiotics (doxycycline, achromycin, and minocin), thiazide diuretics, sulfa drugs, and certain anti-inflammatory drugs. This condition looks like a sunburn and actually involves damage, usually due to the UVA wavelengths.

Skin Damage from Tobacco

Every cell in your body ages faster with every tobacco chew, or cigar or cigarette you smoke. You do get wrinkles faster. Your skin gets thinner and starts to sag <u>years</u> sooner. SO **stop smoking, or never start if you want to keep looking much younger than you really are for a long time.**

Keeping Your Skin Young

Be sure to take your estrogen as you reach menopause (discussed elsewhere in this book).

> *"MEDICAL RESEARCH PROVES: SMOKING CAUSES WRINKLES"* On the day when this is the banner headline appears in the entertainment newspaper Variety every young actor and actress in Hollywood will stop smoking, at least for a little while.

> *I had a set of identical twins, ladies in their early '50s, both of whom had stopped menstruating at about age 44. Their cases are discussed more fully in the chapter on* **Hormone Replacement.** *One of them had started taking supplemental estrogen therapy immediately when she stopped having periods. The other had never taken estrogen supplements. When I became acquainted with them, they were 51 years old. The one who had taken estrogen replacement therapy looked like she was about 45 years old. The other one looked like she was about 65 years old.*

The other beneficial effects of estrogen replacement therapy (ERT) (also sometimes referred to as simply hormone replacement therapy or HRT) are discussed elsewhere in this book.

Don't Get Fat

Avoid sagging skin and non-pregnancy-related stretch marks by never allowing yourself to get fat. If you get fat when you are young, your skin may return to normal elasticity when you lose weight, but the stretch marks won't go away, ever. If you are fat when you are older (as in your forties, which isn't really very old), your skin's elasticity won't be as good as it used to be, and your skin will sag when you lose the weight. High-priced plastic surgery will be a lot of help, but **save money. Don't get fat.**

Liposuction

While we are talking about surgery for fat, please be careful to have your liposuction done only in a real honest-to-goodness surgicenter, with a real operating room and everyone in sterile gowns and gloves, instead of just in someone's office. A lot of office surgery requires little except sterile gloves and drapes. But Liposuction has a very high risk of infection and requires the same attention to sterile precautions as major surgery.

There have been a large number of liposuction deaths from overwhelming infection. Plastic surgeons are routinely well-trained in this procedure, dermatologists less so, and cosmetologists not at all. Maybe they read a manual.

Eat less. Lose weight early in life. Don't be a couch potato. Save money. Don't be a statistic.

CHAPTER 92 -- STAYING FIT MENTALLY

Mental capabilities don't need to tail off as we get older. "Use it or lose it" applies equally to the mind as it does to all parts of the body.

Here are some great activities for keeping your mind sharp: 1) Turn off your TV set for days at a time. 2) Also stay away from your computer when you are home. Don't browse the Internet. 3) Get books of brain-teasing puzzles and work one three times a week. 4) Play games with family and friends that require imagination and problem solving. Bridge and chess are my two favorites. 5) Read all kinds of books, but especially seek authors who stimulate your imagination with word pictures. 6) Practice visualizing something that you want or expect to happen. Include color, smells, the wind, the surrounding sounds of nature, for just five minutes daily. These mental activities will keep the neural synapses open and functioning, while also opening new connections. Even people who already have had a stroke can benefit from these activities.

Sleeping

Getting a good night's sleep.

Insomnia. There are three types of insomnia: 1. Trouble falling asleep 2. Trouble staying asleep 3. Awakening too early.

Trouble falling asleep: I had this for years and years. I just couldn't turn my mind off. My younger son finally suggested that I put a notepad and pen on my bedside table and write down anything that seemed important, thus clearing my mind. It has worked pretty well.

The relaxation exercises that I learned when I was at the Olympic Training Center in Colorado Springs as a member of the United States International Shooting Team helped the most.

I used to be awake half the night before a big match and then lose my stamina in the next day's match about noon. No more. Within three months after my session at the U.S.O.C., I was sleeping like a six-month-old baby.

If you have this type of insomnia, here is what you should do: no caffeine within eight hours before sleep. Or, none at all is even better.

Limit alcohol to 0-1 drink no less than three hours before sleep.

Exercise daily, but not within 3 hours of bedtime if wakefulness is a problem.

Shift workers, such as police, who change shifts every 2-4 weeks are chronically tired. It takes one day for every one-hour change in your sleeping hours to reset your biological clock to the new sleeping pattern. If you try to change your sleeping times on your days off back to where they were, then you will never have a normal biorhythm until you are rotated back to a day shift.

Relaxation Exercises

This is the 10-minute program I have recommended to my patients for the last twenty years. It has been changed a little from time to time, but is mainly a shortened version of the one I devised for myself after going through psychological training in Colorado Springs in 1979. Equally effective and similar programs can be found in psychology textbooks, books on hypnosis, and elsewhere. Feel free to share it with your friends, if it works for you. An addition that I sometimes like to use is to have some soft music playing in the background. Or the sound of rain or surf, which you can purchase at many music stores. I recorded my own personal tape while sitting on the porch overlooking Oak Creek, near Sedona, Arizona. The sound of the water is clearly audible, and it invariably brings to my mind a carefree time and place. You can also purchase relaxation tapes and CDs.

This is your own to memorize and use to prevent stress, as well as when you already feel stress developing.

Take a Quick Break for "Power Relaxation"!

Instructions: 1) do this exercise two times each day, once during the day and once in the evening when you go to bed. 2) Do this exercise every day even on weekends. 3) You can read these exercises to yourself, have someone read them to you, or play them on a tape recorder after you yourself have recorded them. If you record them, do so in a quiet voice, and allow time for yourself to follow the suggestions.

As you do the muscle tightening and relaxing, think of your muscles as being pulled tight as a string. Then mentally cut the string and relax.

Sit or lie quietly in a comfortable position.
Take a deep breath.
Pull your toes toward your head.

Tighten your leg muscles.
Breathe out and let go.

Take a deep breath.
Make a fist with both hands and tighten your arms.
Breathe out and let go.

Take a deep breath.
Bite down with all your might and tighten your jaw muscles.
Breathe out and let the muscle relax.

Close your eyes as tightly as possible, take a deep breath and relax.

Now take a deep, deep breath.
TIGHTEN every muscle in your body.
Feel your body start to tremble.
HOLD the tension.
Breathe out and let go COMPLETELY.

Now repeat what I say mentally or out loud:
I feel very quiet.
I feel very quiet.
I am beginning to feel quiet and relaxed.
My feet feel heavy and relaxed.
My legs feel heavy and relaxed.
My feet and legs are heavy and relaxed.
My ankles, my knees, and my hips feel heavy and relaxed.
My entire lower body is beginning to feel heavy and relaxed.

My hands and arms feel heavy.
They feel heavy and relaxed.
My shoulders feel heavy and relaxed.
My neck is very relaxed.
My neck feels heavy and relaxed.
My entire head, neck, and face are heavy and relaxed.

I feel the tension draining out of my neck, into my shoulders, down my arms, into my hands and out my fingers. My fingers tingle as the tension drains from them.

My breathing is getting deeper and deeper.
My breathing is getting deeper and deeper.

My entire body feels heavy and relaxed.

My whole body feels quiet.
I feel very quiet.
My mind is quiet.
I am quiet.
I am very, very quiet.
I am relaxed.
I am very quiet and relaxed.

(You may stop here if you have reached the quiet and relaxed state.)

My breathing is getting deeper and deeper.
My arms are getting warmer and warmer.
Even my hands feel warmer.
Warmer and warmer.
I am beginning to feel warm all over.
The warmth flows into my left shoulder.
My left shoulder is heavy and warm.
The warmth flows into my right shoulder.
My shoulders feel heavy and warm.

I have nothing else to do at this time except to feel warm, quiet and relaxed.
There are no other thoughts except to feel warm, quiet and relaxed.
It is very pleasant.
It is very pleasant and enjoyable.
It is very pleasant and enjoyable.

Now just sit or lie there in a relaxed state for as many minutes as you can spare. Or even fall asleep. Then just let yourself gradually come back to the here and now.

CHAPTER 93 -- STAYING WELL PHYSICALLY

Wash Your Hands

Hand washing is perhaps the most important single thing you can do to prevent disease both in yourself and members of your family. (Examples include prevention of spread of RSV in hospitals, prevention of spread of the germs that cause boils, and pink eye, plus food poisoning, and many, many more. Washing your hands can even stop the spread of Ebola. The one nurse who survived Ebola at the mission hospital where the index patient was brought in the 1970s outbreak was the only one who washed her hands after caring for each patient after the rubber gloves were gone.)

Wash your hands a lot, several times a day -- particularly before meals and after going to the restroom.

If you get a scratch or scrape somewhere on your skin, don't wait. Wash it out right away thoroughly with soap and water. Then cover it until the end of your workday to prevent contamination, then remove the bandage and wash it again, this time leaving it open. Or leave it open after the first washing. The air is a wonderful germ killer.

The reason for washing it out immediately is to remove as many of the germs as possible before they start to grow in your wound. They begin to grow in a wound within 30 minutes, so clean it quickly. If you think it may need to be stitched up, then still clean it out as much as you can before you head for a doctor, because you almost certainly will have to wait more than 30 minutes before the doctor starts to work on you. In most offices those who are bleeding on the floor get a fast priority -- same for any open wound, because we greatly reduce our infection rate by starting a wound cleanout and repair within 30 minutes. But your location at the time of injury and rush hour traffic may delay your arrival at a medical facility longer than that.

So clean a wound out as best you can before bandaging it to stop the bleeding, even if it is just holding it under running water for 5 minutes. Soap in addition to the water is a valuable addition to your treatment. Just allowing it to bleed is vastly overrated as a method for cleaning out a wound. **Prevention of infection begins with YOU!**

As a general rule try to avoid allowing people with obvious respiratory symptoms to get any closer than three feet away from you, or even in the same room or house if you have that option. Move, when possible, if there is someone coughing behind or beside you in a theater or other gathering.

Flush your nostrils with eight or ten squirts of a saline nose spray, then blow it all out after every time you have been out in a crowd during cold and flu season, also after an airplane flight. *Save money by mixing your own spray solution, 1/8 to 1/4 teaspoonful of table salt to 8 oz water.

Avoid the Things that Can Hurt You, Either Directly or Indirectly

Avoid tobacco.

Always wear a seat belt. Never start the car until it is fastened.

Avoid having casual sex without a condom.

Avoid ever drinking more than two alcoholic drinks in any 24-hour period.

Avoid drinking alcohol more than two days per week. Give your body several days to recover from any alcohol you drink.

Never drive after drinking alcohol.

Never ride with anyone who has been drinking alcohol or using any other drugs.

Never use illegal drugs.

Never share needles if you do use illegal drugs.

Never drive if you use illegal drugs.

Never climb a mountain alone.

Add your own thoughts to this list. There must be at least a dozen more.

Exercise

As noted at length in the chapter on **Exercise**, the Harvard Medical study that has been ongoing since 1929, tells us that we live about an extra two minutes for every minute we exercise aerobically. Get off the couch!

Women

Breast self examination

On one of our exams in medical school was the following question: who finds the most breast cancers? (a) husband (b) boy friend (c) doctor (d) the patient herself. To these today we would have to add (e) girl friend, and (f) mammography. The answer was and still is (d) the patient herself.

Every woman should start examining her breasts once a month, at the conclusion of her menstrual period, from about the age 21 for the rest of her life. These simple instructions will give you an idea how do this accurately, but you should also ask your doctor to give you some additional instruction when you go in for a Pap smear. Most women's breasts have some small lumps or nodules in them. It's best to become acquainted with those that are present normally in your breasts long before you need to worry about cancer. Then if you notice something new or different, you can watch carefully and call it to the attention of your doctor.

Breast self-examination should be done by every woman after about age 21 on about the day after her period is over. The reason for that particular time is that the woman's hormone effect on the breasts is at its lowest at that time and the fluid retention that often occurs in relation to her periods has gone away. Thus there are less likely to be hormone-related lumps or cysts that might be confusing. Also it is easy to remember.

Approach the self-examination in a methodical way. I suggest that you first sit or stand in front of a mirror with a good light and look at how your breasts are supported and how they hang. It is unusual for both to be totally identical and symmetrical, but they should look the same every time. Look for *dimples in the skin*. Look for *irregularities in the skin surface*. These are possible danger signals. Clasp your hands in front of you without blocking your view, and first push the hands together. That causes contraction of the underlying pectoral muscles and may cause a *dimple to appear that wasn't there before* if there is a lump or other tissue in the breast that is attached to the muscle. That is another danger signal. Then clench your fingers together as you try to pull your hands apart to contract slightly different muscles to produce the same result.

Lie down. Place a small pillow under your right shoulder blade. Put your right arm over your head on the bed. That position will flatten your breast as much as possible on your chest wall, making it easier to feel any lumps. First, with the palm of your opposite hand, push firmly down on all parts of the breast, and notice any lumps or unusual sensation of fullness down deep in the breast. Now mentally divide your breast into four parts (as north, south, east, and west). Next with the flats of your fingers start out at the very farthest edge of your breast, which is out at your armpit in the northwest quarter, and push first lightly and then firmly as you go like the spokes of a wheel from the rim to the nipple area (we call it the areola) all around that quarter. Then move to the southwest quarter and do the same. Repeat for the northeast and southeast quarters, and you are done.

Expect to find lumps and nodules (maybe lots) that are perfectly normal. Get acquainted with where they are and how they feel. **What you are looking for is a lump that wasn't there last month.** That needs to be checked by your doctor. Also:

**Anything that feels hard like a rock should be checked by your doctor right away.

In spite of mammography, which is hugely important in picking up early breast cancers, breast self-examination still finds a significant percentage of these tumors. If you are sure that a lump is new (and you will be when you become acquainted with the contents of each breast after a few months of self-examination), see your doctor immediately for a biopsy or aspiration. If your doctor doesn't do these, then he will refer you to someone who does. Don't waste time. **Breast cancer is curable if it is found early enough.**

See the chapter on **Breast Cancer** for additional information.

CHAPTER 94 -- STROKE

Strokes are caused by sudden failure of blood to reach part of the brain. This failure of circulation is most often due to one of the vessels being closed off by too much hardening of the arteries in the vessel wall or by a bit of an arteriosclerotic plaque breaking loose and traveling in the vessel until it reaches a narrow area where it lodges. It can also occur from a bit of blood clot traveling to the brain after breaking loose from a heart that is fibrillating or one that has had a myocardial infarction. (Preventing such an occurrence is why people with heart attacks and atrial fibrillation need to take an anticoagulant such as Coumadin.)

The other cause of interruption of circulation occurs when a vessel breaks open and bleeds into the surrounding brain. People with uncontrolled high blood pressure are especially at risk. This type is more likely to be fatal right away.

Symptoms of Stroke

Weakness, numbness, or paralysis of face, arms, or legs, almost always on only one side. One side of the face may droop. (This also happens in Bell's Palsy, which is caused by a virus and gets well eventually. But you have to find out for sure).

Trouble speaking

Sudden vision disturbances

Lack of, or loss of, coordination

Unsteady walking

Intense headache, perhaps the worst you have ever had, and very different from your usual tension or migraine headache

What to do if symptoms like this suddenly occur? Call 911. Tell them your symptoms so that they will send the paramedics instead of the police. Leave the phone off the hook. You don't need to give your address unless you are using a cell phone. They automatically have the address of any fixed phone you are calling from. Go to the front door, if you can, and leave it open.

Do not drive yourself to the hospital. You may have such poor coordination on the way that you drive into another car or people on the sidewalk and kill others, while eliminating any possible chance of saving yourself.

What Can You Do to Help Prevent Stroke?

You can't do anything about your age, family history, sex, or some heart conditions, all of which are risk factors.

But you can do something about your use of tobacco, life as a couch potato, excessive alcohol consumption, poor control of your diabetes if that applies, high cholesterol and generally unhealthy eating habits, excessive weight, and inadequately-controlled high blood pressure. All of these are risk factors, but use of tobacco and poorly controlled high blood pressure are the two highest. If you have any two risk factors, from either category above, your risk of stroke increases 1000%. See the chapter on **High Blood Pressure** for what constitutes adequate blood pressure control and how to achieve it.

Several years ago, a study group of 25,000 physicians, including yours truly, started taking a number of substances or an identical-appearing placebo (sugar pill). We had our blood tested for a lot of stuff, and we had to fill out extensive questionnaires every year about our lifestyles, exercise, vitamins, what foods we ate, illnesses, and anything else that might have occurred during the preceding twelve months. Part of the study is still ongoing after more than 15 years. However one part was discontinued in less than five years because the data showed conclusively that the group that was taking an aspirin every other day was having significantly fewer heart attacks. So from then on we were all put on an aspirin every other day, if we so wished.

The only problem with that was that there was another finding concerning the aspirin. That was that the aspirin group also had a significantly greater risk of incurring a stroke. The stroke risk was found to be considerably less than the heart attack prevention gain.

But, there may be something inside you that says, "I would rather have a heart attack than a stroke." I personally feel that way -- it's not the physician talking here, but the person. That's the way I feel. My beloved grandmother lived three hellish years after her stroke, and I don't want any part of it for me.

I have put dozens of my patients on a baby aspirin a day instead of the higher dose in the study after sharing this information with them. I do everything I have outlined for you above and in the chapters on **Heart Attacks**, **Exercise**, and **High Cholesterol.** As far as a healthy diet is concerned, the only way I can get red meat into the house is to smuggle it in when my wife is away. And as I am writing this, I am eating a salad containing lettuce, carrots, apples, red grapes, and wheat germ, with a dressing that contains polyunsaturated vegetable fat. It's delicious!

But I don't take aspirin. I might feel different if there were any history of heart attacks in my family, but there isn't. I am telling you <u>what you should do</u> all through this book and in the first paragraphs of this chapter, but I won't advise you here where aspirin is concerned. My personal feelings may be affecting my objectivity.

CHAPTER 95 -- TENNIS ELBOW

The medical terms for this condition are medial or lateral epicondylitis. The most common by far is the lateral, on the outside of the elbow. In my experience only about one of every 100 cases of this are really from tennis (from poor backhand mechanics where the elbow hasn't reached full extension when the racquet strikes the ball). Most of these are caused by repetitive stress, such as lifting heavy objects with the palm down or turned toward mid body with the thumb up; hammering and sawing are common causes; pickers in warehouses, especially in 25 to 50 pound lines. Another frequent cause is bumping your lateral elbow, as on a door frame or anything else you walk too close to.

One man (yours truly) had to shake hands 250 times in a reception line at the annual hospital charity ball when he became president of the medical staff. My elbow felt like it was on fire by the end of the line.

Basically what happens is that the tiny tendons that are attached to the inside or outside knob of the elbow become irritated and inflamed, either from being over stressed or being bumped. The bone becomes tender too where they attach to the periosteum (the tough but thin covering of the bones), and the soreness gradually spreads down the muscles, clear to the hand and even up to the shoulder and neck, if let go long enough.

**<u>This condition does not need a doctor</u> if you take care of yourself soon enough with the following program. If it is work-related however, you <u>will</u> usually need to see a doctor in order to get approval for the modified duty needed to relieve the stress on the elbow until it gets well.

If the cause is a blow, be careful because it seems that a sore elbow gets bumped over and over. I personally bumped mine 22 times one week when I moved into a new house. For some reason I measured the doorways and found they were one inch (!) narrower than the doorways in our old house due to a slightly different door frame construction. I finally put a wrestler's knee pad on the elbow whenever I was at home, and I tried to consciously lead with my elbow and walk through the center of the doorways.

452

Treatment

If the pain is on the outside of the elbow, the first thing is to stop doing what caused it in the first place. That includes also never picking up anything with the palm turned down or facing to the middle. Don't shake hands, use a hammer, or shoot a .45 pistol with that hand. If you really do play tennis, then you must be sure the elbow is fully extended when you hit a backhand stroke. Even better is to switch to a two-handed backhand.

If the pain is on the inside of the elbow, then you must avoid picking up something with the palm up. And if you play tennis, be sure your elbow is fully extended when hitting a forehand. Volleys are tough, but possible if you have the elbow bent about 90 degrees when the racquet contacts the ball on either side.

Second is to apply ice or something very cold out of the freezer for 15 minutes twice a day if possible. It may hurt worse for the first 5-10 minutes, but will then go to sleep the last 5 minutes and usually feel better when it wakes up after the first few treatments. Put a layer or two of cloth between the cold and your skin. We don't want to get frostbite.

Third for both types is to wear a tennis elbow strap tightly around your forearm two fingers below the outside bone whenever you are doing any kind of activity with the hand and forearm.

Fourth, do firm massage <u>across</u> (not up and down) the muscle fibers within the limits of tenderness twice a day before using ice.

Fifth, start an exercise program to strengthen the small muscle fibers surrounding the injured tendons.

The exercise programs are very simple. <u>Lateral type</u> (the most common): Start with gentle stretching. With the palm down and the elbow locked in extension, grab your extended hand just behind the fingers, and pull the hand down to bend and thus stretch the top (extensor) wrist and forearm tendons to the limit of pain for 30 seconds to one minute. <u>Medial type</u>: Pull the hand upward in the same manner to stretch the bottom (flexor) wrist and forearm tendons. This is the only exercise you do with elbow straight.

Then for the lateral one, bend your elbow to exactly 90 degrees with palm down, and support your forearm just behind your wrist, either with the other hand or on a table or counter. Then lift a 1 to 1 1/2 lb. weight with the hand, from neutral position to full extension and relax back to neutral. Start with 10 repetitions. Then do the same stretch again. Increase by one rep every day. By the time you get to 100 reps per day, I almost guarantee you that your elbow will be well. Do not increase the weight to more than 1-1/2 lbs Just increase the reps -- slowly.

The weight lifting is the same for the medial type, except that your palm is up, and you are flexing your wrist instead of extending it. Again the forearm is supported behind the wrist while the elbow is bent 90 degrees.

If you don't have weights, just put a couple of cans of soup in a plastic grocery sack and let the sack hang from your hand as you lift it.

These exercises <u>will</u> make you well if you also modify or discontinue the activity that caused the problem in the first place. In my own case I couldn't stop shooting practice or my considerable skill would have disappeared rapidly. So I increased my reps. My elbow didn't get totally well until I reached 1200 reps per day. But that turned out to be my best year of punching holes in a target.

If you need, ultimately, to see a doctor, an injection with a cortisone medication up to three times two weeks apart can produce dramatic results. But the shots hurt a lot for the rest of the day. It is <u>extremely</u> rare for one with this problem to need surgery. Often, when surgery is being considered, the person will pay much closer attention to doing what is necessary to get well, thus avoiding the knife.

CHAPTER 96 -- THYROID DISEASE

(GOITER, HYPER- AND HYPOTHYROIDISM)

Your thyroid gland is located in the lower part of the front of your neck. It is one of the several endocrine glands which are regulated by the master gland, the pituitary, which is located on the underside of the brain just behind the eyes. The thyroid regulates the metabolism of the body, simplistically the rate at which the various parts of the body burn oxygen and do their thousands of jobs. A slowdown in hormone production by the thyroid means that things soon begin to slow down all over the body.

The pituitary secretes Thyroid Stimulating Hormone (TSH), which keeps the thyroid producing its own hormone, thyroxin, in the correct amounts. Thyroxin then circulates back to the pituitary in a continuous feedback mechanism. If the glandular tissue of the thyroid loses some of its hormone-producing capabilities because of disease, then there won't be as much reaching the pituitary, and so the pituitary puts out more TSH to make the thyroid produce more thyroxine. This often makes the thyroid grow larger and larger because the thyroid cells have been sick, and the only way more hormone can be produced is by growing more cells. This may result in a large growth in the neck known as a goiter.

Sometimes the cells are so damaged that no more can grow, and you have a hypothyroid condition. Then, even though the pituitary sends out a request for more thyroxine, not enough can be produced for the body's needs, and many parts of the body begin to malfunction as the body's metabolism slows down more and more.

Treatment of most goiters, as well as hypothyroidism, is very simple and relatively inexpensive. Just take a small tablet of Synthroid or a related thyroid replacement hormone every day for the rest of your life. It sounds drastic, but it really isn't. The thyroid isn't functioning, so we substitute the pill for the real thing, and our body never knows the difference! While the pill doesn't cure the deficiency, it does beautifully control it. But you have to keep taking the pills.

The hyperthyroid condition occurs when a part, or all, of the thyroid begins to produce too much thyroxine. Sometimes the extra hormone comes from what we often call a "hot" nodule rather than the whole gland. Those lumps must often be examined by biopsy to be sure that they are not cancer. A radioactive iodine scan is usually done to confirm how much of the gland is over secreting.

If you have the hyperthyroid condition and you are a woman who is past menopause, by all means have the condition treated and cured by radioactive iodine. Don't even consider surgery. The risks of surgery are high in this condition because the thyroid gland has a lot more blood vessels than it normally does; so it is a bloody and exceedingly risky procedure. Damage to the nerve that controls your vocal cords is an all too frequent occurrence. So is loss of the tiny parathyroid glands, which control your calcium and bone metabolism and are attached to the much larger thyroid.

After the radioactive iodine course of treatment, there will eventually almost certainly be a time when your thyroid hormone level falls to the hypo state, and you will need to take the small, relatively inexpensive thyroid supplement for the rest of your life, with once a year (after the initial stabilization) lab tests and possible fine tuning.

If you are younger, two drugs, tapazole and propylthiouracil are very effective in depressing the excessive output of thyroid hormone. But they can be tricky to manipulate and may require an endocrinologist's help if your doctor has trouble fine tuning one of them. If you overshoot, it is easy to take a little thyroid hormone supplement, as noted above.

Taking supplemental iodine (the cheapest and the one we have used the longest is SSKI, saturated solution of potassium iodide) is often helpful for better control. It is absolutely mandatory that you take it for at least two to four weeks before surgery if you have to have a thyroid operation.

CHAPTER 97 -- TICK-BORNE DISEASES

These include **Lyme Disease**, which is now the most common and is found mainly in the Northeast and upper Midwest, although I personally have seen one case in Arizona, which was imported from New England in a vacationer.

We have all heard about **Rocky Mountain Spotted Fever** for about a hundred years. Obviously it was first described in the mountain states, but it is actually more common in the Southeast Atlantic coast states and Midwest. It is also found in Central and South America. It shows up with a red spotty rash, severe headache, fever, which may be high, and weakness.

Tularemia, otherwise known as rabbit fever, is transmitted to humans by ticks about 50% of the time. It is seen most in Arkansas, Missouri, and Oklahoma, and anywhere in the Midwest.

Ehrlichiosis

Ehrlichiosis (say air-lick-ee-o-sis) is named in honor of one of the pioneers of modern medicine, Dr. Paul Ehrlich. It is found in two different forms in the whole eastern United States, but has world-wide distribution.

These diseases occur mostly during spring and summer when we are more likely to be outdoors in tick-infested areas, either with work or recreation. The ticks usually wait near the top of grassy plants and low bushes for animals or people to brush up against their perch. Ticks may be on clothes for several hours before finally attaching to the skin.

They seem to love dark spots like the ear. I must have removed at least two dozen ticks from people's ears while I was practicing in Indiana, and a few even in Arizona. That is a tricky business and involves putting some fluid down into the ear to get the tick to disengage and come out on its own. Digging it out is not a good Idea because it is usually attached to the eardrum. When they are feeding, their bodies swell up to three or four times their normal size.

When I was in the 4th grade, my Dad had a successful day of hunting, killing three rabbits. When he cleaned them, he showed me their livers. I remember to this day that they had little yellow dots all over them. He said that meant they had rabbit fever. Because of the possibility of rabbit fever, he told me that a hunter should never shoot a sitting rabbit. If it wasn't able to run, it might be sick with this disease. He said that these rabbits had been running, so he hadn't suspected that they had it. Cooking the meat killed the germs, so we were able to eat the rabbits, a good thing because meat was scarce for us in those days of the Depression.

He washed his hands very carefully, because he said that if the rabbit blood got into any little cuts in his skin, he would get sick with it. First he would get an ulcer at the site of the cut, then big swollen glands up toward the heart, plus a high fever, chills, and aching, just like the flu. Well, in four or five days, Dad did get sick, but not in the way he expected. Since he had had no cuts on the skin and had scrubbed himself so carefully, he had no ulcer and no enlarged glands. But he did have a severe cough and shortness of breath, along with the chills and fever and other flu-like symptoms.

help inspect each other.

When you find one on your skin, try to pick it off with tweezers, catching it on or just in back of the head. We want to try to prevent their excretions from getting into the wound, because we think that their feces (shit) may carry the worst germs.

Before trying with the tweezers, you might try pouring rubbing alcohol on it. Or before using the alcohol, try lighting a match, blowing it out and then applying the still-hot end to the tick's body. Other fluids that have been used include acetone or nail polish remover and lighter fluid. The alcohol is safe to use in the ear, and maybe a drop or two of nail polish remover. It is not a good idea to use a hot match after using most of these fluids, which are flammable.

We do suspect that their saliva may also carry infection in Ehrlichiosis. So scrub the area very hard with soap and water after tick removal, and apply an antibiotic ointment if you have one.

Prevention

Obviously the best prevention is to avoid being bitten by ticks. That is sometimes easier said than done. However, these suggestions will be very helpful.

First, try to avoid areas where ticks are more likely to live, such as wooded, brushy areas. Wear long pants and shirts with long sleeves. Tuck your pant legs into your socks so that they will have to crawl up the outside of your clothes in plain sight. Check your entire body for ticks as soon as possible after being out in tick country. If you are with someone,

Tick repellants are a very good idea. Those containing DEET are safe to apply to the skin. These are also good for warding off mosquitoes. Repellants containing permethrin, on the other hand, may be used on the clothing but aren't safe on the skin.

If you become ill with flu-like symptoms, with or without a rash, within a week or so after being in tick country, **see your doctor right away.** This will enable you to get medication and get well quickly, thus **saving money** in the long run. Unfortunately, Lyme Disease sometimes doesn't produce symptoms for several weeks, so remember that hike of several weeks ago when you see your doctor. Remember, **Flu isn't likely in summer, so what seems like flu might be a tick disease.**

Treatment

All of these conditions respond well to antibiotics. All that is needed is to make the diagnosis in time. Here is where you can **save money by helping the doctor make the diagnosis.** Just tell him or her that you have been in tick country. In the case of Lyme Disease early diagnosis can prevent a disabling nerve condition that may not show up for several weeks or months after the acute phase of the disease is over.

His doctor was mystified. Dad told him that he was sure that he had, perhaps, a rare form of Tularemia, but the doctor wasn't convinced. He knew that Dad had pneumonia and told us that he probably didn't have long to live if he couldn't break the fever. Fortunately we lived only about 25 miles from the Indiana University Medical Center. The doctor had him transferred there by ambulance to the care of Dr. J. O. Ritchey, chief of Medicine. Dr. Ritchey agreed with my Dad's diagnosis (cultures showed it was the rare and deadly pneumonic form) and obtained an experimental drug called sulfanilamide from Eli Lilly & Co. there in Indianapolis. Within 24 hours the fever was falling, and in two weeks Dad was back home, a little the worse for wear but alive!
Sulfanilamide later proved too dangerous to the kidneys to be given internally, though it didn't hurt Dad's, and ultimately was used in World War II as a powder disinfectant in wounds. Dr. Ritchey became my hero, and about 15 years later was my much-beloved mentor in medical school, still as chief of the Department of Medicine at I. U.

CHAPTER 98 -- TOBACCO

This is a very addicting drug. Most tobacco users begin using it long before legal age. It is, right now, causing the worst health epidemic the world has ever known. Worse than the Black Death of the Middle Ages. Worse than AIDS. Worse than Ebola. Worse than all of these combined. Just slower. A World Health Organization study begun during the last two years suggests that within ten years tobacco will be the cause of a full **one-third of all non-war deaths in the world every year.**

It is insidious. If one smokes the equivalent of one-half to one pack of cigarettes per day for 20 years, he or she has a 70 percent chance of developing a serious health condition that may ultimately be the cause of death, not to mention severe morbidity along the way. At two packs the risk goes up to 90%.

For the past several years roughly 500,000 people per year, in the United States alone, have been dying premature deaths from exposure to tobacco and tobacco products. Ten percent of those are innocent bystanders, people who have never smoked themselves, but have inhaled someone else's second hand smoke for years. Two years ago the number of deaths from second hand smoke was reported as approximately 63,000, or 13% of the total deaths caused by tobacco.

In Europe, with about the same population as the United States but far more smokers, 1,600,000 people died in 2001, the last year we have full figures for. The second hand exposure death percentages are probably similar to our country -- at least 160,000 there! Every one of those, and our, premature deaths are totally preventable: **Just don't let non-smokers have to inhale the second hand smoke of those who smoke.**

Second hand, or side stream, tobacco smoke has been recognized for several years by the Environmental Protection Agency to be a serious health hazard in the workplace.

It has classified second-hand smoke as a Group A carcinogen, the most dangerous class of cancer-causing chemicals.

The EPA determination was the basis for eliminating smoking on all domestic airplane flights as a protection for the crews of these planes. Admittedly a lot of passengers complained bitterly about their exposure, but the ultimate argument was the workplace health hazard of the crews. The same EPA determination played a big part in the banning of smoking, even in bars, first in California, and now other states, along with airplanes.

No one can smoke in airplanes. But there are still all too many places where smoke cannot be avoided by those who do not choose to smoke.

Kerry Pearson, a young columnist for *The Lumberjack*, the school paper of Northern Arizona University, wrote in September 2002 about second hand smoke, "If people want to smoke, that is their decision and I respect that. But my decision is to not smoke, and people need to respect that as well."

Several studies have shown that passive smoke exposure by a pregnant woman for as little as two hours per day will double the risk of having a low birth weight baby, with its many complications.

Other studies suggest that harm to the fetus may occur from much less frequent passive smoke exposure. The risk of miscarriage is greatly increased in the first 3 months of the pregnancy with any kind of smoke exposure. Any young woman who works anywhere in a place where smoking is allowed is being exposed to that risk right now if she is pregnant. The risk is there even before she has missed a period and then becomes aware that she may be pregnant. So she has an increased risk even if she quits her job the day she misses her first period.

Asthma is a terrible breathing condition, the incidence of which, in our country alone, has more than doubled in the past ten years to over 5 million kids now afflicted with it, with annual deaths of 50,000 or more. The most recent information (one month old) indicates that infants exposed to second hand smoke within a few months after birth are much more likely to develop asthma as they grow older. As the father of an asthmatic and the physician for many asthmatic kids, I can think of few worse fates! It also causes older children to have more severe and more frequent bouts of asthma.

Recent studies have shown that exposure to second hand smoke increases the risk of Sudden Infant Death Syndrome by 50% to 500%, depending on the study.

It increases the risk of acute and chronic middle ear infections in children and causes children to get many more lower respiratory infections, such as bronchitis and pneumonia.

In conclusion, people with the following conditions should never enter a place, such as a restaurant, where anyone has smoked, and especially not work there, because they have an immediate risk, rather than the slow ticking time bomb of most long-term smoking:

Pregnant women
Newborns and children under 4, or maybe 5, or maybe no children ever
People with coronary artery disease

Asthmatics

People with COPD (emphysema)

People with chronic bronchitis

People with nasal allergies

People with high blood pressure

Diabetics

Do any of us have friends in any of these categories? Of course we do.

Can we do anything to prevent any of these people from harm? **Yes, we can stop all smoking in public places and all places of business.**

Direct Bad Effects of Tobacco

In those who chew, cancer of the mouth, tonsils and throat, esophagus, stomach, intestines, and bladder are frequent, and more common than in those who smoke. High blood pressure, heart disease, stroke, peptic ulcers: all of these are more common in the tobacco chewer than even in those who smoke, and are <u>much worse</u> than in non-tobacco users. The only thing that is better for those who chew over those who smoke is the lack of airway disease in the chewers, such as cancer of the lip, larynx, and lung, and no chronic bronchitis or COPD. All the other conditions are likely to be worse because the areas in the first sentence above get a much more concentrated dose of tobacco in chewers. Chewers say they spit out the tobacco and don't swallow it, but when I question them closely, they admit that they swallow "a few drops" with each chew.

Did you know that the Marlboro Man of cigarette advertising fame died a horrible death with lung disease caused by his cigarettes? His family has sued Phillip Morris, maker of Marlboros, according to the papers.

Cancer of the lung caused by smoking tobacco is the leading cause of all cancer deaths. I heard Dr. Evarts Graham, the man who first discovered that smoking caused lung cancer and who performed the first successful surgical removal of such a cancer, speak in an auditorium that contained 250 people. The room was blue with smoke when he started talking. When he finished 45 minutes later, there wasn't a cigar or cigarette lit anywhere. Many of us, including me, walked out of there and never smoked again. Dr. Graham told us that he had smoked for 50 years but had quit about two years before his talk because he got scared. Unfortunately, he didn't quit in time and later died of lung cancer himself.

We all know or have known someone who has a serious health condition caused by tobacco. Do we continue to smoke or chew because we think it can't happen to us? Read on.

There are perhaps 1,000 chemical compounds in cigarette smoke. Some may cause the **accelerated aging** we see in smokers. The most obvious effect is the reduction in oxygen being carried to every cell in the body. Every puff of tobacco, causes narrowing of every blood vessel in our bodies, so that less total blood volume is carried to the tissues. In addition the smoke carries carbon monoxide into the lungs. Carbon monoxide competes with oxygen for the hemoglobin in your red blood cells and thus each RBC doesn't carry as much oxygen on each trip from the lungs to the cell levels of the body. So there is less total blood flowing to each cell, and what blood that arrives there is depleted in oxygen. And thus every cell in the body ages faster in a smoker than in a non-smoker.

The use of tobacco is a common cause of **impotence** in men, probably mainly because it reduces the circulation to the sex organs as well as to the rest of the body.

Smoking **increases anesthesia risk** enormously in surgery, **slows healing** due to poor circulation, and **increases the risk of post-operative lung infection**, along with **increasing the risk of pulmonary embolus**.

Yet another reason to quit smoking is for protection of your children's teeth against **cavities**. A recent study tells us that second-hand smoke doubles the risk of developing cavities in kids ages 4 through 11. One of the by-products of nicotine (cotinine) encourages certain tooth-destroying bacteria to grow and multiply.

> *"**Smoking Causes Wrinkles,** says noted physician,"-- headline in Variety. No, this headline hasn't appeared in that paper yet, but it should. And even after it does, a high percentage of movie stars will continue to smoke. But they will also age faster, as will you. Of all the places in the world where people want to look young forever, Hollywood is the leader by a wide margin. But they have a lot of company among the rest of us.*

Yet another recent study stated that second hand smoke probably greatly increases the risk of **Sudden Infant Death Syndrome** (SIDS). So don't take your newborn out to a restaurant or country club where smoking is still allowed. And of course don't smoke yourself. If you work in a smoky environment, change from your work clothes out in the garage or someplace before you walk into the house.

COPD (emphysema) is a lung condition caused by tobacco smoke where the tubes become obstructed, then begin to break down till at the end there is very little usable lung left. See the chapter on it.

The latest proven addition to the list of diseases that longtime smokers are more likely than non-smokers to get is **colon cancer.** An American Cancer Society study reported in December 2000 found that those who smoke for 20 years or more are 40 percent more likely to die of this disease.

As a matter of fact several of their studies report that **at least 40 percent of those who smoke die from their addiction**. We all have to die, but dying of any kind of cancer or emphysema are particularly horrible ways to go.

This simply adds to the information first reported more than ten years ago that told us that 70 percent of people who smoke up to one pack of cigarettes a day for 20 years will develop a serious health condition that will probably be the cause of death. The same study said that 90 percent of people who smoke up to two packs of cigarettes per day for 20 years will have the same thing happen.

And those who die from tobacco die much younger than they would otherwise in most cases. **So, if you don't fully intend to commit suicide, quit smoking -- today!**

There are a lot of statistics here, and it has often been said that you can prove anything with statistics. But everything I tell you in this book is true because I personally have either seen it or treated it, or both. I have lost six friends who were particularly close to me from lung cancer because each of them smoked. I had successfully persuaded and helped all but one to quit smoking before the cancer came on. My nurse's husband died in my arms.

My experience with these friends simply illustrates that you are still at risk for lung cancer after you quit, but the good news is that your chances of dying of lung cancer are reduced by 50% ten years after you quit.

Within the first day after your last puff several desirable things begin to happen. The carbon monoxide level in your blood disappears, and your red blood cells begin to operate with a full load of oxygen for the first time since you started smoking. Your blood pressure falls, to normal if you don't already have hypertension, and to definitely lower levels even if you do. (That makes your blood pressure easier to control and you **save money on your drug bills**.) Your risk of having a heart attack decreases. The temperature in your hands and feet rises to as near normal as they ever will be.

Within one month the circulation to your sex organs is noticeably improved, and is as normal as you are ever going to get within three months. If you are still having impotence secondary to erectile dysfunction, then it may be Viagra time. (See the chapter on **Impotence**.)

As far as other conditions caused by smoking are concerned, your lungs begin to clean themselves out within 24 hours after you quit. The little hairlike cilia that beat to move out mucus in the lungs begin to regain their normal motion that is paralyzed for eight hours by just one puff of a cigar or cigarette. Within 6 to 9 months your lung function tests improve by up to 50 percent from their pre-quit levels. That doesn't mean that they return to normal. Unfortunately there is a lot of lung damage that occurs after just five to ten years of smoking, and much of that is permanent.

Your sinuses begin to clear out also, and you may notice the improvement there even before your shortness of breath and morning cough begin to get better.

Having those organs starting to cleanse themselves again reduces the frequency and severity of infections, thus **saving you even more money**, and making life more enjoyable.

Within a month after quitting you will probably notice that the bluish tinge to your toes and fingers has improved. Whether you notice it or not, your circulation definitely begins to improve within 24 hours after your last chew or puff.

The good news is that people with chronic bronchitis (and coughing up phlegm every morning is the first symptom of that bad disease) can improve enough to perhaps totally quit coughing, and quit having lung infection after lung infection, within just a few short months away from tobacco smoke.

This was certainly the case with one of my dear lady friends who had smoked for 40 years (her husband was one of the best poker players I know of -- I wouldn't play against him, or anyone else for that matter, as I've had to work too hard for my money -- but I sure enjoyed watching him). After we almost lost her with pneumonia, she decided that, since she already hadn't smoked for ten days in the oxygen tent, she could manage to last the next four days till the nicotine was out of her system and she wasn't addicted anymore. She did quit, and six months later her cough had stopped; her lung function had improved by 50%, and she was able to continue to live and play with her grandchildren at the 7,000 foot elevation of Flagstaff, despite having already bought a house at lower elevation while still smoking.

And boy, was she a recruiter! She got up a little group of her smoking girl friends and made them quit too. She was only 5 feet tall and weighed about 95 pounds soaking wet, but they were all afraid to say "no" to her. She remains to this day one of my most grateful patients.

If she can do it after 40 years, so can you!

HOW TO QUIT SMOKING

** If you quit smoking now, it will save you more money than almost all the other ideas in this book put together.

Smokers are risk takers, most with the attitude that "it can't happen to me." When it one day dawns that maybe "it *can* happen to me," then you are ready for this part of the chapter.

All kinds of ways have been tried to quit smoking (And most of these also apply to those who chew tobacco, although we will be mostly referring to smoking as we go on here). I've had two smokers who were also former cocaine addicts. They both told me that stopping smoking was harder than quitting the cocaine. So you can be <u>very</u> proud of yourself when you successfully quit using tobacco.

It is not unusual for a smoker to try to quit and fail the first *several* times. Keep trying. You will learn from each failure. The Great American SmokeOut in November every year is a great time to always try quitting. Another is as a New Year's resolution. Another is on your birthday.

When you set a quit date, start doing some things to help to reinforce your decision. Deliberately keep a small notebook in your pocket and each time you have a cigarette, write it down with the time of day. Also write down a number from 1 to 10, which tells how much you really want that cigarette. Start keeping your cigarettes in a different place, so that you can't just unconsciously reach for one and have it lit before you even know it. You will soon find that you are smoking less without even trying.

Draw a line down the middle of a clean sheet of paper. On one side of the line write down all the reasons you can think of to stop smoking. Feel free to use any ideas from this book that you wish. Be sure to include the amount of money you will have saved at the end of one year (**a tax-free gift of more than fifteen hundred dollars per year** if you smoke one pack a day.) Write down the amount of money you expect to save on medical bills as your immune system improves your resistance to infections. Write down what you are going to do with that money.

On the other side of the page write down all the reasons you can think of to continue smoking. That will help to convince you of what you already know in your heart, that the benefits of quitting tobacco far outweigh the benefits of continued usage.

The most important single thing, if you're going to be successful, is to make up your mind that you're going to quit. When you quit, I suggest that you take the money you're currently spending on tobacco, and put that money in a savings account. Then reward yourself for quitting: at the end of a year spend that money on something you really want. When you have something to look forward to, that will help you stay away from tobacco.

** Just remember, it takes only 14 days after your last puff of tobacco or from your last patch, or last chew of Copenhagen or Nicorette gum to get the tobacco unplugged from your body's chemical (enzyme) system so that you're no longer addicted.

After you quit, you must stay away from second hand smoke or you will soon be addicted all over again.

It may, however, take two years before you quit wanting a smoke or a chew. Something that helps you through the withdrawal period is avoiding some of the activities that you often do when you smoke. Like having a cup of coffee, or a beer. Going to a smoky bar while you are quitting will set you back because of the second hand smoke that you inhale there. It will be another 14 days from that exposure until you are no longer addicted. Also, because alcohol dulls your inhibitions, you are more likely to think "Aw, I'll just have one; it won't hurt." But all it takes is one puff, then one cigarette, then one pack, then one carton to start the addiction again.

So, practice saying, "No, thank you, I don't smoke." In front of a mirror, to your family, in your car. When you do that, also visualize yourself in a situation where you would have smoked before but are saying "no" this time and from now on.

If you have a friend who has quit, call him or her up and use that person as a support system. I have encouraged my patients to call me at any hour, day or night, before taking that first puff. They have, and each one who did call was ultimately successful. I'm happy to also be able to say that none (yet) has called me at three o'clock in the morning!

It is important to avoid so-called high risk situations where you know you will not only be exposed to second hand smoke but also feel a strong urge to smoke because you always have before under those conditions.

When you reach your quit day, flush all your old cigarettes down the toilet. Wash all the ashtrays. Have the carpet steam-cleaned. Send the drapes to the dry cleaner, along with your suits and dresses. Wash all your clothes that you don't dry-clean.

Be as physically active as possible, so that you aren't constantly thinking about smoking. Hobbies help.

Every time you want a cigarette, drink a glass of cold water instead.

Force fluids for two weeks, one 8-10 oz glass of water at least. Some studies suggest that using cranberry, blueberry, pomegranate or other juices high in anti-oxidants will greatly accelerate the detoxification of the body. In Germany they also take a tsp. of baking soda in water three or four times a day during the two week washout period to help neutralize acids and tars. I'm not totally sure about some of these, but they have some good anecdotal reports, are inexpensive, and they "can't hurt."

Greatly reduce or totally avoid coffee and alcohol.

Don't make the mistake of eating candy whenever you want a smoke or a chew. A good doctor friend of mine finally was able to quit, He gained 20 pounds in a few weeks because he ate a horehound drop every time he wanted a cigarette. The good news is that he lost the weight, didn't resume smoking, and is still alive and well now 40 years later. Good work, Bill!

I know several people who resumed smoking because they gained weight from snacking and eating too much at mealtime. Here is what you have to remember. Within days after you quit the taste buds on your tongue will begin to wake up. Food will taste better than it has for years. Also you are used to putting a cigarette or chew into your mouth frequently every day, so you may decide to substitute food. Don't do it! Not only will you be more likely to succeed but also you won't gain weight. So drink a glass of cold water instead -- no calories there. If you absolutely have to munch, then do it on celery, or chew sugarfree gum for the first few days. One of my lady patients successfully chewed on swizzle sticks.

Other people I have known went back to smoking because they felt that it made them relax. The truth of the matter is that it is the *ritual* that you go through when you smoke that produces a sort of relaxation, especially on breaks at work. Think about it. You suspend all thoughts about problems momentarily while you concentrate your thoughts on the simple tasks of opening the pack, shaking out part of a cigarette, pulling it out, placing it in your mouth, lighting it, and taking a deep breath.

This is very much like we do in the chapter on **Staying Well Mentally,** with its relaxation exercise sample. Basically you are changing your focus of attention, taking a deep breath, and letting your muscles relax.

Actually tobacco is a stimulant and is much more likely to keep you "wired" all day than to help you relax. Three cigarettes are about equivalent to one cup of highly caffeinated coffee in stimulative effect on your body. The caffeine in three cups of coffee is equivalent to the amount we used to use by injection to try to awaken someone who had taken an overdose of sleeping pills. Interesting, eh? Make you think about all that coffee you are drinking too?

When you quit smoking, I suggest that you use at least a short version of the exercise in that chapter several times a day, including at breaks. You won't feel the need to smoke for "relaxation."

Tell your family and friends not to take anything personally after you reach your quit date. You may feel ouchy, grouchy, yell at the cat, try to kick the dog. Try going out in the yard and yelling at a tree, if that will make you lose some tension. Then go back and apologize to the tree later (trees have feelings, according to several studies done by -- are you ready for this? -- plant psychologists. I know it must be true because my wife talks to her roses -- tells them how beautiful they are -- and they just bloom their little hearts out for her).

Using the <u>patches</u>: nicotine patches come in three sizes: 21 milligram, 14 milligram, and 7 milligram. Those who smoke a pack a day or more should start with the 21 mg, putting it on in the morning and taking it off at bedtime, for 14 days. Then do the same with the 14 mg patch for 14 days, and the 7 mg patch for 14 days then stop. Never smoke while you're using the patches, or **you could die.**

Using the <u>gum</u>: using the gum merely substitutes chewing tobacco for smoking tobacco and rarely works. I had a patient last week who told me he had been chewing the gum for *ten years!*

Progressive filters are another aid. Actually most of the quit smoking aids out there have the same 50% rate of success. The next one does a little better because it also helps the withdrawal symptoms.

<u>Zyban or Wellbutrin</u>. These are the same drug, made by the same drug company. But Zyban costs more. So if you use this approach, ask your doctor to order the Wellbutrin. This will save a little money for your insurance company also if your plan covers it. Many plans don't. But the money you save from not smoking will more than make up the difference if you have to pay for it out-of-pocket. Recent good news is that some insurance companies are finally paying for quitting smoking programs.

This medicine is used for depression, among other things. According to the story of its discovery for tobacco withdrawal, it was on the formulary at a big Veterans Hospital where it was being used for post-traumatic depression after some of our recent short wars. (I don't know if you have any idea how many veterans smoke in a VA hospital, but it's a lot!)

After awhile one of the doctors and/or nurses noticed that a lot of these patients were giving up cigarettes. When asked why, many of the quitters said that they had begun to lose their desire soon after being started on Wellbutrin. The doctors then compared the medications of those who quit with those who were still smoking and found that Wellbutrin was the only medicine which seemed to have that effect. The doctors told the drug rep, who relayed this news to his company. Soon a full study funded by the pharmaceutical company was underway. "Zyban" was the result.

With this method, you set a "quit date" and seven days before that you start the medication, one tablet daily for three days. From the fourth day on you take a dose twice daily. A few people develop some mild side effects on the higher dose, which usually soon wear off. If they don't, drop back to the lower dose, because even one daily is likely to be helpful. Also, in the meantime, reduce your smoking as much as you can so it won't be as much of a shock when quit day arrives. Tell all your friends that you are quitting and when. Start thinking of yourself as a nonsmoker.

At the end of seven days stop all tobacco. The medication will reduce some of your desire, as well as eliminating most of your withdrawal symptoms. Continue the medication for four weeks (that's two weeks past the date when you have no more tobacco in your body). If you are still severely craving tobacco, then continue the medicine until the craving goes away and then cut it to one daily for another week or two. I've used this on many people. It really does help to reduce the craving in many people and especially helps the withdrawal symptoms in almost everyone.

Cold turkey. This is more likely to be permanently successful than the other methods. It requires the strong desire to quit (which the lists of reasons to quit will help you with). You may have to change your friends if they all smoke and continue to do so when you are around.

One of my friends in Flagstaff (another poker player) was a *five pack a day* smoker! Now the only way he could go through that many cigarettes in a day was to have one going constantly from ten seconds after he awoke in the morning until the instant that he turned out the light on his bedside table at night. The other thing was that he slept only about 4 hours per night.

One night he saw one of those cancer of the larynx commercials that were put out by the Cancer Society, where the person who had had his larynx (voice box) and upper trachea removed for cancer. The patient could breathe only through the tracheostomy hole below where his larynx had been. He was smoking by putting the cigarette in the opening and then pinching the skin closed around it so that he could draw in the air through the cigarette. I saw a real patient doing it, so I can testify that it was pretty revolting.

Well, my friend saw that and decided then and there that he didn't want to die of cancer, even though he was already in the highest possible risk category. So he just quit, then and there. He told his wife that he was through. And he was. Cold turkey! He later swore to me that he hadn't any withdrawal symptoms at all. He was (and is) a pretty tough hombre, and I know that if he made up his mind that he would have no withdrawal symptoms, then he wouldn't. That's been 10 years now and no lung cancer, so maybe he'll make it after all. [Unfortunately the rest of the story is that his wife also smoked, to a lesser degree on her own, but also got a lot of his second hand smoke and died of emphysema (COPD) only two or three years after her husband quit.]

What this story illustrates is that withdrawal symptoms don't have to get you down if you won't let them. Just make up your mind that you are going to quit the tobacco, come hell or high water. **And you can do it!**

CHAPTER 99 -- TRAVEL TIPS FOR STAYING WELL

On the trip: Take one aspirin every day to reduce the risk of blood clots in the legs from sitting still so long at a time. Wiggle your toes and move your ankles up and down every few minutes. Take some foam shooter's ear plugs to wear on the plane; it reduces your fatigue. The MAX brand is probably the most comfortable. Just roll them tightly and insert them into your ear canals, pointing them toward your nose, as that is the direction the ear canals run. Also an inflatable neck support is helpful in sleeping, but the most help is some Valium 5 mg or Ambien 10 mg (I recommend this one most) taken just after you take off. Avoid caffeine for 24 hours before you leave.

In the airplane: Remove the magazines from the pouch on the back of the seat in front of you to get an additional inch or more of leg room.

After you arrive: For third-world countries, be very careful to eat no raw fruits or vegetables unless you have personally peeled them. And don't even think of eating raw fish, other sea food, or meat of any kind.

Drink only bottled water or bottled soft drinks (no ice), or boiled drinks such as tea. Be sure that you personally open the bottled water. Use it to brush your teeth. Don't accept it if it has been opened before it reaches you, no matter how upscale the hotel or restaurant seems. I personally saw a restaurant employee filling "bottled" water out of the tap when I went to inspect the kitchen in one third world country I visited when I was on the U. S. International Shooting Team.

For third-world countries, get a gamma globulin shot before you go, if you can, to help protect against hepatitis. Even better is to get the hepatitis A and B series of shots starting about eight months before you are to leave. And take Doxycycline or Cipro, along with Lomotil or Imodium with you. If you do get diarrhea, just take a lot of safe fluids to keep up with the loss for the first several hours so that the bacteria and/or toxins will be mostly flushed out of your system. After 8 hours though, if you aren't getting better, start the Lomotil or Imodium. (Imodium AC is available over the counter, but you have to take two at a time to achieve a therapeutic dose). And if you aren't a lot better by the next day, start the antibiotics. Take two for the first dose, and one twice a day thereafter for both of them. Cipro is more versatile, but Doxycycline is a lot cheaper.

Drink a <u>lot</u> (juice and bottled water) on the plane over. Remember when you get back on the plane for home, that beautiful salad came from that third world country, no matter what country's airplane you are on.

Traveler's diarrhea is usually caused by bacteria in the local water supply. It may be caused by several different bacteria, parasites, or viruses. Our old enemy E. coli, however, is the most common culprit. The reason is inadequate local water purification.

In 2002 a number of cruise ships became contaminated with Norwalk virus, which caused hundreds of passenger and crew illness with diarrhea. Walt Disney's ship, **Magic**, as I am writing this, has been pulled from service for total prow to stern disinfection.

Most of us know "don't drink the water," but we forget and take a soft or alcoholic drink with ice in it.

Another thing we do is to brush our teeth with a toothbrush rinsed in the local water. Or eat fresh fruits and vegetables rinsed in local water.

On the Airplane

That noted medical periodical, *The Wall Street Journal*, in their article <u>How Safe is Airline Water?</u> on November 1, 2002, printed the results of their survey of 14 airline flights, in which they took samples of water from the galleys and lavatories of each plane for laboratory analysis by good labs. The flights were a randomized sample all the way from Atlanta to Sydney, Australia. They were looking for possible disease-producing contamination. And boy did they find it! Their idea to do this was triggered by some poorly publicized studies from Japan and The Netherlands in which E. coli and the Legionnaire's disease germ have been found. Apparently U.S. studies have had "mixed results." The WSJ samples produced "a long list of microscopic life you don't want to drink, from *Salmonella* and *Staphyloccus* to tiny insect eggs. Worse, contamination was the rule, not the exception."

Federal regulations require that the tanks of airplanes are supposed to contain drinkable water. Many, perhaps most, airlines dispense bottled water initially, but on long flights, when they run out of the bottled variety, they turn to the taps.

Lessons to be learned from these tests: When you drink water on an airplane, drink only that which is bottled. Bring your own bottled water, maybe several bottles, for overseas flights for use when the bottled water from the airlines runs out. Use bottled water for brushing your teeth, as you would in any third world country. Bring some disposable towelettes for washing your hands before eating.

Never eat any fruits or vegetables that you have not personally peeled. Don't eat salads.

For traveling, particularly to a third world country, take the items from the chapter on **First Aid** but add a few things, listed on page 472, some of which you will have to have a prescription for or get from your doctor. The reason for some of these is that many of these countries are so poor that they reuse syringes and needles without sterilizing them, especially in Africa.

1. Several sterile disposable syringes, 3 ml and 5 ml, with both 25 gauge 5/8 inch and 21 gauge 1 1/4 inch needles.
2. A 30 ml bottle of 1% Xylocaine for local anesthetic.
3. Lomotil, 2.5 mg tablets, 25 or 30, to be taken in a dose of 2 every four hours for diarrhea. The generic ones work well and are cheaper.
4. Doxycycline, 100 mg tablets or capsules. These can be taken prophylactically, one daily for diarrhea prevention, or up to twice daily after you are infected.
5. Cipro 500 mg. These are somewhat stronger, perhaps, and certainly more expensive, than doxycycline, but cover other types of infection besides diarrhea too.
6. Acidophilus or lactobacillus pills. These are good bacteria to be taken to help restore normal GI function after you are infected, or if antibiotics have destroyed too many of your good bacteria. Probiotica is a good brand, as is Lactinex.
7. Some pain pills.

CHAPTER 100 -- ULCERS

Peptic Ulcers

These are much less of a problem now than they were even as recently as ten years ago. We used to x-ray people with heartburn and tenderness in the pit of the stomach (the epigastric area of the abdomen below the breast bone), find an ulcer in the duodenum (the first part of the small intestine, you remember, just beyond the stomach), and treat it with antacids, probanthine, and a really bland progressive diet for several months. Sometimes a gastroenterologist would have you swallow a long straight tube with a light on the end of it and take a biopsy of the ulcer. Then fiber optics came along, and the sword swallowing became snake swallowing.

Tagamet, which greatly reduces the acid production by the stomach, came along 20 years or so ago and suddenly people were getting well in two or three months.

But people who resumed or continued to smoke or drink coffee or alcohol would soon relapse, especially with the changes of season in March and September.

Zantac, Pepcid, and others are better than Tagamet because Tagamet has too many drug interactions. Also they can be taken just twice a day instead of four times per day for Tagamet. A newer one, Prilosec, which just became available in the much cheaper "generic" form, has been used especially for those with GERD to relieve the nighttime acid reflux symptoms. It is also good for ulcers, but is so much more expensive than these others, and still requires a prescription.

So now with heartburn, take two Zantacs (a total of 150 mg in the OTC dose -- OTC drugs always come in half the usual prescription dose sizes) twice a day for up to two weeks before consulting your doctor if you aren't too sore.

Stop coffee (decaf too -- coffee has two things that bother ulcers -- caffeine and an acid -- decaf still has the acid and some "decafs" still have as much as 14 percent caffeine), stop alcohol, stop tobacco in all forms. These three things cause more acid production in the stomach than everything else put together.

After some pathologists, using special new stains, saw some strange new bacteria under the microscope in some of the biopsy specimens, the biopsies continued. But soon one, then many, doctors began to culture the biopsies to see if any bacteria were there. Then some blood tests were developed for the bacteria. Low and behold, now we do blood tests for H. Pylori (the H. stands for Helicobacter, if anyone is interested) often before we even consider x-rays in people with chronic heartburn and tenderness in the pit of the stomach (the epigastric area, remember). If the test is positive, then a two-week course of three antibiotics, or two antibiotics and Pepto-Bismol or Prilosec (or one of the Prilosec family of drugs) will cure you about 90 percent of the time.

If this is no help in two weeks, go to your doctor and surprise him by asking for an H. Pylori (pronounced pie-lor-eye) test.

There are two main types of ulcers: first, those that occur in the duodenum just past the exit from the stomach (the pylorus), which are the most common and also the hardest to heal, but are almost always benign. Second are those that occur in the stomach which usually heal quickly with the proper treatment but are occasionally malignant. NSAIDs (anti-inflammatory drugs), such as ibuprofen, Motrin, Advil, Nuprin, Aleve, Naprosyn, Relafen, Oruvail, Voltaren, and many others, cause GI inflammation in 15 to 20 percent of people who take them. Many of those people are likely to develop stomach ulcers if they continue to take these medications after heartburn, diarrhea, or other GI symptoms develop. Ulcers caused by NSAIDs aren't malignant, but they can bleed, sometimes severely. Most ulcers usually cause what most people describe as a burning sensation in the pit of the stomach just below the breastbone. This is usually relieved by an antacid or milk and made worse by tobacco in any form, coffee (with or without caffeine), alcohol, and caffeine-containing sodas. Usually, but not always, there is tenderness to palpation in the pit of the stomach if there is an ulcer.

The same symptoms can be felt a little higher up under the breast bone in many, if not most, cases of GERD and also may be simply felt as a pressure. In that location differentiating GERD and ulcer symptoms from heart disease becomes very important. Only a doctor can make that differentiation usually, and sometimes even he can have trouble sorting out the life-threatening from the merely uncomfortable.

The best key to the correct diagnosis is that the discomfort of heartburn is likely to be relieved by a dose of antacid (e.g., two tablespoons of plain Mylanta or Maalox, or two tsp. of Mylanta II, or chew two tablets of these or others) in GERD or peptic ulcer disease due to hyperacidity. Pancreatitis, gallbladder disease, and heart disease will not usually be affected by antacids. Also the pit of the stomach won't be tender to your pushing on it in heart disease. (Unless some poor guy has an ulcer in addition to his heart disease!)

Other conditions that can cause pain in the epigastric area include pancreatitis, which usually comes on suddenly with very severe pain that may also be felt in the back. Gall bladder disease may be felt there, but more often the pain is centered under the right edge of the ribs. If inflamed, there may be pain around the tip of the right shoulder blade. Pneumonia in a very few cases may produce pain there, but there are usually a cough, fever, or other symptoms along with the unusual pain location. The pain of appendicitis often begins in the epigastrium before gradually moving to the right lower side of the abdomen.

One of the best ways to tell whether you have peptic disease (or something else just caused by hyperacidity), is to take some doses of antacid. If you get relief pretty quickly, then peptic disease is a strong bet. In that case go on the program outline above.

CHAPTER 101 -- URINARY TRACT INFECTIONS (UTIs)

Urinary tract infections are infections which involve the bladder, the urethra, the kidneys, and/or the prostate (in men). Our blood is filtered by our kidneys. Except in the rare instances when there are bacteria (germs) in the blood, the urine made by our kidneys does not contain any germs.

Signs and symptoms of urinary tract infections are as follows: burning pain during urination, frequent urge to urinate, passing small amounts of urine frequently, urge to urinate even when the bladder is empty, blood in the urine, cloudy or foul-smelling urine (pee into a clear glass and hold it up to the light; normal uninfected urine is almost crystal clear), back pain under the lower ribs, discomfort in the lower abdomen just above the pubic bone. Fever and/or chills along with any of the above symptoms are likely to mean that the kidneys are involved (pyelitis or pyelonephritis) or that the prostate is infected (especially if there is pain down there just in front of the rectum during intercourse), and <u>in those cases you need a doctor very soon</u>.

Diagnosis is very simple with one of the cheapest tests in medicine, the urinalysis. Every doctor can do this in his office, using just a chemical strip (dipstick) with 3-12 tests on it which is dipped into fresh urine and then each test's color change (or no color change) is compared to a chart for abnormal findings (these tests cannot be done if you are taking pyridium, or AZO, because its orange color messes up the colored spots on the test strip).

With these infections we are particularly interested in whether there is an abnormal amount of albumin in the specimen. If there is, then the kidneys are probably infected to some degree. And that means that we really need to get hot after the illness. The urine is always tested for sugar (glucose). Diabetics tend to get many more infections in the urine than others, simply because a lot of bacteria grow much faster if there is sugar in the fluid they are living in. So people who didn't suspect they were diabetic are frequently diagnosed as such when they go to their doctor with a urine infection.

In addition to the dipstick chemical tests most of us still spin the specimen in a centrifuge and look at the residue at the bottom of the tube under the microscope, particularly for red blood cells and white blood cells in the case of urine infections. The dipstick color tests do test for cells, but they aren't as accurate as looking with a microscope.

Most of the time the bacteria causing urinary tract infections come up the urethra from the opening just above the vagina in women or in the penis in men. Then if the urethra becomes infected, you have urethritis.

The most common causes of urethritis in men are two sexually transmitted diseases (STDs) called gonorrhea and chlamydia. The same germs, along with other types of germs from the bowel and vagina, cause this condition in women. Non-bacterial causes of urethral inflammation in women include irritating soaps such as bubble baths and certain deodorants.

Cystitis (infection of the bladder) is the most common urinary tract infection. If germs that get in the urethra spread upward into the bladder and aren't flushed out soon enough by urination (before they begin to multiply), then a bladder infection may result.

Women (at least 25 percent of all women get least one bladder infection in their lives) are much more likely to get urinary tract infections than men because the urethra (the tube from the outside to the bladder) is very short, only one to two inches long. It is also located close to the rectum, and bacteria from bowel movements can easily travel up the urethra into the bladder. Well over 95 percent of bladder infections in women are caused by E. coli, the normal bacteria found in our bowels.

Hormone changes in pregnancy often cause incomplete emptying of the bladder. Loss of support of the bladder following childbearing or menopause may also interfere with complete bladder emptying. This means that there is always some urine in the bladder for bacteria to multiply in, if any are present. Insertion of a diaphragm for contraception may squeeze any bacteria present in the urethra into the bladder. Sexual intercourse or female masturbation may do the same.

A U. S. Air Force study done several years ago with a blue dye (methylene blue) in the bath water showed that up to forty percent of women who take tub baths have water from the tub in their bladders at the end of the bath. (Their urine came out blue when they voided after their baths.) Naturally there are a lot of bacteria washed off the skin, particularly around the rectum, floating in that bath water. So it is a good idea to empty your bladder after taking a bath in the bathtub, just in case you are part of the 40 percent.

Prevention of urinary tract infections is two-fold: (1) keeping bacteria out of the bladder and (2) flushing bacteria out as soon as possible after they get into the bladder so that they don't have time to multiply enough to cause an infection.

(1) Practice good hygiene. Keep your genital area clean and dry. Always wipe from front to back after a bowel movement to keep bacteria away from the opening into the bladder.

(2) Up to several hours before sexual intercourse women should wash the vaginal area with soap and water to reduce the number of bacteria in the area. After sexual intercourse empty your bladder soon to flush out any bacteria that may have been squeezed up the tube into the bladder before they can reproduce.

(3) Try to drink at least 8 glasses of water per day and try to empty your bladder at least every two or three hours to keep the urine flowing through. Think of a small creek or stream of water. The water in the middle of the stream where it is flowing freely is so clear that you can see the bottom. The water along the edges that is hardly moving, however, is murky with growing things. The same thing happens in your bladder. So keep the urine flowing through. If you are drinking enough water, your urine will be almost colorless.

Most women won't get bladder infections even if they ignore these suggestions. But if you ever get the first bladder infection, then these rules will become very important in preventing further infections.

In men over 50 an enlarged prostate gland (benign prostatic hypertrophy or BPH) may prevent the bladder from emptying completely when you urinate. If there are any bacteria left in the bladder after urination, they may grow and multiply and cause an infection. Medications such as Flomax, Hytrin, and Cardura may be taken to help contract the muscles of the prostate to make it smaller. If the prostate is very large, then Proscar may help it to stop growing and reduce its size. Currently these medicines must be obtained from your doctor by prescription. **Saw palmetto** is an herbal remedy that is proving probably as effective as these prescription drugs, at a much lower price.

If the germs spread upward from the bladder to the kidneys, then you have a kidney infection, which may be referred to as pyelitis or pyelonephritis. When the infection involves the kidneys, you may become very sick with high fevers and will always require antibiotics to get well.

Recurring UTIs often take some detective work to figure out why the infection keeps coming back. Is it contaminated water from the bathtub? Is it soilage while wiping after having a bowel movement? Is it from bacteria squeezed from the urine tube (urethra) up into the bladder during lovemaking? Is it from bacteria that weren't all killed by the antibiotics the last time the UTI was treated (in a case like this you might have quit taking them too soon, or not enough were prescribed)? Or some other source?

One other possible source that I haven't seen in the medical literature was suggested by my wife after she read the first draft for this chapter. She noted that many toilets splash a little water on the exposed body parts of one seated on the toilet seat. Obviously, in the case of one who has had a bowel movement as well as urinating, that water is contaminated with bacteria from the bowel. This then is another possible source of the bacteria that cause recurring infection.

The solution to this last is simple. Just don't flush the toilet until you stand up and have your clothes back in place.

Treatment

Treatment of most UTIs involves the use of antibiotics. My usual approach is to begin with one which will kill E. coli bacteria. If my patient is not better in 48 hours after the first dose, or gets worse, then I want a "urine culture and sensitivity" to identify what bacteria other than E. coli may be involved and what antibiotics it is sensitive to (what will kill it). Because the culture usually takes 48 to 72 hours to be reported, an additional antibiotic may be added to the first one for those three days, and yet a third one may wind up being used when the sensitivity tells us what should work the best. Fortunately the extra time and expense are rarely needed because the organism is almost always E. Coli, particularly in women.

When you are given medicine by your doctor, be sure to always take it for the full number of days he or she has prescribed. Continue taking it <u>even after you start feeling better.</u> If the germs in the urine (or anywhere else in the body, as we discuss more fully elsewhere) are not <u>completely</u> removed, the infection may come back, with bacteria that have now developed some resistance to antibiotics and are more difficult to kill the second time around. Always remember, **germs cannot mutate and become resistant to antibiotics if they are all killed the first time.**

In order to eliminate as many bacteria as possible by just flushing them out of the bladder almost as you would flush the toilet, you must drink a lot of non-sugar containing, non-alcoholic fluids, at least twelve 8 ounce glasses per day, until a week or more after your infection is completely gone as shown by urinalysis.

Your doctor may want to save you some money and not require that you return for a urinalysis after you finish your medicine. This is one time when it is best to spend a little more and return for a urine exam in no more than ten days to two weeks just to be sure you got them all. Otherwise relapses may occur.

I have known of a significant number of women who started drinking large quantities of cranberry juice at the first sign of burning and got better. I have examined their urines under the microscope before and after using that approach and seen the bacterial count fall dramatically in just a couple of days. It seems to work best in cases where there are a lot of bacteria but not many pus cells (RBCs) and no red blood cells (RBCs). Some recent studies have finally confirmed what our grandmothers told us, that cranberry juice really does interfere with the reproduction of bacteria. So feel free to use cranberry juice instead of, or in addition to, water to help flush out the infection.

Then keep your urinary tract flushed out by drinking plenty of water-based fluids every day.

CHAPTER 102 -- VOMITING, DIARRHEA, AND DEHYDRATION IN CHILDREN

Vomiting and diarrhea in children, particularly little ones, is a difficult problem for a parent. Many, perhaps most, cases are due to a rotavirus, especially in those who spend their days in daycare. Most cases, just as in adults, may be due to food poisoning. They are usually self-limiting but may last three or four days, or even more, before subsiding. During that time it is necessary to get enough fluids and electrolytes (sodium and potassium) into the youngster to keep it well hydrated and prevent dehydration from occurring. Antibiotics usually don't work.

You can buy Pedialyte (the best option) for fluid replacement, or use 1/4 to 1/3 strength of the child's favorite flavor of Gatorade, which is not optimally formulated for childhood electrolyte (blood minerals) replacement. Or you can mix your own, the fluids we used before the commercial ones were available. We call it the "1-2-3 Solution." The recipe is as follows:

1 cup orange juice (for the potassium)

2 cups water

3 tbsp sugar

1/2 teaspoon table salt (NaCl)

Chill and start with 1 teaspoon, then in 10 minutes give 2 teaspoons, then in another 10 minutes give 3 teaspoons, and keep increasing the amount by a teaspoon at a time until you get up to two oz Then just give 2 oz every 30 minutes to one hour. If the child vomits after one of the doses, drop back to the next lower one where it didn't vomit at the next 10 minute dose.

Preventing dehydration while the stomach upset passes is <u>very</u> important. Little ones can get in trouble in just a few hours if you aren't careful.

The best single way to get an idea of whether the little one is getting and retaining enough fluids is by observing whether the youngster continues to urinate. This may be somewhat difficult when diarrhea is involved, but you can usually tell whether the front or the back of the diaper is more wet. Urination should occur at least every couple of hours to be adequate.

After hydration is achieved, you can use other fluids that are usually well tolerated by little stomachs. These include 7-Up, ginger ale (both with fizz mostly gone), clear Jell-O, bouillion, clear soup broth, salty crackers, then later rice cereal with water. No milk, because an inflamed stomach doesn't produce the necessary digestive juices for milk until about three days after the vomiting ends.

Lactinex, which you can get without a prescription, contains lactobacilli, which are good bacteria to replace the bad germs causing the problems. It can be mixed with applesauce and given, one or two capsules or spoonfuls 3 times a day at mealtime. I firmly believe that approach will speed recovery.

CHAPTER 103 -- WATER SAFETY in LAKES AND STREAMS

Drowning is the leading cause of injury-related deaths for children from one to fourteen years of age. Then the automobile takes over.

You can greatly reduce the chances of one of your own children becoming a statistic by following these safety tips, which are in addition to those already presented in the chapter on **Pool Safety**.

Learn to swim. Take lessons yourself, and for your children age 4 years or older.

To prevent choking, never chew gum while swimming, diving, or just playing in the water.

Learn CPR.

Never drink alcohol during or up to several hours before swimming, boating, or water-skiing. Teach your teenagers and their friends about the dangers of drinking alcohol while engaging in these activities, just as you must do with driving and drinking.

Never swim alone or in unsupervised places. Children must always swim with a buddy, even in a pool. Check the water depth before entering. A nine-foot minimum is recommended by the American Red Cross for jumping or diving.

In open water:

Know the local weather forecast before swimming or boating. Call the Coast Guard where possible. Strong winds and thunderstorms can be very dangerous. Small boats should not be on the water when there are white caps on the waves.

Restrict swimming activities to designated areas, which are usually marked by buoys.

When you go to the beach, always note where the nearest lifeguard is located. It's not a bad idea to set up your base camp fairly near one. Be cautious, even with lifeguards present. You are responsible for the safety of yourself and your loved ones. When a lifeguard is needed, it may already be too late.

If caught in a riptide or undertow, swim parallel to the shore until you reach an area where the outflow is weak enough for you to swim against the current toward shore.

Open water usually has limited visibility, and conditions can change from hour to hour.

Currents are often unpredictable. Watch for dangerous waves and signs of rip currents. This may be water that is discolored, unusually choppy, or filled with debris.

Always carry U. S. Coast Guard-approved life jackets, enough for every person on the boat when out on the water, regardless of the distance to be traveled, the size of the boat, or the swimming ability of the passengers. Not only carry them, but wear them! Especially non- or inexperienced swimmers. I know this flies in the face of those macho people who think just having life jackets in the boat is enough, but I have lived around water for a good part of my life and have yet another story to tell.

I have known of all kinds of boating mishaps where there was a collision, or the boat overturned because of a strong wake or waves that were unexpected, or a sudden wind. So: *When you go out in a boat, put on a life jacket before the motor starts, just as you would (or should) fasten your seat belt before starting your car.**

The son of some friends of mine dived into a pool in Oak Creek, near Sedona, Arizona, one year. He and his friends had dived there before, so they thought nothing of doing it again. Unfortunately, the winter rains had changed the depth of the pool, and he struck his head and broke his neck, paralyzing himself from the neck down. Another acquaintance of mine in college at Indiana University was swimming at a limestone quarry outside of town. In the spring a lot of students take a break at the quarries on sunny days to swim and soak up some rays of sun. If you saw the movie Breaking Away then you know what those quarries are like. They are supposed to be off limits, but fence climbing comes easy to goal-oriented college students. Also these breaks are inevitably accompanied by several six-packs of beer, which proved to be fatal to this young man. He got drunk, resisted the efforts of those friends who were sober enough to be alarmed, and dove into the still-icy waters, striking his head on a boulder at the bottom, and drowning right there in front of everybody.

We all know that sitting in a closed garage with the car motor running is a great way to commit suicide. People do it all the time.

A friend of mine who was the president of a bank in Warsaw, Indiana, took his beloved grandchildren out on his boat for a little troll around Winona Lake one summer evening. They had life jackets in the boat and all could swim, at least after a fashion. None had a life jacket on. Their boat speed was only about 5 miles per hour, but suddenly as his little granddaughter stood up to change seats in the small boat, a large powerboat zoomed by with a waterskier in tow, creating enough of a wake that the little girl was knocked overboard. My friend threw her a life jacket, but she couldn't quite reach it. He, old and fat and out of shape, jumped in to try to save her, while his grandson called desperately for help across the lake. Grandpa wasn't able to get to her, and she disappeared for the last time below the darkening surface of the water.

Just as my friend was going down for the last time himself, help came, and he was pulled from the water in a near-drowning condition. Artificial respiration was administered, and he was brought to the hospital emergency room, where I met him. His blood electrolytes (sodium and potassium) were quite low, and his lungs were still somewhat waterlogged, but these could be successfully taken care of with oxygen, an IPPB breathing machine, and IV fluids. But I couldn't heal his spirit. Even several years later he still wished that he had died that evening along with his darling granddaughter.

At Lake Powell in Arizona in 2001, officials first became aware of deaths caused by inhalation of carbon monoxide from the exhausts of boat motors. Some people swimming off the back of houseboats with the motors running drowned. Then some people in the water under a pier drowned. Then some people being pulled along close to a boat on modified water-skis were overcome and drowned. Review of deaths at the lake over a period of several years revealed many more, previously inadequately explained, losses of life which seemed to fit the pattern of close exposure to a motor's exhaust pipe just before the person collapsed.

Remember, carbon monoxide is invisible and has no odor, thus giving no warning of possible exposure. Exhaust fumes contain other substances besides carbon monoxide, and those are what produce the odors we smell. Also remember that some exhausts are vented under the water, but the fumes still rise immediately to the surface and contaminate the surrounding air. The water may filter out some of the odor-producing substances, thus reducing the warning smells. But the deadly carbon monoxide is still there.

You get better protection from toxic levels of the gas if the boat is moving rapidly, and if the swimmer or water skier is 30 or 40 feet at least from the boat when the motor is running.

Just sitting in the back of the boat with the motor idling puts you at potential risk. And sitting at the pier, or working on the rear of the boat with the motor running prior to loading it onto the boat trailer puts you at high risk, especially if there is no wind that day.

The rangers at Lake Powell now have warning fliers that they hand out to everyone who puts a boat into the water, but there have been still more deaths. So be aware of the high risks, especially in boats with big motors.

> *When I was an intern, I was called to pronounce dead two beautiful young people who had been necking in a car in a warm garage in the dead of a cold winter in South Bend, Indiana. They had been dead for several hours, and the car had run out of gas. They were dead in each others' arms.*

> *A friend of mine, who was the manager of a Flagstaff savings and loan, was said to have probably gotten drunk and fallen from his boat into the lake at night. The problem with that theory was that those of us who knew him well had never known him to take more than two drinks in a whole evening, and usually it was only one or none at all. And no one else on the boat had noted his intake of more alcohol than usual. In retrospect he had been seen sitting at the back of the houseboat before he disappeared and may have been overcome by the exhaust fumes before falling overboard.*

Follow these few safety hints, and enjoy the water for a long, long time.

CHAPTER 104 -- WHIPLASH

The classic whiplash injury often occurs when someone who hasn't been paying attention to his or her driving because of using a cell phone, dropping a lipstick or nail file on the floor, turning around to yell at the kids, looking at the pretty girl or handsome guy walking down the street, looking in the mirror while shaving or putting on lipstick, thinking that the car ahead was going to go through the stoplight on the yellow, and he didn't -- or whatever -- slams into the back of your vehicle. That causes your head to first be thrown backward, then forward, like the lash on the end of a whip, then backward again to a lesser degree.

The headrest behind you, if at proper height (a big if), will reduce the backward motion, especially if you see the car coming and put your head back before the impact. Shorter backward motion means also less forward snap. The muscles and ligaments that hold the neck portion of your spine together and support your head are suddenly overstretched, sometimes to the extent of being partially torn, at least microscopically. The degree of overstretching depends on several things: the speed of the car that hit you, obviously, whether you had any warning and could brace backward at least a little, how old you are (our tissues are not nearly so elastic as we advance in age), how big the muscles are in your neck (athletes of many sports who lift weights and have really big trapezius muscles do much better), and gender (like it or not, women tend to have more severe injuries because most don't have neck muscles as strong as most men).

So the injuries usually include a combination of ligament damage (sprain) and muscle and tendon injury (strain). The best situation is when you have no pain at the scene of the accident but develop pain, usually more in the back of the neck, sometimes in the sides, and sometimes also in the lower back, a few hours later. That almost always means that there was not any severe tearing of tissue, and the outlook is good for a quick recovery . . . **if you follow these simple instructions.**

Saving Money

First, put ice on the back of your neck as soon as possible after the wreck. You do not have to go to the doctor or any Emergency Room right away unless you have immediate and fairly severe (for you) pain, and maybe won't need to see a doctor at all. Keep in mind that everyone has a different pain threshold (some feel more or less pain than others with identical injuries). By all means see a doctor if you have been thrown against the door handle and bruised your left lower rib cage where your delicate, blood-filled spleen is located, or if you have any doubts at all about the severity or your injuries. Do not go to the doctor just because your attorney says to. Use your own best judgement. My experience has been that one doesn't get well for about two years if he or she sees an attorney before going to the ER.

Second, start doing some simple shoulder shrugs, gently, even while you are at the scene. Just stand or sit at attention. Look at something on the wall or in the distance and make sure it doesn't move. If the spot moves, that means your head moved, and it is better if just your shoulders move, first one and then the other. Bring your shoulder up as close to your ear as possible, hold it for a couple of seconds, and then relax. Repeat ten times on each side and quit for the time being.

As time passes work up to where you are doing three sets of ten on each side two or three times a day. Work within the limits of discomfort. Due to stiffness and muscle spasm the shrugs may produce some tenderness with the first few, but as the muscles are used, the spasm will go away. If the muscle discomfort then comes back while you are still exercising, quit for the time being and put some ice on the sore areas. When you are able to do three sets of ten on each side, then it is time to add weight. Start with 2-3 lbs, if you are a woman, or 5 lbs if you are a man and do the exercise once every day. Again work up to where you are doing three sets of ten, alternating sides till you get up to 30 with each arm and shoulder. Gradually increase the weight until you reach at least 15 lbs for women and 20 to 25 lbs, for men.

This simple exercise accomplishes several things. It relieves pain caused by spasm of the injured muscles (or by severe tightening of uninjured muscles to limit the motion of and guard injured ligaments) because a muscle that is moving and being used, even lightly, won't go back into spasm for several hours. And we all know that muscle spasms hurt. Exercise also prevents the development of muscle atrophy (which begins within hours of an injury). And it strengthens the supporting muscles of the neck, thus protecting the injured tissues even more.

Third, do Isometrics: 1) Lock your fingers together and place your hands against your forehead as you sit upright with your chin tucked in. Bring your hands up to your head; don't lean forward into them. Push your hands against your forehead while you prevent your head from moving by resisting with your neck muscles. Do this for a slow count of twenty. 2) Lock your hands behind your head without moving your head. Push against your head while you resist with your neck muscles, again for a slow count of twenty. 3) Bring one hand up to the side of your head and push against it while the neck muscles again resist it for a slow count of twenty. Repeat it for the other side. Each time pick a spot on the wall or outside and make sure that spot doesn't move. For if the spot moves, then your head has moved, and it isn't isometric. Be gentle. Use no more force than is comfortable each time. Do these twice a day.

As noted above injured muscles start to atrophy, or wither away, after not being used for about three days in the absence of injury, but within a few hours after an injury. Therefore, if we start the shrugs the same day, then little or no atrophy occurs, and healing is much faster. That is why I never recommend using a neck collar for an uncomplicated whiplash injury. The collar supports the neck, so the muscles don't have to work and quickly wither.

Neck roll. Some medical supply places have foam neck rolls you can buy. But without spending a penny you can simply fold a bath towel in half, then roll it up fairly tightly and tie strings or rubber bands around it so that it is about 3 inches in diameter. Place that under your neck as you lie on your back, and even sleep in that position if possible. A good alternative to the neck roll is tying a string around the middle of a pillow, so that there is a narrow crotch to put your neck in and support from the ears of the pillow on the sides.

ICE. Always start all injuries off with ice for 15-20 minutes at least twice a day on the sore areas. After 5-7 days you can add medium heat ("medium" on your heating pad rather than "high" because we just want to warm the area, not cook it) for 10-15 minutes at a time. Another good way, after 5-7 days, is to use ice for 10 minutes, medium heat for 10 minutes, and always end up with ice for 10 minutes. The use of ice obviously draws blood to the area and reduces swelling. There are also some beneficial effects that are poorly understood. The thing to keep in mind is to always start with ice.

NSAIDS. Non-steroidal anti-inflammatory medications are available over the counter as Advil, Ibuprofen, Nuprin, Naproxen, and others. They are half the therapeutic strength of a prescription. They reduce the inevitable inflammation that follows an injury to some degree and also help relieve pain. Their side effects can be severe, however.

The worst side effect is bleeding from the stomach, and I have had three patients in my practice that I had to hospitalize with bleeding from the stomach caused by taking one of these medications on their own. I have also had one patient who started bleeding from the stomach within six hours of taking his first (and only) dose of Oruvail, a prescription from the same drug family. Diarrhea and stomach cramps are frequent. Always take them with food. If you are allergic to aspirin, then you may also be allergic to one or more of these. They can also cause drowsiness. Another long term problem in people who take them for arthritis is a bad effect on the kidneys. High doses of Tylenol can be toxic to the liver. So for pure pain relief, you may need a prescription from your doctor, and he will probably have to see you before he can prescribe a narcotic.

Three newer anti-inflammatory drugs are Bextra, Celebrex and Vioxx (see page 489 for how to save money on Vioxx). Whereas in the older NSAIDs about 15-20% cause GI upsets, these new ones seem to cause similar problems in less than 5% of people.

I don't recommend chiropractic manipulations initially because the soft tissue injury is often made worse by manipulation at this stage. About 18% of these may involve some mild subluxation, and these can be reduced by manipulation by an osteopath or chiropractor, or the occasional family doctor, after the soft tissue inflammation has subsided. If manipulation is needed, it will be successful after only one or two sessions. Further manipulations simply keep the delicate injured tissues irritated and slow down the healing process.

Be very careful in your driving, with an eye on your rear view mirror every time you stop. An insurance company source of mine told me that their statistics indicate that having one rear end collision greatly increases the risk for a second, and even a third within the next three years.

Continue your neck muscle strengthening for at least six months after the initial injury. You can reduce the frequency to three times a week after you reach your weight and repetition goals, but stay with them. This would become especially important if you should have a second accident because strong muscles are less likely to be injured severely.

When You Need to See a Doctor:

1) if you have instant and severe neck pain. 2) If you have pain or numbness, or tingling down one or both arms. 3) If you have loss of feeling or loss of muscle function in any part of your body, even if it doesn't last. 4) If you have had any loss of consciousness. These cases usually require X-rays and/or other types of evaluation.

Vioxx, as in many other medications, is available in a larger double dose size at, or only slightly more, than the size of the smaller one. The usual dose of Vioxx is 25 mg once or twice daily. Ask your doctor to prescribe the 50 mg size, and just cut them in half with a razor, or a pill-cutter that some pharmacies carry.

See the **Drug Savings** chapter for more of these possibilities.

CHAPTER 105 -- WORK-RELATED INJURIES AND COMPENSATION

Every state has laws governing this type of injury. The laws vary a lot, but the basic thing is that the injured worker is entitled to have his or her medical bills paid until he or she is well *or medically stationary.*

In most states the law allows your employer to select a physician or clinic specializing in workers comp injuries for the initial visit. If your employer makes such a choice and you are satisfied with your care there, then stay with that person or group. Most states allow you to switch care to a physician of your choice at any time after the first one to three visits. If you feel for any reason that you want to switch, then do so. There will be some, but probably not much, additional paperwork. Be aware, however, that using a physician who does not deal with workers comp cases on a regular basis may complicate matters for you as far as scheduling physical therapy, arranging for consultations, and dealing with the industrial insurance carrier is concerned. The other side of the coin is that your personal physician may, on a few occasions, more closely represent your interests in the case.

If you have an injury on the job, it is important for you to report it <u>immediately</u> to your supervisor and fill out an accident report. This does not necessarily mean that you have to see a doctor right away. Use your own judgement unless the company insists that you go at that time. Most companies now require that a drug test be performed at the time of the injury, and thus will send you somewhere for evaluation of the injury along with the testing on a urine specimen.

In addition to medical care, the worker is entitled to receive some compensation if off work for an extended period of time as a result of the injury. In Arizona one has to be off for a week before beginning to qualify for 2/3 of the employee's <u>base</u> salary. No matter how much overtime you have been receiving, that isn't counted in what you will receive.

Therefore it is a really good thing if your physician and employer will work together to let you do some kind of modified duty within the limits of your injury. At the present time most employers are aware of the numerous studies done on recovery times for work-related injuries. People recover <u>much</u> <u>faster</u> if they can return to almost <u>any</u> kind of activity back on the job, even if it's just pushing a pencil. And you don't lose a week's wages, nor have the reduced pay rate that might cause you to miss a payment on your house or car. Again, doctors familiar with the workers comp system of care will be more likely to make these arrangements for you.

When the case is closed, not by full recovery but by becoming medically stationary, you may receive a cash settlement, the amount prescribed by law, for any permanent disability. There is a national standard for determining permanent disability percentage of the body part and the whole man. Any physician who cares for worker's comp cases will probably have the AMA disability manual and can make a determination. If the insurance carrier thinks that percentage is too high, then they may send you for an IME (Independent Medical Evaluation) by a physician who has had to take a course, pass an examination, and obtain a certificate. Insurance companies have to pay big bucks for these exams, so the insurance company will often just accept your doctor's percentage.

If you disagree anywhere along the line, there are various appeals processes in each state, most *requiring* no attorney. But you personally, and anyone (such as a union representative) will have to get all the information available from the state industrial commission or comparable body for your state.

Often there will be a lady there who will be only too happy to help you in every way if you just go in with a smile on your face and ask for help. The insurance companies are often another matter. (See the chapter on **HMOs**.)

If the amount of potential money is only a few hundred dollars, you will have trouble getting an attorney to represent you except on an hourly basis. That gets pretty expensive when they charge you for every time someone in the firm even *thinks* about pulling the file, and inevitably the senior partners involve one or more of the kids just out of school to pad the billable hours. Not all firms operate that way, but my stepson is an attorney, and he has told me some real horror stories. John Grisham's book, *The Firm,* isn't so far off base in some respects.

If the possible amount is in the thousands, you can easily find an attorney (they advertise on television every day) who will take your case on what is called a *contingency* basis. That means that the attorney won't charge you for his or her time but instead will take a percentage of the amount of money awarded to you after the case is settled. The percentage to the attorney is <u>always</u> negotiable. The attorney may have a "standard" fee of anywhere from 20% to 60% of the settlement. It may vary upward if you have to go to trial. Thirty percent is usually a fair percentage if the attorney has to do quite a bit of work. The figure should be lower if all he has to do is write a threatening demand letter.

If you can't agree on a figure you both can live with, let your fingers do the walking till you find an attorney you are pleased with. Also, be prepared for the first attorney to turn down your case for one of several reasons: he feels you have no chance to win; he thinks your case has no merit; he won't generate enough billable hours to pay his office staff;

the case will require too much time for too little pay; he doesn't like your hairdo; or fill in your own reason.

If you don't have a winnable case, the attorney isn't going to take it on a contingency basis, and the average worker has no further recourse than to exhaust the appeals prescribed by law and the take the final settlement offer. In some states that's all the attorneys do anyway, so you'll wind up saving money.

So before you actually sign anything with an attorney, consider whether you can and want to pursue the case yourself. It is much easier for someone who has been there before -- if the fees are reasonable and you are happy with your attorney. It is also often possible that the attorney will get you enough additional money to more than pay for his fees. But don't just sign up with someone before you learn all you can about the process. **Be an informed consumer!**

Types Of Work-Related Injuries

25% of all work-related injuries are backs. Most back injuries occur in people who are in relatively poor physical condition, and/or use poor body mechanics for lifting. See the chapter on **Back Injuries** for a complete discussion of this very common problem.

More work-related injuries occur on Mondays and Fridays (or the day before a holiday). The reasons for these seem to be that on Mondays, people are tired, hung-over, or still thinking about the weekend's activities, while on Fridays our minds wander, and our concentration tends to be on what we are going to do on our days off. Also, on Fridays we may be tired from lots of overtime. The most dangerous hours are the first hour on Monday and the last hour on Friday.

Workers compensation insurance in all states pays for all medical and surgical expenses for work-related injuries. This includes all drugs, supplies, and equipment, as well as specialist care, if needed, and physical therapy. In addition, the insurance carrier is required to pay a percentage of the employee's regular wages if the injured worker is off work for more than a few days.

This varies considerably from state to state. In one state that I am familiar with the employee doesn't start receiving money until he or she has been off work for five consecutive days. In another state where I have practiced, it is three days.

At the end of the initial time off, then paper work is filled out by the employer and the attending physician. Then those papers are processed, and in a few weeks (plan on 5-6 weeks) your checks begin to come in. Unfortunately, those checks are usually for much less than your normal wages. In Arizona, the state I am most familiar with, the injured person receives only about 2/3 of his base salary. This doesn't include the

> *Advice: When you get overtime pay, don't plan on always getting it. Take it and put most of it in a savings account. Most of all <u>never</u> buy something new and plan to use your overtime to make the payments for it!*

weekly overtime pay that many of us come to depend on. So the money you bring in if you are off work completely is just subsistence pay, something you can barely live on.

Most physicians who see very many of this type of injury are well aware that many studies have shown that workers who return immediately to some kind of modified duty at the work place will recover faster from almost *any* injury than someone who just sits around the house.

There are a number of reasons for this. One, of course is the economic one where the injured person continues to have a weekly paycheck, and thus does not fall into a depressed state from lack of money to pay the bills.

Another is also a mental thing: where you are under foot with your spouse at home, bickering may occur that disturbs your mental health.

Another is that continued physical activity of any amount will help prevent the muscle and other tissue atrophy (atrophy means the muscles shrivel up and get weak) which slows down recovery and makes for a longer rehab time. Not only that but making the muscles actively move reduces spasm and therefore reduces pain. Couch potatoes don't get well as fast as those who are physically and mentally active.

The opposite of the last paragraph is that some people who aren't supposed to do a particular physical activity (or their spouses) find chores they have been putting off around the house, some of which may not be what their doctor or physical therapist have in mind for their rehab program.

Computer-Related Injuries

Many of these involve repetitive stress as well as improper keyboard-monitor-mouse-chair ergonomics (or just relationships to your body mechanics.)

Sore neck

Probably your monitor is not at the proper level, or the material you are reading from is not either. The

> *One recent patient of mine had sore and swollen knees. He was supposed to give them some rest. Well, he felt so much better in three days that he decided he could put on the new roof, which he had been putting off, over the weekend before he saw me again on Monday. He hauled the asphalt shingles up the ladder all by himself, squatted and knelt down all day for two days, and guess what? When he saw me on Monday, he said, "Gee, I'm not any better." After a little discussion, the story came out, bit by bit. So I sent him back to regular duty, figuring that he would strain his knees a whole lot less at work than at home.*

monitor should be at eye level, and the material you are reading from should be close enough to eye level so that you don't have to move anything but your eyes when inputting on the keyboard. Especially you don't want to have to tilt your head back and forth all day.

Sore shoulders, arms, elbows, forearms, wrists, and hands

Symptoms may include a burning sensation, cramping, numbness or tingling, pain, swelling, and weakness in these areas, as well as your neck, and even your back. These are especially related to your posture at the keyboard. Usually you aren't sitting properly in relation to your keyboard, mouse and monitor.

You should be sitting so that your elbows bend at right angles (90 degrees) as the hands work on the keyboard. For this you may have to raise or lower your keyboard or your chair.

The wrists should be supported with a slightly spongy support, and there should be a similar smaller padded mouse support attached to the mouse pad. 3-M makes the best of these that I have seen, but there are lots on the market.

You should be able to rest your elbows on the arms of your chair without disturbing the 90-degree angle.

Sore back

Ideally you should be sitting upright with the small of your back supported by a small lumbar support. If you are slouching, or your chair doesn't give enough support, you might try a small pillow in the small of your back, or get one that you can strap to the chair from a physical therapy supply store. Or just roll up a towel and put a couple of rubber bands around it to hold the roll.

Sometimes putting one or both of your feet on a footrest will cause the hips to bend just enough to change your lumbar angle and relieve the strain.

Numbness in legs or feet

This may be caused by too much pressure on the blood vessels of your legs from two or three possible causes: the angle of flexion of the hips, same for the knees, or pressure on the thighs just above the knees. Again, a footrest might be helpful, or a chair with the front part of it sloping downward a little.

Sore bottom

This is caused by too much pressure on the portion of the posterior pelvic bone called the ischial (is-key-al) tuberosities. We all know what those are, especially of us with pretty bony behinds. The way to relieve that is to transfer much of your weight to the backs of your thighs. So ideally you should have a soft enough chair that supports at least the top 6 or 8 inches of the backs of your thighs as well as your bottom end. Just be sure it doesn't go far enough out to press on the blood vessels behind the knees, as noted above. A swivel chair that tilts may be a good solution because you can then easily change positions when you notice a hot spot developing.

The perfect workstation chair is not easily found! I once spent over two hours checking out all the chairs in a business furniture warehouse before I found one that would fit the measurements I took on my receptionist. I'm happy to report that she loved it.

INDEX

H

I